# Cardiac Sodium Channel Disorders

*Editor*

HUGUES ABRIEL


# CARDIAC ELECTROPHYSIOLOGY CLINICS

www.cardiacEP.theclinics.com


*Consulting Editors*

RANJAN K. THAKUR

ANDREA NATALE


December 2014 • Volume 6 • Number 4

**ELSEVIER**

1600 John F. Kennedy Boulevard • Suite 1800 • Philadelphia, Pennsylvania, 19103-2899

http://www.theclinics.com

**CARDIAC ELECTROPHYSIOLOGY CLINICS Volume 6, Number 4**
**December 2014 ISSN 1877-9182, ISBN-13: 978-0-323-32640-7**

Editor: Adrianne Brigido
Developmental Editor: Barbara Cohen-Kligerman



*Cardiac Electrophysiology Clinics* (ISSN 1877-9182) is published quarterly by Elsevier Inc., 360 Park Avenue South, New York, NY 10010-1710. Months of issue are March, June, September, and December. Subscription prices are $200.00 per year for US individuals, $293.00 per year for US institutions, $105.00 per year for US students and residents, $225.00 per year for Canadian individuals, $331.00 per year for Canadian institutions, $285.00 per year for international individuals, $354.00 per year for international institutions and $150.00 per year for Canadian and international students/residents. To receive student/resident rate, orders must be accompanied by name of affilliated institution, date of term, and the signature of program/residency coordinator on institution letterhead. Orders will be billed at individual rate until proof of status is received. Foreign air speed delivery is included in all Clinics subscription prices. All prices are subject to change without notice. **POSTMASTER:** Send address changes to Cardiac Electrophysiology Clinics, Elsevier Health Sciences Division, Subscription Customer Service, 3251 Riverport Lane, Maryland Heights, MO 63043. **Customer Service: 1-800-654-2452 (US and Canada). From outside of the US and Canada, call 314-477-8871. Fax: 314-447-8029. E-mail:** JournalsCustomerService-usa@elsevier.com **(for print support);** JournalsOnlineSupport-usa@elsevier.com **(for online support).**

*Reprints.* For copies of 100 or more of articles in this publication, please contact the Commercial Reprints Department, Elsevier Inc., 360 Park Avenue South, New York, NY 10010-1710. Tel.: 212-633-3874; Fax: 212-633-3820; E-mail: reprints@elsevier.com.

# Contributors

## CONSULTING EDITORS

**RANJAN K. THAKUR, MD, MPH, MBA, FHRS**
Professor of Medicine and Director, Arrhythmia Service, Thoracic and Cardiovascular Institute, Sparrow Health System, Michigan State University, Lansing, Michigan

**ANDREA NATALE, MD, FACC, FHRS**
Executive Medical Director, Texas Cardiac Arrhythmia Institute, St. David's Medical Center, Austin, Texas; Consulting Professor, Division of Cardiology, Stanford University, Palo Alto, California; Adjunct Professor of Medicine, Heart and Vascular Center, Case Western Reserve University, Cleveland, Ohio; Director, Interventional Electrophysiology, Scripps Clinic, San Diego, California; Senior Clinical Director, EP Services, California Pacific Medical Center, San Francisco, California

## EDITOR

**HUGUES ABRIEL, MD, PhD**
Professor of Pathophysiology; Director, Department of Clinical Research, Ion Channel and Channelopathies Research Group, University of Bern, Bern, Switzerland

## AUTHORS

**HUGUES ABRIEL, MD, PhD**
Professor of Pathophysiology; Director, Department of Clinical Research, Ion Channel and Channelopathies Research Group, University of Bern, Bern, Switzerland

**RONG BAI, MD**
Cardiologist, Department of Cardiology, Beijing An Zhen Hospital, Capital Medical University, Beijing, China

**YANGYANG BAO, BS**
Department of Pharmacology, University of Michigan Medical School, Ann Arbor, Michigan

**JULIEN BARC, PhD**
Department of Experimental Cardiology, Academic Medical Center, Amsterdam, The Netherlands

**D. WOODROW BENSON, MD, PhD**
Department of Cardiology, Children's Hospital of Wisconsin; Professor of Pediatrics and Director, Congenital and Pediatric Cardiac Research, Medical College of Wisconsin, Milwaukee, Wisconsin

**CONNIE R. BEZZINA, PhD**
Department of Experimental Cardiology, Academic Medical Center, Amsterdam, The Netherlands

**LIA CROTTI, MD, PhD**
Center for Cardiac Arrhythmias of Genetic Origin and Laboratory of Cardiovascular Genetics, IRCCS Istituto Auxologico Italiano, Milan, Italy; Department of Molecular Medicine, University of Pavia, Pavia, Italy; Helmholtz Zentrum München, Institute of Human Genetics, Neuherberg, Germany

**DAWOOD DARBAR, MD**
Director, Vanderbilt Arrhythmia Service and Cardiac EP Fellowship Program; Associate Professor of Medicine, Division of Cardiovascular Medicine, Vanderbilt University, Nashville, Tennessee

**SERGEI DZEMESHKEVICH, MD, PhD**
Professor, Director, Head of Heart Surgery Department, Petrovsky Russian Research Centre of Surgery, Moscow, Russia

**ALICE GHIDONI, PhD**
Laboratory of Cardiovascular Genetics, IRCCS Istituto Auxologico Italiano, Milan, Italy; Department of Molecular Medicine, University of Pavia, Pavia, Italy

**JEAN-BAPTISTE GOURRAUD, MD**
Reference Centre for Hereditary Arrhythmic Diseases, Cardiologic Department and INSERM U1087, l'institut du thorax, CHU de Nantes, Nantes, France

**ROBERTO INSOLIA, PhD**
Department of Molecular Medicine, University of Pavia, Pavia, Italy

**LORI L. ISOM, PhD**
Professor of Pharmacology and Professor of Molecular and Integrative Physiology, Department of Pharmacology, University of Michigan Medical School, Ann Arbor, Michigan

**ANDRE G. KLEBER, MD**
Visiting Professor, Department of Pathology, Beth Israel Deaconess Medical Center, Harvard Medical School, Boston, Massachusetts

**JOSHUA R. KOVACH, MD**
Assistant Professor, Pediatrics, Cardiology, Children's Hospital of Wisconsin, Medical College of Wisconsin, Milwaukee, Wisconsin

**JOHN W. KYLE, PhD**
Senior Scientist, Division of Cardiovascular Medicine, Department of Medicine, University of Wisconsin, Madison, Wisconsin

**FLORENCE KYNDT, PharmD, PhD**
Reference Centre for Hereditary Arrhythmic Diseases and INSERM U1087, l'institut du thorax, CHU de Nantes, Nantes, France

**HERVÉ LE MAREC, MD, PhD**
Reference Centre for Hereditary Arrhythmic Diseases, Cardiologic Department and INSERM U1087, l'institut du thorax, CHU de Nantes, Nantes, France

**NIAN LIU, MD**
Clinical Cardiologist and Research Scientist, Department of Cardiology, Beijing An Zhen Hospital, Capital Medical University, Beijing, China

**JONATHAN C. MAKIELSKI, MD**
Professor of Medicine, Division of Cardiovascular Medicine, Department of Medicine, University of Wisconsin, Madison, Wisconsin

**ARGELIA MEDEIROS-DOMINGO, MD, PhD**
Department of Cardiac Electrophysiology, University Hospital of Bern, Bern, Switzerland

**YUKA MIZUSAWA, MD**
Department of Cardiology, Heart Center, Academic Medical Center, Amsterdam, The Netherlands

**CARLO NAPOLITANO, MD, PhD**
Associate Professor, Molecular Cardiology, IRCCS, Fondazione Salvatore Maugeri, Pavia, Italy; Cardiovascular Genetics, Leon Charney Division of Cardiology, New York University, New York, New York

**SEAN O'ROURKE, MD**[†]
New York University, New York, New York

**PIETER G. POSTEMA, MD, PhD**
Department of Cardiology, Heart Center, Academic Medical Center, Amsterdam, The Netherlands

**SILVIA G. PRIORI, MD, PhD**
Professor of Medicine, Molecular Cardiology, IRCCS, Fondazione Salvatore Maugeri; Department of Molecular Medicine, University of Pavia, Pavia, Italy

**VINCENT PROBST, MD, PhD**
Professor of Cardiology, Reference Centre for Hereditary Arrhythmic Diseases, Cardiologic Department and INSERM U1087, l'institut du thorax, CHU de Nantes, Nantes, France

[†]Deceased.

**RICHARD REDON, PhD**
Reference Centre for Hereditary Arrhythmic Diseases and INSERM U1087, l'institut du thorax, CHU de Nantes, Nantes, France

**CAROL ANN REMME, MD, PhD**
Department of Experimental Cardiology, Academic Medical Center, University of Amsterdam, Amsterdam, The Netherlands

**DAN M. RODEN, MD**
Departments of Medicine and Pharmacology, Vanderbilt University School of Medicine, Nashville, Tennessee

**YANFEI RUAN, MD**
Clinical Cardiologist, Department of Cardiology, Beijing An Zhen Hospital, Capital Medical University, Beijing, China

**ELEONORA SAVIO-GALIMBERTI, MD, PhD**
Research Fellow in Cardiovascular Medicine, Division of Cardiovascular Medicine, Vanderbilt University, Nashville, Tennessee

**JEAN-JACQUES SCHOTT, PhD**
Reference Centre for Hereditary Arrhythmic Diseases and INSERM U1087, l'institut du thorax, CHU de Nantes, Nantes, France

**PETER J. SCHWARTZ, MD**
Center for Cardiac Arrhythmias of Genetic Origin and Laboratory of Cardiovascular Genetics, IRCCS Istituto Auxologico Italiano, Milan, Italy

**HANNO L. TAN, MD, PhD**
Department of Cardiology, Heart Center, Academic Medical Center, Amsterdam, The Netherlands

**CARMEN R. VALDIVIA, MD**
Center for Arrhythmia Research, University of Michigan, Ann Arbor, Michigan

**RAYMOND L. WOOSLEY, MD, PhD**
Arizona Center for Education and Research on Therapeutics (AZCERT), Oro Valley, Arizona; University of Arizona, College of Medicine-Phoenix, Phoenix, Arizona

**ELENA ZAKLYAZMINSKAYA, MD, PhD**
Professor, Head of Medical Genetics Laboratory, Petrovsky Russian Research Centre of Surgery, Moscow, Russia

# Contents

**Foreword: The Sodium Channel: One Gene, Many Diseases!** xiii

Ranjan K. Thakur and Andrea Natale

**Preface: Cardiac Sodium Channel Disorders: One Gene with Many Genetic Variants Leading to Many Cardiac Phenotypes** xv

Hugues Abriel

**Role of the Cardiac Sodium Current in Excitability and Conduction** 657

Andre G. Kleber

The theoretic and experimental work discussed in this review demonstrates that the role of $Na^+$ inward current in cardiac excitability and propagation cannot be discussed independently of $Ca^{2+}$ inward current, the discontinuous structure of cellular network, and cell-to-cell coupling. The contribution of all these variables to propagation is interdependent. Moreover, all these variables may change in a specific pathologic setting, helping to explain the different behavior of electrical propagation and responsiveness to pharmacologic drugs of diseased hearts.

**Role of Rare and Common Genetic Variation in *SCN5A* in Cardiac Electrical Function and Arrhythmia** 665

Julien Barc and Connie R. Bezzina

Commensurate with the central role of the cardiac sodium channel in cardiac electrical function, mutations in *SCN5A* have been associated with a broad spectrum of cardiac rhythm disorders associated with sudden cardiac death. Recent work dealing with the effect of noncoding genetic variation at the *SCN5A* locus has now extended insight into *SCN5A* disease mechanisms beyond the coding region of the gene. Work in this regard is expected to grow as insight concerning the regulatory noncoding regions of the genome continues to increase.

**$Na_V1.5$ and Regulatory β Subunits in Cardiac Sodium Channelopathies** 679

Yangyang Bao and Lori L. Isom

Voltage-gated sodium channels (VGSCs) are critical for impulse initiation and propagation in excitable cells. The ion-conducting VGSC α subunits are modulated by 2 β subunits. This article discusses β subunit tissue distribution and subcellular localization in the heart, the anatomic basis of β subunit–linked cardiac disease, β subunit electrophysiologic function, cardiac disease–related β subunit gene mutations, and clinical phenotypes. Possible mechanisms of β subunit–mediated cardiac arrhythmias are presented. The pathophysiologic implications of simultaneous expression of β subunit gene mutations in heart and brain are considered. Future directions for therapeutic intervention and personalized medicine are discussed.

**Pharmacology and Toxicology of $Na_v1.5$-Class 1 Antiarrhythmic Drugs** 695

Dan M. Roden

Although cardiac sodium channel blocking drugs can exert antiarrhythmic actions, they can also provoke life-threatening arrhythmias through a variety of mechanisms.

This article addresses the way in which drugs interact with the channel and how these effects translate to clinical beneficial or detrimental effects. A further understanding of the details of channel function and of drug-channel interactions may lead to the development of safer and more effective antiarrhythmic therapies.

**Congenital Long QT Syndrome Type 3** 705

Yanfei Ruan, Nian Liu, Rong Bai, Silvia G. Priori, and Carlo Napolitano

Long QT syndrome type 3 (LQT3) is caused by mutations of the *SCN5A* gene encoding the α-subunit of the human cardiac sodium channel. Specific ST-T wave patterns, triggers, and risk for cardiac events are associated with this LQT syndrome variant. Bench studies have gathered enough knowledge to allow devising of gene-specific therapies to specifically counteract the effects of the mutations. In this article, the authors delineate the LQT3 pathophysiology and epidemiology. They also discuss the clinical management with a focus on the appropriate use of gene-specific therapy.

**Brugada Syndrome and $Na_V1.5$** 715

Vincent Probst, Jean-Jacques Schott, Jean-Baptiste Gourraud, Richard Redon, Florence Kyndt, and Hervé Le Marec

The sodium channel and its regulatory subunits play a central role in the pathophysiology of Brugada syndrome (BrS). The identification of rare and common variants that modify the sodium current involved in the development of BrS favors the predominant role of conduction abnormalities. Even if the sodium current is a key factor in the development of BrS, the relationship between *SCN5A* mutations and BrS is weak and does not allow the use of molecular tests for genetic counseling for families. Improved genetic knowledge about this syndrome should help elucidate the pathophysiology and perhaps better define patients at high arrhythmic risk.

**Conduction Disorders and $Na_V1.5$** 723

Joshua R. Kovach and D. Woodrow Benson

The heritability of cardiac conduction disease has been observed and reported for decades. These diseases frequently manifest as progressive and variable degeneration of the cardiac conduction tissues at young ages. Recently mutations in the SCN5A gene encoding the $Na_V1.5$ channel have been identified as causes for these conduction abnormalities, improving the ability to diagnose and understand this disease process. Additionally, there has been increased detection of overlap syndromes characterized by varied phenotypic manifestations of certain mutations beyond conduction disease. Although the understanding of these heritable disorders continues to improve, treatment options remain limited to pacemaker support.

**Dilated Cardiomyopathy and $Na_V1.5$** 733

Elena Zaklyazminskaya and Sergei Dzemeshkevich

Dilated cardiomyopathy (DCM), a progressive cardiac muscle disease, is the most common reason for heart transplantation. Over 40 genes have been associated with DCM. In 2004, a new genetic form of cardiomyopathy, DCM 1E (MIM: *601154) associated with mutations in the *SCN5A* gene, was identified. *SCN5A* encodes the $Na_V1.5$ sodium ion channel protein responsible for the inward current of sodium. This type of DCM is accompanied by progressive conduction disturbances, and atrial and ventricular arrhythmias. We outline and analyze the various $Na_v1.5$ sodium channel genetic variants, molecular mechanisms of myocardial remodeling, phenotypic manifestations of known mutations, and potential implications of gene-specific treatment.

**Atrial Fibrillation and *SCN5A* Variants** **741**

Eleonora Savio-Galimberti and Dawood Darbar

Although atrial fibrillation (AF) is clinically and genetically a highly heterogeneous disease, recent studies suggest that the arrhythmia may arise because of interactions between genetic and acquired risk factors—the so called "double-hit" hypothesis. Genome-wide association studies have identified common AF susceptibility loci, and linkage analysis and candidate gene approaches have identified mutations in genes that encode for cardiac ion channels and signaling proteins; however, most of the heritability of AF still remains unexplained.

**The Role of the Cardiac Sodium Channel in Perinatal Early Infant Mortality** **749**

Lia Crotti, Alice Ghidoni, Roberto Insolia, and Peter J. Schwartz

The cardiac sodium channel gene *SCN5A* plays an important role in arrhythmias of genetic origin. With exceptions, loss-of-function mutations become more important in adult life, whereas gain-of-function mutations can manifest their clinical impact as early as the perinatal period. The best-known disease caused by the latter variants is long QT syndrome type 3, which tends to manifest in adolescence. However, when symptoms appear in the first year of life the likelihood of cardiac arrest and sudden death is very high.

**Cardiac Sodium Channel Overlap Syndrome** **761**

Carol Ann Remme

Mutations in the *SCN5A* gene encoding the cardiac sodium channel are associated with a wide range of arrhythmia syndromes, which potentially lead to fatal arrhythmias in relatively young individuals. In recent years, an increasing overlap in clinical presentation and biophysical defects of associated mutant sodium channels has been reported, a presentation known as "cardiac sodium channel overlap syndrome." Here, an overview is provided of our current knowledge about *SCN5A* mutations associated with sodium channel overlap syndromes. In addition, the underlying genetic and biophysical mechanisms and the clinical and genetic determinants of variable disease expressivity and severity are discussed.

**Cardiac Sodium Channel $Na_v1.5$ and Drug-Induced Long QT Syndrome** **777**

Hugues Abriel

Genetic factors and acquired pathologies, such as cardiac ischemia and heart failure, may lead to an increase in the late sodium current carried by the cardiac sodium channel $Na_v1.5$. As a result, cardiac action potential repolarization is delayed, which in turn reduces the cardiac repolarization reserve of afflicted patients. This repolarization alteration may cause polymorphic ventricular arrhythmias called Torsades de pointes. This review summarizes the genetic and molecular mechanisms explaining why such patients are more susceptible to drug-induced long QT syndrome when taking QT-prolonging drugs.

of sodium current disorders. Identification of the underlying genetic variants has improved understanding of the pathophysiologic mechanism. Genetic tests allow physicians to diagnose concealed/borderline cases, perform risk stratification, and select gene-specific and/or mutation-specific therapies. Appropriate selection of candidates for genetic screening is essential to optimizing the cost/benefit ratio.

# CARDIAC ELECTROPHYSIOLOGY CLINICS

## FORTHCOMING ISSUES

***March 2015***
**Frontiers in Non-invasive Cardiac Mapping**
Ashok Shah, Michel Haissaguerre, and Meleze Hocini, *Editors*

***June 2015***
**Arrythmias in Cardiomyopathies**
Mohammad Shenasa, Martin Maron, and Mark Link, *Editors*

***September 2015***
**Interpretation of Complex Arrhythmias: A Case-Based Approach**
Melvin Scheinman, *Editor*

## RECENT ISSUES

***September 2014***
**Electrocardiography of Complex Arrhythmias**
Mohammad Shenasa and Edward P. Gerstenfeld, *Editors*

***June 2014***
**Implantable Devices: Design, Manufacturing, and Malfunction**
Kenneth A. Ellenbogen and Charles J. Love, *Editors*

***March 2014***
**Stroke in Atrial Fibrillation**
Samuel J. Asirvatham, Ranjan K. Thakur, and Andrea Natale, *Editors*

# Foreword
# The Sodium Channel: One Gene, Many Diseases!

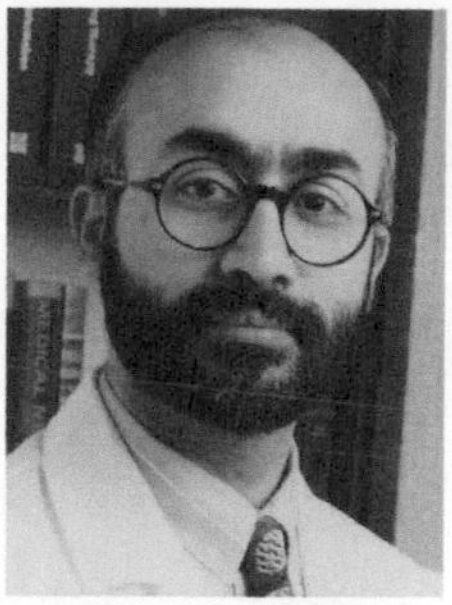

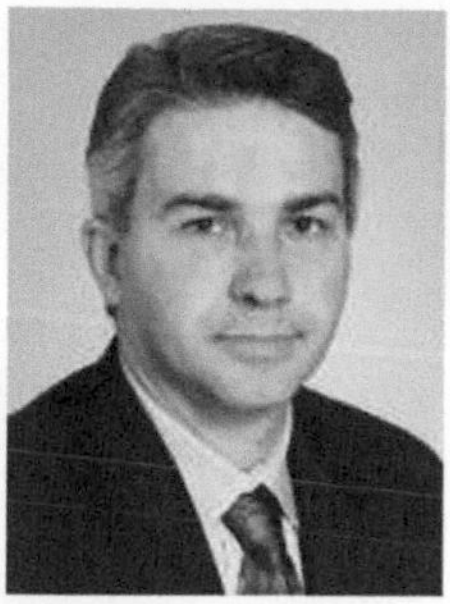

Ranjan K. Thakur, MD, MPH, MBA, FHRS    Andrea Natale, MD, FACC, FHRS
*Consulting Editors*

The cardiac $Na^+$ channel is a voltage-gated channel that consists of assemblies of proteins: α-subunit, the pore-forming component, and one or two β-subunits, which modulate the function of the pore or channel. The structure of these proteins is encoded by genes.

A mutation is defined as any change in a DNA sequence away from normal. This implies that there is a normal allele that is prevalent in the population and the mutation changes it to a rare and abnormal variant. In contrast, genetic polymorphism is a DNA variation that is "common" in the population. The arbitrary cutoff point between a mutation and a polymorphism is 1%. Mutations occur in less than 1% of the population, whereas genetic polymorphisms are defined as variants that occur at a frequency greater than 1%.

Polymorphisms may be caused by insertion/deletion, single-nucleotide polymorphisms, or short-simple-sequence repeats. Polymorphisms located within the coding region of a gene can directly influence the structure and function of its protein, whereas changes within the regulatory sequences of a gene can influence the level of expression of the protein. Genetic variations may also alter phenotypic expression under certain conditions, such as electrolyte disturbance, ischemia, and so on. However, DNA variation may also be inconsequential and may not have a clinical manifestation.

The $Na^+$ channel plays a critical role in cardiac conduction because it initiates the action potential ($I_{Na}$) and, via gap junctions, determines the velocity of conduction and impulse propagation. Mutations/polymorphisms in these genes underlie many clinical arrhythmias and conditions, such as the Brugada syndrome, long QT syndrome, sudden infant death syndrome, conduction abnormalities, sick sinus syndrome, dilated cardiomyopathy, and atrial fibrillation.

Molecular understanding of arrhythmias is proceeding at a breakneck pace, and most clinical electrophysiologists don't have a comprehensive understanding of this field. This is due in large part to a lack of direct translation of molecular understanding into daily practice of clinical medicine. But this is the next frontier.

We want to congratulate Dr Abriel for editing this issue of the *Cardiac Electrophysiology Clinics* and assembling contributors leading this field to give us expert summaries of the important advances to date. This issue of the *Cardiac Electrophysiology Clinics* will be of interest to clinical electrophysiologists as well as experts

Card Electrophysiol Clin 6 (2014) xiii–xiv
http://dx.doi.org/10.1016/j.ccep.2014.08.010
1877-9182/14/$ – see front matter 

in the field who may need to catch up with advances outside of their own focused research interest.

Ranjan K. Thakur, MD, MPH, MBA, FHRS
Sparrow Thoracic and Cardiovascular Institute
Michigan State University
1200 East Michigan Avenue; Suite 580
Lansing, MI 48912, USA

Andrea Natale, MD, FACC, FHRS
Texas Cardiac Arrhythmia Institute
Center for Atrial Fibrillation at
St. David's Medical Center
1015 East 32nd Street, Suite 516
Austin, TX 78705, USA

E-mail addresses:
thakur@msu.edu (R.K. Thakur)
andrea.natale@stdavids.com (A. Natale)

# Preface
# Cardiac Sodium Channel Disorders: One Gene with Many Genetic Variants Leading to Many Cardiac Phenotypes

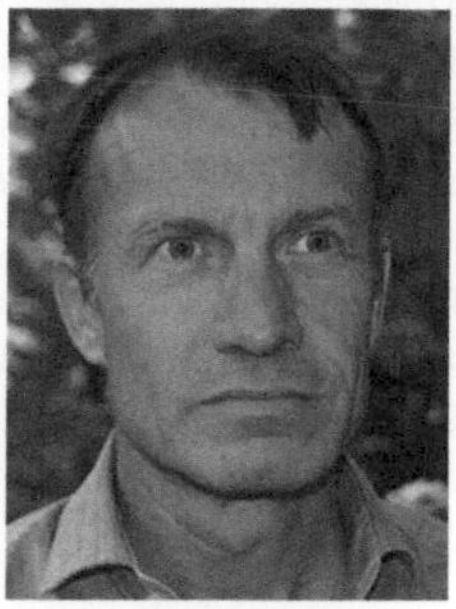

Hugues Abriel, MD, PhD
*Editor*

The field of molecular arrhythmology has progressed at an impressive pace during the past 20 years. This is mainly the result of outstanding collaboration between cardiologists, arrhythmia specialists, molecular and medical geneticists, biophysicists, and physiologists from many different countries.[1,2] Throughout the years, we have learned more and more about the genetic factors and molecular mechanisms underlying electrical abnormalities of the heart,[3] such as congenital long QT syndrome (LQTS) and Brugada syndrome. In several cases (ie, risk stratification of LQTS patients), this new knowledge has led to a clear clinical benefit.[4] Since, in most cases, the genes that are found to be mutated are encoding either the pore-forming subunit of cardiac ion channels or of ion channel regulatory proteins, the term "genetic cardiac channelopathies" has been used to define these disorders.

Among the still-growing list of genes that lead to genetic cardiac channelopathies, the role of the gene *SCN5A*, is truly unique. The gene *SCN5A* encodes the pore-forming subunit of the cardiac sodium channel $Na_v1.5$, which is the main channel responsible for the cardiac sodium current. The history of the discovery of this current and channel has been discussed by Dr Fozzard in a classic review article.[5] Since 1995, beginning with the seminal work of the group of Dr Keating,[6] hundreds of genetic variants (many of them being pathogenic mutations) have been reported by geneticists and cardiologists. The striking point here is that these variants were found in patients with a long list of distinct clinical manifestations ranging from delayed repolarization (in LQTS) to structural abnormalities (in the case of patients with dilated cardiomyopathies).

Together with many colleagues, we felt that there was a clear need to summarize this rapidly expanding field in a series of reviews, and we were encouraged by the Consulting Editors of *Cardiac Electrophysiology Clinics*. Bench scientists and clinical scientists have written reviews in this volume that are each dedicated to one of the distinct phenotypes linked to variants in *SCN5A*. The introductory articles introduce the role of this channel in pathophysiology and genetics. Final articles are the views of geneticists and clinicians about how to deal with patients who have (or are

Card Electrophysiol Clin 6 (2014) xv–xvi
http://dx.doi.org/10.1016/j.ccep.2014.08.009
1877-9182/14/$ – see front matter 

suspected to have) a cardiac sodium channel channelopathy.

As Guest Editor, I am indebted to all of the authors of this series for writing timely and didactic review articles on the many phenotypes caused by variants of *SCN5A*. I would like to warmly thank them for their time and effort. It is my hope that this series will be a useful medium for basic and clinical scientists who are looking for an updated presentation of this clinically important topic.

Hugues Abriel, MD, PhD
Department of Clinical Research
Ion Channel and Channelopathies Research Group
University of Bern
Bern, Switzerland

E-mail address:
hugues.abriel@dkf.unibe.ch

## REFERENCES

1. Cerrone M, Priori SG. Genetics of sudden death: focus on inherited channelopathies. Eur Heart J 2011;32(17):2109–18.
2. Napolitano C, Bloise R, Monteforte N, et al. Sudden cardiac death and genetic ion channelopathies. Circulation 2012;125(16):2027–34.
3. Abriel H, Zaklyazminskaya EV. Cardiac channelopathies: Genetic and molecular mechanisms. Gene 2013;517(1):1–11.
4. Priori SG, Schwartz PJ, Napolitano C, et al. Risk stratification in the long-QT syndrome. N Engl J Med 2003;348(19):1866–74.
5. Fozzard HA. Cardiac sodium and calcium channels: a history of excitatory currents. Cardiovasc Res 2002;55(1):1–8.
6. Wang Q, Shen J, Splawski I, et al. SCN5A mutations associated with an inherited cardiac arrhythmia, long QT syndrome. Cell 1995;80(5):805–11.

# Role of the Cardiac Sodium Current in Excitability and Conduction

Andre G. Kleber, MD

**KEYWORDS**

• Sodium current • Propagation velocity • Safety factor • Discontinuous propagation
• Propagation block

**KEY POINTS**

- The role of the $Na^+$ inward current in cardiac excitability and propagation is discussed in the context of the other variables affecting normal propagation: the $Ca^{2+}$ inward current, the discontinuous structure of the cellular network, and cell-to-cell electrical coupling.
- These variables and their interaction may change in a specific pathological setting, which explains why diseased hearts can have a different electrical behavior and responsiveness of propagation to pharmacological agents.

## HISTORY OF SODIUM CURRENT MEASUREMENTS IN THE HEART

In 1952, Hodgkin and Huxley published seminal papers in the *Journal of Physiology*[1–3] describing the dependence of the upstroke of the action potential in nerve on external $Na^+$ and defining activation and inactivation kinetics of inward $Na^+$ current and their dependence on membrane potential. In 1949 Coraboeuf and Weidmann, when working in the laboratory of Huxley and Hodgkin, profited from the fact that the dog "false tendons" became available in the laboratory[4] to record the first cardiac transmembrane action potential.[4,5] Whereas the very first recording did not show any overshoot, probably for technical reasons, subsequent recordings showed an overshoot expected from the reversal potential of $Na^+$ ions. In subsequent seminal papers, Silvio Weidmann[6,7] provided quantitative parameters of cardiac action potential shape and the dependence of the upstroke velocity of the cardiac action potential on the resting potential. This work already showed a large conductance dependent on external $Na^+$ during the upstroke, and the so-called availability of the membrane elements to carry sodium current. In modern terms, this corresponded with the first inactivation curves of $Na^+$ channels, long before the existence of protein membrane channels had been shown. Although early work on cardiac $Na^+$ inward current, using the so-called sucrose gap technique to measure inward $Na^+$ current, were exposed to significant problems (related to the control of the clamped membrane potential), they yielded the approximate kinetic variables determining flow through $Na^+$ channels.[8] With the introduction of the patch clamp technique,[9] it became possible to more accurately measure whole cell current and to define the kinetics and magnitude of single channel openings. Because $Na^+$ inward current was defined early on as the major charge carrier driving impulse propagation, numerous publications have appeared looking at structure, molecular function, and pharmacologic blockers of cardiac Na* channels (for review see Sheets[10] and Fozzard and Hanck[11]).

Disclosure: Consultant for Schiller Inc., Baar, Switzerland.
Department of Pathology, Beth Israel Deaconess Medical Center, Harvard Medical School, Dana 752, 330 Brookline Avenue, Boston, MA 02215, USA
*E-mail address:* akleber@bidmc.harvard.edu

Card Electrophysiol Clin 6 (2014) 657–664
http://dx.doi.org/10.1016/j.ccep.2014.07.004
1877-9182/14/$ – see front matter 

## Na⁺ INWARD CURRENT AND THE ACTION POTENTIAL UPSTROKE IN HEART

Because $I_{Na}$ is responsible for the fast portion of the action potential upstroke in most cardiac regions, the maximal upstroke velocity of the action potential upstroke, $dV/dt_{max}$, is often taken as a simple, indirect measure for inward sodium current flow. Although this relationship holds true for a cell or multicellular preparations with uniform membrane potential (voltage clamp condition), it is not true for a propagated action potential. In the case of a propagating action potential, only a part of the electrical charge flowing through $Na^+$ channels discharges membrane capacitance and thereby produces depolarization of the membrane potential. The other portion flows into the nonexcited cells downstream of the propagating wave where it delivers stimulatory current to drive propagation forward. This so-called axial or electrotonic current changes the relationship between $dV/dt_{max}$ and $I_{Na}$. The axial current depends on the impedance to electrical current flow downstream, it is high at sites were axial current is dispersed into a so-called sink, and low where axial current meets a resistive obstacle, for instance at sites of collision with a tissue boundary. Accordingly, the relation between action potential upstroke and $I_{Na}$ changes with changing resistive load downstream.[12,13]

A further point related to the relationship between the upstroke of the transmembrane action potential and $I_{Na}$ relates to the instant of local activation. The determination of the time point of local activation is necessary to establish 2-dimensional or 3-dimensional maps of propagation. Often this moment is taken as the moment of occurrence of $dVdt_{max}$. However, owing to the complexities related to the balance between charge delivered to membrane capacitance and charge delivered to downstream current, as explained, the time instant at the half amplitude of the transmembrane action potential seems a more accurate measure of maximal $Na^+$ current flow and local activation.[13–15]

## Na⁺ INWARD CURRENT AND THE SAFETY FACTOR OF PROPAGATION

An important issue in physiology and pathophysiology of propagation relates to the question of "propagation reserve" of safety of propagation. Over the past years, several algorithms have been published to define safety of propagation. A definition that has proven to be very useful and to provide theoretical results in close agreement with experimental findings was published by Shaw and Rudy[16] and follows the formalism:

$$\frac{\int_A I_c dt + \int_A I_{out} dt}{\int_A I_{in} dt} \qquad (1)$$

The numerator in this equation bears 2 terms and stands for the charge flow across depolarizing ion channels ($I_{Na}$ and/or $I_{Ca,L}$; see below). The first term corresponds with the charge flow into the membrane capacitance, *c*, which determines the action potential upstroke. The second term corresponds with the electrotonic or axial charge flow, flowing "out" of the cell, as described previously. The denominator corresponds to the electrical charge flowing into the cell ("in") and needed to drive the cell to threshold for excitation. *A* denotes the time window during which electrical current is integrated. Using this algorithm, propagation is successful if the safety factor (*SF*; dimensionless) of propagation is greater than 1, or—in simpler terms—if a cell produces more electrical charge flowing through depolarizing ion channels than charge needed to excite the same cell. Normally, SF is about 1.5,[16] and accordingly, the margin of safety (or "propagation reserve") is 0.5 above threshold of block. Although this biophysical definition is straightforward, it does not include the molecular contributors to propagation (ion currents, intercellular conductance, cell size, geometric cell arrangement). Investigating the contribution of these various molecular or geometric determinants of propagation to conduction safety requires detailed computer modeling.[16] A second point relates to the time window of integration, *A*, in equation 1. It may be difficult to determine in multidimensional tissue with heterogeneities in the geometric network or in expression of the molecular components.[17]

## Na⁺ INWARD CURRENT, PROPAGATION SLOWING, AND PROPAGATION BLOCK

Circulating excitation with reentry, often abbreviated 'reentry', is among the major mechanisms underlying arrhythmogenesis. The basic electrophysiologic changes leading to reentry have already been defined at the beginning of the last century (see Kleber and associates[18] and Kleber and Rudy[19]). For reentry to occur, the electrical excitation wave needs to be blocked at a given site and propagate unidirectionally around a zone of functional or anatomic block (so-called unidirectional block; see Kleber and Rudy[19] for a review). A second condition predicts that the wave length of propagation, which is defined as the product of the effective refractory period and propagation velocity has to be smaller than the reentry path. **Fig. 1** depicts the change in propagation velocity with decreasing availability of $I_{Na}$ and its comparison with the change caused by increasing cell-to-cell electrical conductance.[16] This comparison shows an essential characteristic of the role of $I_{Na}$ in propagation: With increasing block of $I_{Na}$, represented by the decreasing percentage of relative Na conductance, $g_{Na}$, there is an abrupt occurrence of block at relative high propagation velocities, in the order of 20 cm/s.

This signifies that reentry caused by blocking of $Na^+$ channels alone produces relatively large reentry circuits. Indeed, such large circuits can be observed, for instance, in the early phase of acute myocardial ischemia,[20] a condition characterized by resting membrane depolarization and decrease of $I_{Na}$ availability as the primary change. In contrast, propagation is very resistant to an increase in intercellular or junctional resistance, which has to increase by more than 100-fold for block to occur at very low propagation velocities (**Fig. 2**B). These results obtained in theoretical models are in close accordance with experimental studies.[21–23] They demonstrate that very slow electrical propagation, necessary to explain very small local reentry circuits, cannot occur with inhibition of ion channels alone; instead, either a very low degree of cell-to-cell coupling or a highly discontinuous architecture of the myocytes network is required.[22–24]

Even at normal sodium inward current flow and excitability at the level of individual cells, propagation block can occur at sites of so-called source sink mismatch, or structural discontinuities, caused the geometry of the myocardial cellular network. Myocardium contains numerous sites of source-to-load mismatch owing to the organization of the myocardium into layers "wrapped around" the left ventricle,[25,26] which are bridged by myocardial strands. With myocardial fibrosis, increasing with age or in pathologic settings, sites of mismatch between the upstream source (excited tissue) producing axial current and the downstream sink (cells in resting state) are added to these physiologic discontinuities. Three different geometric models have been used to investigate propagation across sites of source-to-load mismatch in experimental and theoretical studies[1]: The geometric expansion,[2] the pivoting point,[3] and the isthmus. Propagation across these discontinuities shares common biophysical principles.

**Fig. 2** illustrates propagation across a so-called tissue expansion (corresponding, for instance, with a myocardial cell bundle emerging into a large tissue layer). In the case of forward propagation, the small cell mass in the narrow bundle produces the axial or excitatory current flow during the action potential upstroke, which has to excite the large cell mass in the expansion downstream. This mismatch and dispersion of excitatory current decreases the current density flowing into the resting cells. As a consequence, a propagation delay develops and propagation blocks at a critical diameter of the strand. Very similar phenomena have been simulated or experimentally observed at a so-called tissue isthmus, that is, at a narrow cleft within a separation of 2 tissue layers (caused, for instance, by a gap in a connective tissue septum), and at a so-called pivot or end of an obstacle around which the propagation wave is forced to turn.[12,15,27,28] Such structures many also represent initiation sites for spiral waves (so-called vortex shedding).[29]

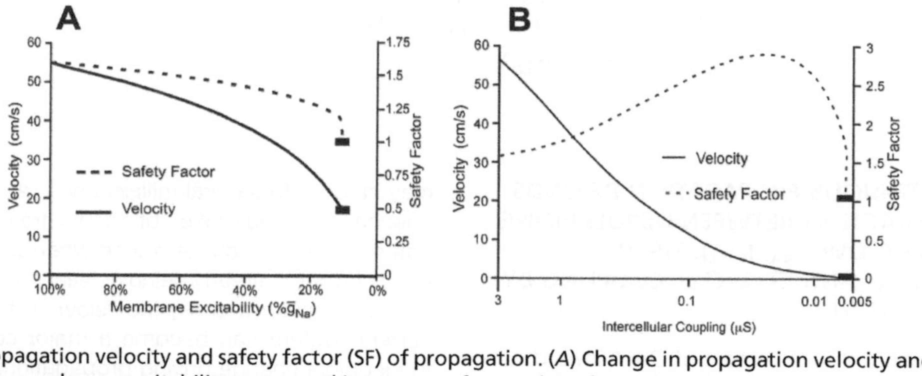


**Fig. 1.** Propagation velocity and safety factor (SF) of propagation. (*A*) Change in propagation velocity and SF with decreasing membrane excitability, expressed in percent of normal Na channel conductance, $g_{Na}$. Note continuous decrease of SF and velocity. There is a rapid transition from relatively high-velocity values (>10 cm/s) to block at approximately 90% of Na channel inhibition. (*B*) Change in propagation velocity and SF with decreasing intercellular electrical conductance expressed in microSiemens. Note logarithmic scale on the abscissa. (*From* Shaw RM, Rudy Y. Ionic mechanisms of propagation in cardiac tissue. Roles of the sodium and L-type calcium currents during reduced excitability and decreased gap junction coupling. Circ Res 1997;81:727–41; with permission.)

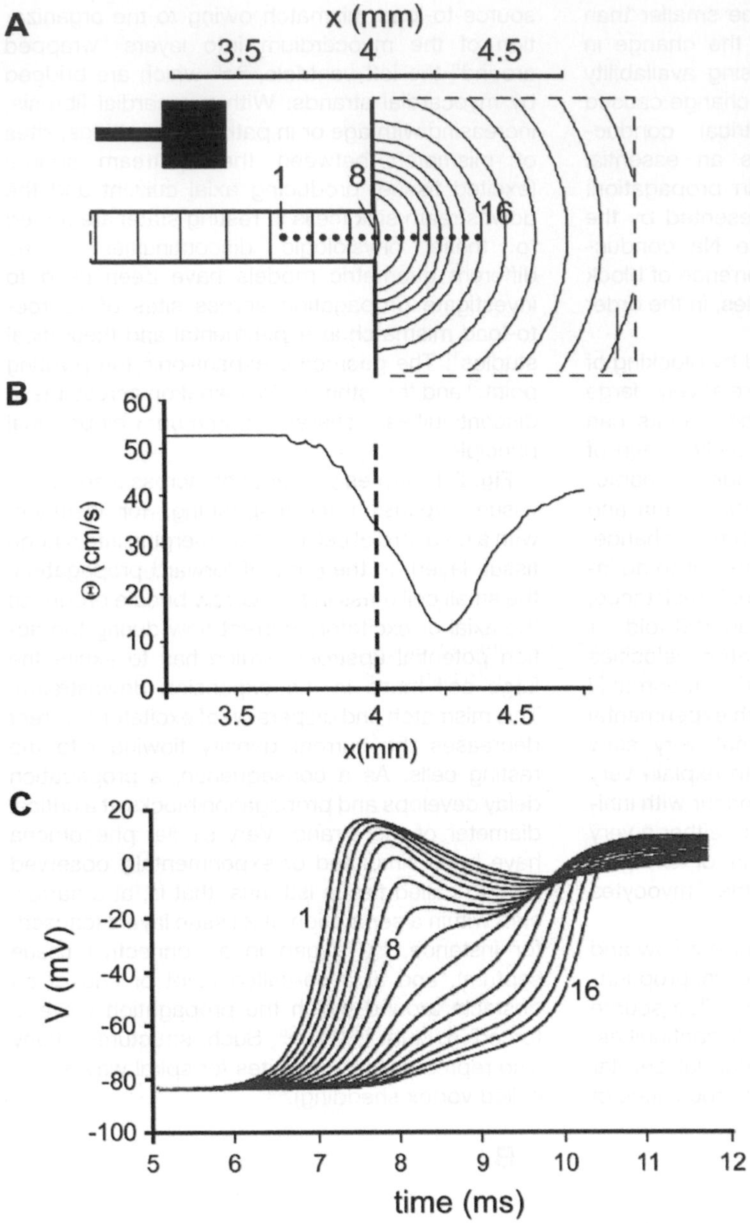


**Fig. 2.** Source-to-sink mismatch at a geometric expansion of cardiac tissue. (*A*) *Inset* shows scheme of cardiac strand emerging into a bulk of cells (*black*). Isochrones (connecting points of simultaneous activation) are shown together with 16 points defining locations from which action potential upstrokes are depicted in C. The isochrone lines become curved, indicating dispersion of local current flow, and crowded, indicating propagation slowing at the transition. (*B*) Local propagation velocity along the midline of the structure (to which the point in *A* is aligned). Note marked decrease of local propagation velocity at the transition. This decrease depends on the width of the strand and can develop to unidirectional block, if the strand width is decreased below a critical threshold. (*C*) Action potential upstroke of the signals computed at points 1 to 16 in *A*. As an expression of dispersion of local current, the upstroke and amplitudes of the action potentials decrease locally. Moreover, the signals beyond the transition show an upstroke with 2 components typical for discontinuous propagation. (*Adapted from* Fast VG, Kleber AG. Block of impulse propagation at an abrupt tissue expansion: evaluation of the critical strand diameter in 2- and 3-dimensional computer models. Cardiovasc Res 1995;30:449–59; with permission.)

## DISCONTINUOUS PROPAGATION DEPENDS ON INTERACTION BETWEEN DEPOLARIZING CURRENT FLOW ($I_{NA}$, $I_{CA,L}$), TISSUE STRUCTURE, AND CELL–CELL COUPLING BY GAP JUNCTIONS

The question of involvement of $Ca^{2+}$ inward current, $I_{Ca,L}$ in propagation, which starts to flow late during the normal action potential upstroke with slower kinetics than $I_{Na}$, drew the attention of electrophysiologists in the 1960s.[30] At sites of conduction discontinuities, local delays in propagation may amount to several milliseconds. As a consequence, the upstroke of downstream action potentials may occur at a time when the $Na^+$ inward current is already being at least partially inactivated. In such a case, the "slow" $Ca^{2+}$ inward current system can become a major contributor to electrical change driving propagation. The role of $I_{Ca,L}$ in propagation has been quantified in studies involving action potential transfer in cell pairs[31] and in experimental and theoretical studies in multicellular preparations.[16,23] It is also predicted to play a role in tissue with low degrees of cell-to-cell coupling, in which very large local delays have been observed at a cellular level using multisite, high-resolution optical mapping.[23,32] Importantly, specific inhibitors of $I_{Ca,L}$ can produce propagation block at sites of local conduction delays, although no such effects are observed during normal continuous propagation.[33] It is often stated that slow propagation in structures such as the atrioventricular node would be caused by $I_{Ca,L}$ as the main charge carrier. The studies discussed in this section suggest that highly discontinuous structures showing a low degree of cell-to-cell coupling, such as the atrioventricular node, require a match between the a "slow ion current system" ($I_{Ca,L}$) and the "slow" structural elements for conduction to occur.

If local current, produced by upstream cells, disperses from a small source into a large downstream sink (see **Fig. 2**B), it crosses multiple cell-to-cell junctions, and (in 2 dimensions) the flow of local current delivered by the terminal portion of the small bundle will occupy a certain downstream area. The electrical conductance of the gap junctions between the cells affects the degree of dispersion. In case of partial cell-to-cell uncoupling, reduced dispersion decreases the dispersion area on one hand, but increases the density of transmembrane stimulatory current flow within this area on the other. This effect can decrease the time delay across a tissue discontinuity (see **Fig. 2**C) and even reverse unidirectional block to bidirectional conduction.[34] This seemingly paradoxic improvement of propagation by partial cell-to-cell uncoupling in discontinuous propagation stands in contrast to linear continuous propagation where increasing cell-to-cell coupling leads to a continuous decrease of conduction velocity (see **Fig. 1**B).[16] Thus, the complexity of interaction between ion current flow, tissue structure, and cell-to-cell coupling challenges the concept that rescuing gap junctional electrical conductance, for instance by a drug, would generally be expected to exert an antiarrhythmic effect.

## CELL-TO-CELL PROPAGATION ACROSS GAP JUNCTIONS VERSUS EPHAPTIC IMPULSE TRANSMISSION: THE ROLE OF THE $Na^+$ INWARD CURRENT

The idea that cardiac impulse propagation from cell to cell would result from local circuit currents at the intercalated disk and not necessitate the presence of low-resistance gap junctions was expressed in the 1960s.[35] At that time the main argument to postulate this mechanism, termed *ephaptic* or capacitive electrical impulse transmission, was based on the observation of the absence of electrotonic current spread after intracellular current injection. Already early on, this hypothesis was controversial and was opposed by demonstration of current spread from cell to cell by others and the analysis of cell-to-cell diffusion of radiopotassium suggesting low resistance pathways (see Weidmann[36] for discussion). Recently, the idea that ephaptic impulse transmission could at least assist electrical transmission via gap junctions was revived. It emerged mainly from findings showing that relatively high propagation velocities could be measured in mice ventricles, in which Cx43 was ablated to a very high degree (cardio-specific germline Cx43 knockout).[37,38] The basic mechanism of ephaptic impulse transmission was assessed in 2 theoretical studies[39,40] and is shown schematically in **Fig. 3**.

**Fig. 3** shows 2 models of cellular arrangement of membrane $Na^+$ channels. In the simple model (see **Fig. 3**A), $Na^+$ channels are located in the surface membrane, whereas the membrane of the intercalated disc (ID) contains the gap junction channels as elements contributing to propagation. In the "ephaptic" model, a fraction of $Na^+$ channels is facing the extracellular space of the ID. Importantly, the narrow ID cleft facing the ID fraction of the channels has a larger extracellular resistance than the normal extracellular space. As a consequence, a voltage gradient between the ID cleft and the extracellular space is built up during inward $Na^+$ current flow. This voltage gradient is expected to depolarize the ID membranes, thereby driving the $Na^+$ channels of the juxtaposed cells to threshold and the juxtaposed cell to electrical excitation. Whereas the voltage gradient between the ID cleft and the extracellular space favors ephaptic transmission, the associated depletion of $Na^+$ ions in the narrow cleft of the ID space opposes it. This depletion reduces the chemical $Na^+$ gradient and, consequently, $I_{Na}$ across the cleft channels.[39]

Although ephaptic transmission can be demonstrated in theoretical simulations indeed,[39,40] it depends crucially on the setting of several variables in the models. A first important variable is the fraction of $Na^+$ channels present at the ID. Ephaptic transmission requires that large majority of $Na^+$ channels are clustered in the ID ($\geq$90%). However, experimental work has shown in adult mice ventricular myocytes that approximately 50% of $Na^+$ channels are located at the ID and distinct from the surface fraction by a specific anchoring protein.[41,42] A further variable is the resistance of the ID cleft, determined by cleft width. Recent work by Rhett and colleagues[43] suggests that the $Na_v1.5$ channels locate around the gap junctional plaques (so-called perinexus), which show a very

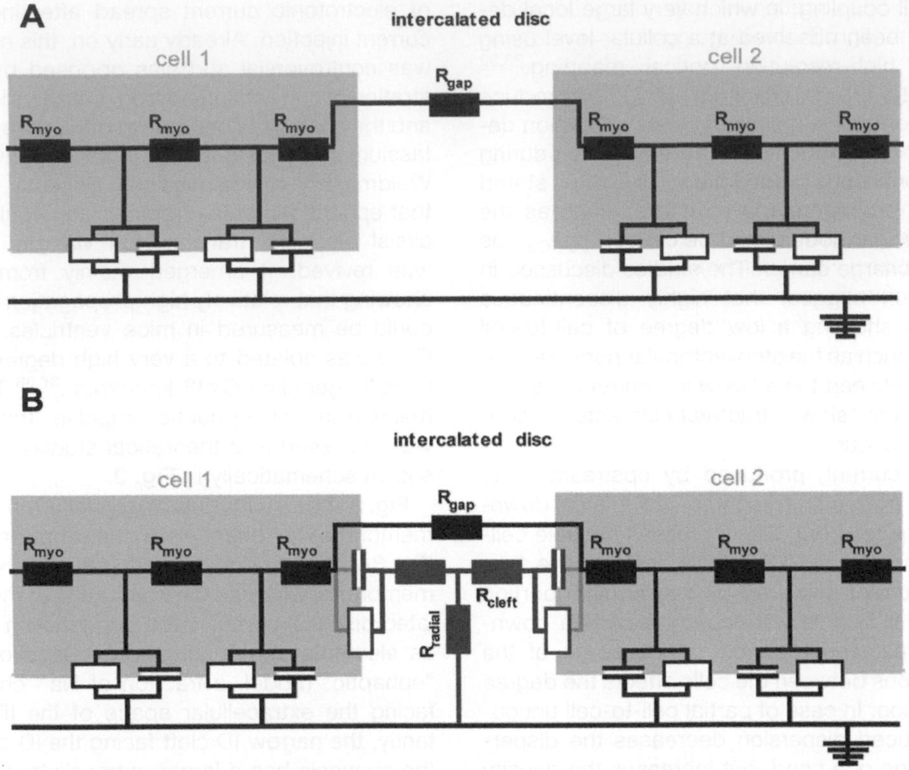


**Fig. 3.** Ephaptic transmission in the heart. The model shows 2 cells (*green*) with an intercellular space (ID). For explanation purposes, this cleft is enlarged. In reality it is a very narrow cleft in the nanometer range. (*A*) Normal model with electrical equivalent circuit showing myoplasmic resistors ($R_{myo}$), which are linked with the extracellular space by membrane elements. Each membrane element consists of a resistor (*white square*). The resistors are connected in parallel with membrane capacitors. This membrane resistor symbolizes the lumped resistance produced by flow through ion channels. Both cells are interconnected by a gap junction resistor ($R_{gap}$). (*B*) Model used to simulate ephaptic transmission. In addition to the circuit elements described in *A*, elements are added (*red*) for simulation of ephaptic transmission. These elements consist of a "membrane element" facing the narrow cleft of the ID, the resistance of the ID ($R_{cleft}$), and the resistance connecting the ID cleft to the extracellular space ($R_{radial}$).

narrow apposition of the cellular membranes in the order of a few tenths of nanometers.

As aforementioned, the observation that propagation velocity was found to decrease only by approximately 50%, even with a marked decrease of Cx43 immunofluorescence signal has revived the former hypothesis, that propagation would not require gap junction channels. However, other explanations exist to explain these phenomena. In cardiac ventricular strands engineered from mixtures of Cx43-expressing and Cx43-deficient cells, it has been shown that the percentage of Cx43 is not a direct measure of the proportion of Cx43-expressing cells and that relatively fast meandering propagation can occur in tissue with markedly reduced Cx43 fluorescence, which does not require ephaptic transmission.[32] Moreover, it has been shown that low electrical coupling exists in absence of detectable Cx43 immunofluorescence, whereas electrical intercellular conductance is approximately proportional to the Cx43 immunofluorescence signal for normal degrees of electrical coupling.[44] Further experimental evidence for absence of ephaptic transmission was obtained in experiments in which very low electrical coupling owing to the presence of Cx45 was observed with full genetic ablation of Cx43. The remaining portion of coupling was immediately abolished by a gap junction channel blocker (although cells remained excitable by field stimulation), demonstrating that ephaptic transmission was not able to substitute for absence of gap junction coupling.[24] Taken all these findings together suggests that ephaptic transmission does not play a major role in cardiac ventricular propagation, at least not in experimental models using cultured cells. Experimental work in adult cell pairs, which differ from neonatal cells with respect to the location of gap junctions, might bring further light in this ongoing controversy.

## SUMMARY

The theoretical and experimental work discussed in this review demonstrates that the role of $Na^+$ inward current in cardiac excitability and propagation cannot be discussed independently of $Ca^{2+}$ inward current, the discontinuous structure of cellular network, and cell-to-cell coupling. The contribution of all these variables to propagation is interdependent. Moreover, all these variables may change in a specific pathologic setting and explain the different behavior of electrical propagation and responsiveness to pharmacologic drugs of diseased hearts.

## REFERENCES

1. Hodgkin AL, Huxley AF. A quantitative description of membrane current and its application to conduction and excitation in nerve. J Physiol 1952;117:500–44.
2. Hodgkin AL, Huxley AF. The components of membrane conductance in the giant axon of Loligo. J Physiol 1952;116:473–96.
3. Hodgkin AL, Huxley AF. The dual effect of membrane potential on sodium conductance in the giant axon of Loligo. J Physiol 1952;116:497–506.
4. Weidmann S. Cardiac action potentials, membrane currents, and some personal reminiscences. Annu Rev Physiol 1993;55:1–14.
5. Coraboeuf E, Weidmann S. Potentiels d'action du muscle cardiaque obtenus a l'aide de microélectrodes intracellulaires. Présence d'une inversion de potentiel. CR Soc Biol Paris 1949;143:1360–1.
6. Draper MH, Weidmann S. Cardiac resting and action potentials recorded with an intracellular electrode. J Physiol 1951;115:74–94.
7. Weidmann S. Effect of current flow on the membrane potential of cardiac muscle. J Physiol 1951; 115:227–36.
8. Pelzer D, Trautwein W. Currents through ionic channels in multicellular cardiac tissue and single heart cells. Experientia 1987;43:1153–62.
9. Neher E, Sakmann B. Single-channel currents recorded from membrane of denervated frog muscle fibres. Nature 1976;260:799–802.
10. Sheets MF, Fozzard HA, Lipkind GM, et al. Sodium channel molecular conformations and antiarrhythmic drug affinity. Trends Cardiovasc Med 2010;20:16–21.
11. Fozzard HA, Hanck DA. Structure and function of voltage-dependent sodium channels: comparison of brain II and cardiac isoforms. Physiol Rev 1996; 76:887–926.
12. Fast VG, Kleber AG. Block of impulse propagation at an abrupt tissue expansion: evaluation of the critical strand diameter in 2- and 3-dimensional computer models. Cardiovasc Res 1995;30:449–59.
13. Spach MS, Kootsey JM. Relating the sodium current and conductance to tho shape of transmembrane and extracellular potentials by simulation: effects of propagation boundaries. IEEE Trans Biomed Eng 1985;32:743–55.
14. Maglaveras N, De Bakker JM, Van Capelle FJ, et al. Activation delay in healed myocardial infarction: a comparison between model and experiment. Am J Physiol 1995;269:H1441–9.
15. Fast VG, Kleber AG. Cardiac tissue geometry as a determinant of unidirectional conduction block: assessment of microscopic excitation spread by optical mapping in patterned cell cultures and in a computer model. Cardiovasc Res 1995;29:697–707.
16. Shaw RM, Rudy Y. Ionic mechanisms of propagation in cardiac tissue. Roles of the sodium and L-type calcium currents during reduced excitability and decreased gap junction coupling. Circ Res 1997; 81:727–41.
17. Kucera JP, Rudy Y. Mechanistic insights into very slow conduction in branching cardiac tissue: a model study. Circ Res 2001;89:799–806.
18. Kleber A, Janse M, Fast V. Normal and abnormal conduction in the heart. In: American Phsyiology Society, editor. The Handbook of Physiology, The Cardiovascular System, The Heart. Bethesda (MD); 2002. p. 455–530.
19. Kleber AG, Rudy Y. Basic mechanisms of cardiac impulse propagation and associated arrhythmias. Physiol Rev 2004;84:431–88.
20. Janse MJ, Wit AL. Electrophysiological mechanisms of ventricular arrhythmias resulting from myocardial ischemia and infarction. Physiol Rev 1989;69: 1049–169.
21. Kleber AG. Conduction of the impulse in the ischemic myocardium–implications for malignant ventricular arrhythmias. Experientia 1987;43: 1056–61.
22. Kucera JP, Kleber AG, Rohr S. Slow conduction in cardiac tissue, II: effects of branching tissue geometry. Circ Res 1998;83:795–805.
23. Rohr S, Kucera JP, Kleber AG. Slow conduction in cardiac tissue, I: effects of a reduction of excitability versus a reduction of electrical coupling on microconduction. Circ Res 1998;83:781–94.
24. Beauchamp P, Choby C, Desplantez T, et al. Electrical propagation in synthetic ventricular myocyte strands from germline connexin43 knockout mice. Circ Res 2004;95:170–8.
25. LeGrice IJ, Smaill BH, Chai LZ, et al. Laminar structure of the heart: ventricular myocyte arrangement and connective tissue architecture in the dog. Am J Physiol 1995;269:H571–82.
26. Pope AJ, Sands GB, Smaill BH, et al. Three-dimensional transmural organization of perimysial collagen

in the heart. Am J Physiol Heart Circ Physiol 2008; 295:H1243–52.
27. Cabo C, Pertsov AM, Baxter WT, et al. Wave-front curvature as a cause of slow conduction and block in isolated cardiac muscle. Circ Res 1994;75:1014–28.
28. Fast VG, Darrow BJ, Saffitz JE, et al. Anisotropic activation spread in heart cell monolayers assessed by high-resolution optical mapping. Role of tissue discontinuities. Circ Res 1996;79:115–27.
29. Cabo C, Pertsov AM, Davidenko JM, et al. Vortex shedding as a precursor of turbulent electrical activity in cardiac muscle. Biophys J 1996;70:1105–11.
30. Cranefield P. The conduction of the cardiac impulse. Mount Kisco (NY): Furura Publishing Company; 1975.
31. Joyner RW, Kumar R, Wilders R, et al. Modulating L-type calcium current affects discontinuous cardiac action potential conduction. Biophys J 1996; 71:237–45.
32. Beauchamp P, Desplantez T, McCain ML, et al. Electrical coupling and propagation in engineered ventricular myocardium with heterogeneous expression of connexin43. Circ Res 2012;110:1445–53.
33. Rohr S, Kucera JP. Involvement of the calcium inward current in cardiac impulse propagation: induction of unidirectional conduction block by nifedipine and reversal by Bay K 8644. Biophys J 1997;72:754–66.
34. Rohr S, Kucera JP, Fast VG, et al. Paradoxical improvement of impulse conduction in cardiac tissue by partial cellular uncoupling. Science 1997; 275:841–4.
35. Tarr M, Sperelakis N. Weak electrotonic interaction between contiguous cardiac cells. Am J Physiol 1964;207:691–700.
36. Weidmann S. The diffusion of radiopotassium across intercalated disks of mammalian cardiac muscle. J Physiol 1966;187:323–42.
37. Danik SB, Liu F, Zhang J, et al. Modulation of cardiac gap junction expression and arrhythmic susceptibility. Circ Res 2004;95:1035–41.
38. Gutstein DE, Morley GE, Tamaddon H, et al. Conduction slowing and sudden arrhythmic death in mice with cardiac-restricted inactivation of connexin43. Circ Res 2001;88:333–9.
39. Kucera JP, Rohr S, Rudy Y. Localization of sodium channels in intercalated disks modulates cardiac conduction. Circ Res 2002;91:1176–82.
40. Mori Y, Fishman GI, Peskin CS. Ephaptic conduction in a cardiac strand model with 3D electrodiffusion. Proc Natl Acad Sci U S A 2008;105:6463–8.
41. Milstein ML, Musa H, Balbuena DP, et al. Dynamic reciprocity of sodium and potassium channel expression in a macromolecular complex controls cardiac excitability and arrhythmia. Proc Natl Acad Sci U S A 2012;109:E2134–43.
42. Petitprez S, Zmoos AF, Ogrodnik J, et al. SAP97 and dystrophin macromolecular complexes determine two pools of cardiac sodium channels Nav1.5 in cardiomyocytes. Circ Res 2011;108:294–304.
43. Rhett JM, Ongstad EL, Jourdan J, et al. Cx43 associates with Na(v)1.5 in the cardiomyocyte perinexus. J Membr Biol 2012;245:411–22.
44. McCain ML, Desplantez T, Geisse NA, et al. Cell-to-cell coupling in engineered pairs of rat ventricular cardiomyocytes: relation between Cx43 immunofluorescence and intercellular electrical conductance. Am J Physiol Heart Circ Physiol 2012;302:H443–50.

# Role of Rare and Common Genetic Variation in *SCN5A* in Cardiac Electrical Function and Arrhythmia

Julien Barc, PhD, Connie R. Bezzina, PhD*

**KEYWORDS**

- *SCN5A* • Mutation • Common variants • Rare cardiac disorders • Channelopathy • GWAS • Polymorphisms • Noncoding region

**KEY POINTS**

- Mutations in the *SCN5A* gene have been associated with a broad spectrum of cardiac rhythm disorders associated with sudden cardiac death.
- Recent work dealing with the effect of noncoding genetic variation at the *SCN5A* locus has now extended insight into *SCN5A* disease mechanisms beyond the coding region of the gene.
- Work in this regard is expected to grow as insight concerning the regulatory noncoding regions of the genome continues to increase.

## INTRODUCTION

The *SCN5A* gene (80 kb, located on human chromosome 3) encodes the major sodium channel in heart ($Na_v1.5$).[1,2] The sodium channel is a critical mediator of cardiac conduction, because it conducts the fast depolarizing sodium current ($I_{Na}$) that mediates cardiomyocyte depolarization (phase 0 of the cardiac action potential). The first mutation in *SCN5A*, underlying long QT syndrome (LQTS) type 3, was identified by the group of Mark Keating almost 20 years ago.[3] Following this initial discovery, mutations in *SCN5A*, most of which are associated with autosomal dominant inheritance, were identified in a broad spectrum of cardiac disorders associated with sudden cardiac arrest (SCA).[4] Advances in genetic and molecular technologies have recently allowed a more comprehensive assessment of the role of this gene in cardiac disease, allowing investigation of not only the coding-region variants but also variants in noncoding regulatory regions that affect *SCN5A* gene transcript levels. Overall, the *SCN5A* locus is now known to harbor a broad range of functional genetic variants that range in frequency from common to rare and that carry mild to severe effects on cardiac electrical function.

## RARE *SCN5A* CODING-REGION VARIANTS UNDERLYING THE INHERITED CARDIAC DISEASES

### *Long QT Syndrome*

Congenital LQTS is an inherited disorder of abnormal myocardial repolarization. It is characterized clinically by an increased risk of potentially fatal ventricular arrhythmias, especially torsades de pointes, and prolongation of the QT interval on the surface electrocardiogram (ECG).[5,6] Coding-region mutations in *SCN5A* are found in about 5% to 10% of probands with the disorder.[7,8] Although the first *SCN5A* mutation that was linked

The authors have nothing to disclose.
Department of Experimental Cardiology, Academic Medical Center, Amsterdam, The Netherlands
* Corresponding author. Department of Experimental Cardiology, Heart Failure Research Center, Academic Medical Center, Room L2-108.1, Meibergdreef 15, Amsterdam 1105 AZ, The Netherlands.
*E-mail address:* c.r.bezzina@amc.uva.nl

Card Electrophysiol Clin 6 (2014) 665–677
http://dx.doi.org/10.1016/j.ccep.2014.07.001
1877-9182/14/$ – see front matter 

to LQTS involved an in-frame deletion of 3 amino acids, most LQTS-causing mutations in *SCN5A* are missense mutations.[7] About 85 missense mutations or small in-frame insertion/deletion mutations have been identified so far with a predominance in the intracellular segments of the channel (**Fig. 1**).[9] No large *SCN5A* gene rearrangements were detected in 2 studies that screened 42 and 93 patients with LQT respectively.[10,11] Electrophysiologic studies on LQTS-causing *SCN5A* mutations have uncovered disruption of fast channel inactivation causing an abnormal sustained sodium current (often referred to as a gain-of-function defect) as a common pathophysiologic mechanism.[12] Other less common mechanisms by which *SCN5A* mutations cause LQTS include an increased window current, slower inactivation, faster recovery from inactivation, and larger peak $I_{Na}$ density.[13] Patients with LQTS harboring a mutation in *SCN5A* often present with clinical features that distinguish them from patients with LQTS with a different genetic cause, such as a tendency for cardiac events to occur during sleep or rest.[14]

### *Conduction Disease*

As for LQTS, strong evidence exists for the involvement of *SCN5A* gene mutations in the pathogenesis of cardiac conduction disease, also referred to as Lenègre-Lev disease. The first report identified mutations in 2 families, one of which was large and allowed implication of the *SCN5A* chromosomal locus by linkage analysis.[15,16] Cardiac conduction disease is characterized by slowing of cardiac conduction within the different cardiac subcompartments, including the specialized conduction system. This slowing of cardiac conduction is reflected on the surface ECG as a prolongation of the P wave and the PR and QRS intervals. The disease may present from birth but may also be exacerbated with increasing age, culminating in atrioventricular block and various degrees of right or left bundle branch block, which may lead to syncope and sudden death. *SCN5A* mutations causing cardiac conduction disease lead to loss of sodium channel function. They include splice-site, frameshift, and nonsense mutations that cause the disease through a mechanism of haploinsufficiency, as well as missense mutations that result in decreased $I_{Na}$ through effects on the folding and trafficking of the channel and/or by affecting the biophysical properties of the channel.[9,13]

### *Brugada Syndrome*

Loss-of-function mutations in *SCN5A* are also found in around 20% of probands with Brugada syndrome (BrS),[17] a disorder associated with sudden death along with the signature ECG pattern of ST segment elevation in the right precordial leads.[18–20] The mechanisms by which *SCN5A* mutations cause BrS are similar to that in conduction disease, involving haploinsufficiency or biophysical defects leading to a decreased current. Thus, patients with BrS harboring *SCN5A* mutations show prolonged conduction indices on the ECG.[21] However, why loss of sodium channel function leads to conduction disease in some patients and BrS in others remains unknown. The same mutation in *SCN5A* can lead to lone conduction disease or BrS even in individuals from the same family, whereas other family members can present both phenotypes.[22,23] In total, about 300 distinct *SCN5A* mutations have been described in patients with the disorder; about two-thirds are missense variations and one-third are nonsense mutations, splice-site mutations, and small insertion-deletions that lead to a truncated channel protein.[17] Although one report identified a large *SCN5A* gene deletion causing the disorder, such mutations do not seem to be a common cause of the disease.[24] In one study it was shown that patients with BrS or conduction disease with premature truncation of the protein or missense mutation with a drastic peak $I_{Na}$ reduction (>90%) present significantly more with syncope compared with patients with incomplete loss of function of the $Na_V1.5$ channel.[25]

### *Sick Sinus Syndrome*

Mutations in *SCN5A* are also a cause of sick sinus syndrome (SSS) (see **Fig. 1**), a disorder characterized by dysfunction of the sinoatrial node. Like conduction disease and BrS, *SCN5A* mutations causing SSS are associated with loss of sodium channel function. Sinus node dysfunction is often part of the clinical picture in families affected by conduction disease and/or BrS harboring mutations in *SCN5A*.[26] Although several autosomal dominant mutations leading to SSS have been described,[27–30] compound heterozygous mutations in line with an autosomal recessive inheritance have also been uncovered both in young children[31,32] and in utero (20–38 weeks' gestation) during Doppler-echocardiographic evaluation.[33] An autosomal recessive mode of inheritance in SSS is supported by a recent study in which a missense homozygote mutation was found in 4 siblings of a German family.[34]

### *Sudden Infant Death Syndrome*

The *SCN5A* gene has also been screened in several cohorts of patients who died of sudden

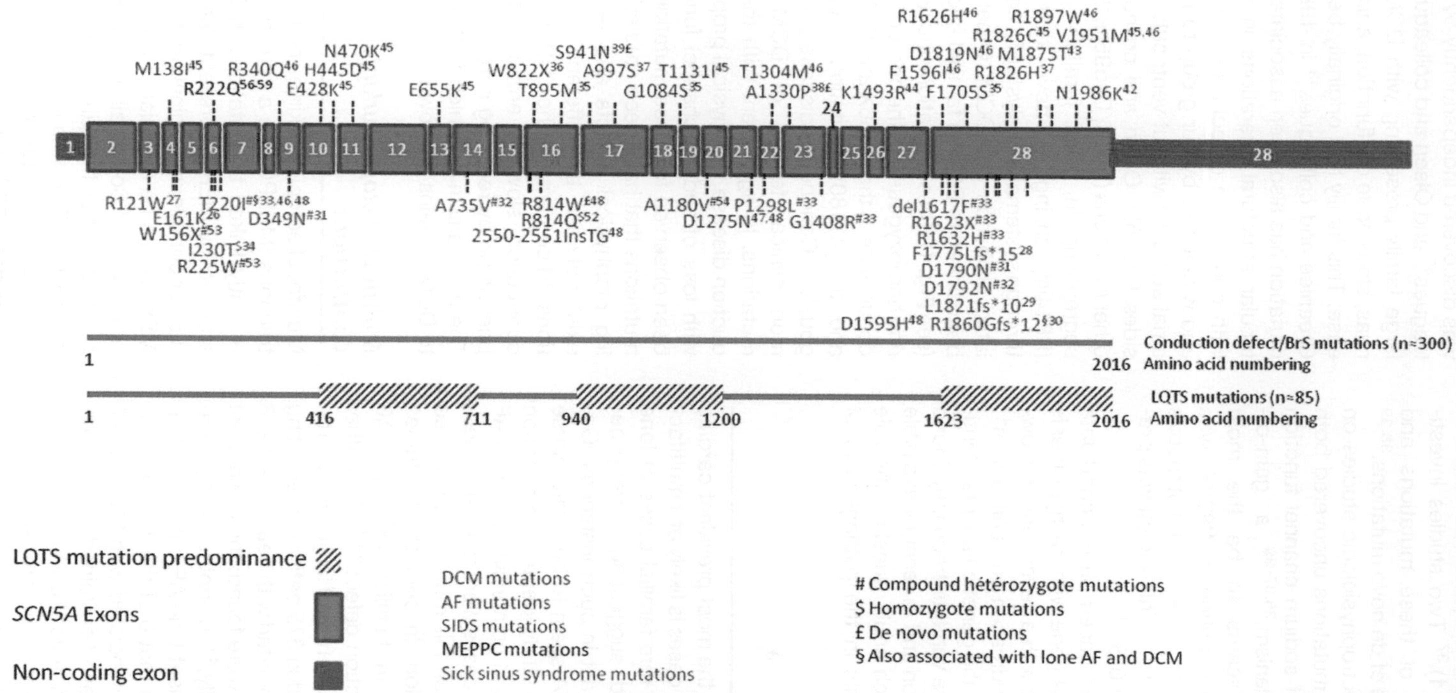


**Fig. 1.** The *SCN5A* gene annotated with the rare coding variants identified in the *SCN5A*-associated cardiac disorders. AF, atrial fibrillation; BrS, Brugada syndrome; DCM, dilated cardiomyopathy; MEPPC, multifocal ectopic Purkinje-related premature contractions; SIDS, sudden infant death syndrome.

infant death syndrome (SIDS), defined as a sudden death of an infant less than 1 year old without any symptom preceding the death.[35–39] *SCN5A* mutations have been reported to explain 2% to 10% of SIDS cases (see **Fig. 1**).[37] Two studies investigated the inheritance of these mutations and showed the occurrence of de novo mutations.[38,39] Although functional electrophysiologic studies on some of the identified mutations uncovered both loss as well as gain of sodium channel function as a possible mechanism,[35,37–39] a gain-of-function mechanism seems to be the most common. A nonsense mutation, p.W822X, was discovered in a singular case of simultaneous SIDS in monozygotic twins.[36] This variant was previously associated with BrS.[40]

These discoveries are based on the candidate screening of the *SCN5A* gene with the hypothesis of identifying mutations with a severe effect. However recent work by Andreasen and colleagues[41] showed that several of the genetic variants identified in these studies are variants frequently found in the general population and in recently available public databases, which could question the role of some of the variants in the pathogenesis of SIDS.

## *Atrial Fibrillation*

Atrial fibrillation (AF) is the most prevalent cardiac arrhythmia and in most cases is likely of a multifactorial origin. However, rare familial cases of lone AF have been reported, suggesting a strong genetic component at least in such instances. Genetic variants in *SCN5A* seem to be a rare cause of AF (see **Fig. 1**). One study identified a mutation in 1 patient from a cohort comprising 189 lone AF probands, of which 57 cases were familial.[42] Electrophysiologic studies on this mutation uncovered loss of channel function. In contrast, 2 studies identified a mutation in families with lone AF showing a gain-of-function defect.[43,44] Two other articles describe the screening of large AF cohorts. In one study conducted in 375 patients presenting with lone AF or AF associated with heart disease, 8 novel *SCN5A* variants were found; these were not investigated functionally.[45] In another study, conducted in 192 early-onset lone AF cases, 10 variants were found. Note that 6 of the 10 mutations had previously been associated with LQTS and 5 variants showed increased sustained sodium current. However, other variants show loss of function of the cardiac sodium current, proving that both gain-of-function and loss-of-function alterations can lead to the development of AF.[46] In one report, a truncating *SCN5A* mutation was associated with SSS and AF in a family.[30]

## *Dilated Cardiomyopathy*

The first *SCN5A* mutation implicated in dilated cardiomyopathy (DCM) was D1275N. This mutation was discovered independently by McNair and colleagues[47] and Olson and colleagues[48] in the same large family presenting with DCM, atrial arrhythmias, sinus node dysfunction, and conduction disease. This family had originally been described by Greenlee and colleagues[49] in 1986. The D1275N mutation has also been associated with mild ventricular structural alterations in a Finnish family with conduction defects and atrial arrhythmias[50] and was linked by our group to the phenotype of atrial standstill without ventricular dilatation.[51] Besides D1275N, Olson and colleagues[48] reported other mutations (T220I, D1595H, 2550–2551insTG) segregating in small families and 1 mutation (R814W) arising de novo that they identified through systematic analysis of a cohort of 156 unrelated probands with DCM. Other mutations have been linked to DCM in familial and sporadic cases (see **Fig. 1**). These mutations include R814Q occurring homozygously,[52] the compound heterozygous occurrence of the W156X and R225W mutations,[53] and the A1180V mutation occurring heterozygously.[54] Conduction disease seems to be a common clinical feature of DCM-related *SCN5A* mutations. In agreement with the observed conduction disease, biophysical properties consistent with loss of sodium channel function have often been observed for these mutations. However, the mutations that have been studied also show varying biophysical defects and few commonalities exist between the different DCM-related mutations. Mice carrying the D1275N variant showed conduction slowing, arrhythmias, and a DCM phenotype by reducing cardiac sodium current.[55] The mechanism by which *SCN5A* mutations lead to DCM remains unknown.

## *Multifocal Ectopic Purkinje-related Premature Contractions*

Multifocal ectopic Purkinje-related premature contractions (MEPPC) are a cardiac arrhythmia entity recently linked to mutations in *SCN5A*. Patients affected by MEPPC present with premature ventricular complexes originating from Purkinje tissue. MEPPC can be associated with atrial arrhythmias or DCM.[56–59] So far, all 5 families described with MEPPC harbor the same mutation in the voltage sensor (see **Fig. 1**) in domain I of $Na_V1.5$, namely the p.R222Q mutation,[56,57,59] showing dominant inheritance and a remarkable complete penetrance. Electrophysiologic studies on the mutated p.R222Q-$Na_v1.5$ channel revealed an increase of the cardiac sodium channel excitability, which could explain the premature ventricular action potentials.

### *Overlap Syndromes*

As described earlier, mutations in *SCN5A* can lead to a large spectrum of different arrhythmia disorders. Multiple overlapping clinical manifestations, including conduction disease, BrS, and sinus node dysfunction, are often encountered in the setting of mutations associated with loss of sodium channel function; in families they may occur in isolation or in combinations thereof.[60] More surprisingly, within a large Dutch kindred carrying the *SCN5A* mutation 1975InsD, we reported on the occurrence of both BrS and LQTS, which are disorders known to be caused respectively by a sodium channel loss-of-function defect and a gain-of-function defect. Functional studies in cellular systems and mice on the mutation in this family uncovered a multidysfunctional sodium channel that could explain the coexistence of both phenotypes.[61,62] Extensive clinical investigation in the family also uncovered bradycardia and conduction disease. A similar heterogeneous clinical phenotype was also reported for the delK1500[63] and the E1784K[64] mutations. Although the multiple biophysical defects of the underlying *SCN5A* mutation can explain the occurrence of multiple clinical phenotypes as a consequence of sodium channelopathy,[62,64] it is also likely that other factors, including additional genetic factors as well as acquired or environmental factors, also contribute in determining the ultimate clinical disease manifestation in the individual patient.

## CHALLENGES IN INTERPRETATION OF *SCN5A* GENETIC TEST RESULTS

Substantial challenges may arise in the interpretation of *SCN5A* genetic test results in the setting of DNA diagnostics. As for most genes, this is largely caused by the large degree of allelic heterogeneity observed in the *SCN5A* gene, which has become increasingly clear in the past 2 years as exome and genome sequencing projects, such as the 1000 Genomes Project[65] and the National Institutes of Health Heart, Lung, and Blood Institute's Exome Sequencing Project,[66–68] have generated extensive maps of genetic variation in thousands of human exomes and genomes. The availability of these databases has brought with it the realization that genomes of control individuals could also contain rare or private genetic variants in arrhythmia-associated genes such as *SCN5A*. In contrast, particular genetic variants, previously deemed pathogenic from their absence in a few hundred control individuals, are present in the general population, as observed in these large samples.[69] In the absence of genetic datasets encompassing large families for extensive and robust cosegregation analysis, which is usually the case, distinguishing deleterious disease-causing variants from innocuous variants remains a major challenge.[70]

## REDUCED PENETRANCE AND VARIABLE DISEASE EXPRESSION

Like most mendelian disorders, the cardiac sodium channelopathies show the phenomenon of reduced penetrance and variable disease expression.[71] The penetrance of a disease is defined as the percentage of individuals possessing the mutation who develop the associated clinical manifestations. Variable expression is defined as the variation in clinical disease severity among carriers of the same mutation; this can range from mildly affected to severely affected individuals. Variable disease severity is probably best appreciated in large pedigrees segregating the same causal mutation or in multiple families harboring founder mutations, because effects on clinical severity that stem from mutations of different severity are excluded.[72,73] Particular mutation carriers might not show clinical signs of the disease (such as ECG abnormalities), even though they carry the familial mutation, whereas others who are affected have variable disease severity.[72] However, only a fraction of mutation carriers develop life-threatening arrhythmia. Although factors such as age and sex are expected to play a role in modulating disease penetrance and severity, the inheritance of other genetic factors alongside the primary genetic defect is also thought to play a role. The identification of genetic modifiers is of considerable interest, because it is expected to contribute to improved risk stratification.

## COMMON VARIANTS IN THE *SCN5A* CODING REGION

The screening of the coding region of *SCN5A* in patients with cardiac rhythm disorders as well as controls revealed the occurrence of missense genetic variants that are common in the general population. These variants have drawn considerable interest because they could potentially modulate the severity of the clinical phenotype in patients with sodium channelopathy. This modulation could occur because they affect the biophysical properties of the wild-type channel (when they occur in trans to the causal *SCN5A* mutation) or they could aggravate or temper the biophysical defect of the *SCN5A* mutation when they occur in cis (ie, on the same allele).

The most frequent of such polymorphisms is the p.H558R missense variant, which has a minor allele frequency of about 25% in populations of European descent and African descent.[68,74] The frequency in the Asian population seems to be lower.[74]

Viswanathan and colleagues[75] were the first to introduce the concept that the interaction of polymorphisms and mutations may exert relevant effects on the functional consequences of the mutation. These investigators studied the biophysical properties of the *SCN5A* T512I mutation, which was found in a proband with conduction disease who was also homozygous for the H558R polymorphism in the same gene. By comparing the biophysical properties of wild-type $Na^+$ channels, $Na^+$ channels carrying the T512I mutation alone, and $Na^+$ channels carrying both the T512I mutation and the R558 variant, these investigators showed that the biophysical defect associated with the mutation was mitigated by the presence of the polymorphism occurring in the same channel molecule. Similar observations of intramolecular complementation were obtained by Ye and colleagues[76] who, through in vitro studies, showed that the plasma membrane–targeting defect associated with the *SCN5A* M1766L mutation was rescued when it was expressed in the setting of a $Na^+$ channel also carrying R558. Later, Poelzing and colleagues[77] also provided evidence for a transcomplementation effect of the R558 variant. They showed that, in heterologous cells, expression of the BrS R282H mutant $Na^+$ channels alone did not produce any $Na^+$ current, whereas coexpression of R282H channels together with channels carrying the R558 variant produced significantly greater current compared with coexpression with channels carrying the H558 variant. This finding showed that the polymorphism rescues the cell surface expression of the mutation; however, the molecular mechanism remains unknown.

The common polymorphisms p.R34C and p.S1103Y show a differential allele frequency between the European-descent and African-descent populations. Both are rare (<1%) among individuals of European descent but are present in 8.9% and 7.3%, respectively, among individuals of African descent.[68] The p.S1103Y polymorphism has been associated with arrhythmia both in case-control studies as well as in families.[78,79] It was also found to be enriched in a set of SIDS cases of African American descent.[80,81] This variant is thought to promote arrhythmia susceptibility during exposure to extrinsic factors such as QT-prolonging medication or acquired cardiac disease, in line with a multihit pathogenesis for cardiac arrhythmia. Collaborative studies led by the groups of Professors Ackerman and Makielski show the biophysical consequences of this polymorphism.[82,83] Another ethnic-specific polymorphism in *SCN5A* is the p.R1193Q variant, which is mainly found in Asian people.[74] However, the functional effect of p.R1193Q on the $I_{Na}$ current remains unclear because 2 studies reported contradictory consequences in the setting of the BrS and the LQTS.[84,85] This discrepancy could be explained by the use of different *SCN5A* isoforms in the two studies: the effect of p.R1193Q variant in the BrS study was evaluated with the isoform containing the glutamine residue in position 1077, whereas in the LQTS study Wang and colleagues[85] used the 2015 amino acid isoform lacking the p.Q1077 residue. Alternative splicing of a single amino acid of *SCN5A* at the beginning of exon 18 causes insertion of glutamine at position 1077 (Q1077), resulting in 2 splice variants: one that forms a 2016 amino acid protein designated Q1077 and a 2015 amino acid protein designated Q1077del.[86] Both splice variants exist in the heart, with a 65% predominance of the shorter 2015 amino acid variant Q1077del.[86] The trafficking defect associated with the BrS mutation G1406R was shown to depend on the background splice variant in which it was expressed, being worse in the Q1077 variant. Although no evidence exists, it is possible that conditions that upset the normal 2:1 ratio of the Q1077del and Q1077 variants could also modulate the phenotype associated with specific *SCN5A* mutations.

## COMMON VARIANTS IN THE *SCN5A* NONCODING REGION

Recent candidate gene and genome-wide association studies (GWASs) have highlighted the role of genetic variation in the noncoding regulatory regions of *SCN5A* in modulation of cardiac electrical function both in samples of the general population as well as in BrS. Genetic variation in these regions of the *SCN5A* gene is expected to modulate the phenotype through effects on the level of expression of the *SCN5A* transcript and ultimately the abundance of the channel protein present on the cardiomyocyte sarcolemma.

The first noncoding *SCN5A* region that was explored for the presence of common genetic modifiers was the promoter region of *SCN5A*. In an analysis covering 2.8 kb spanning the *SCN5A* promoter (including 2.2 kb upstream of exon 1, exon 1, and the proximal 439 bp of intron 1) our group identified a haplotype encompassing multiple polymorphisms that was common in Asian people. This haplotype was associated with a decreased reporter activity in an in vitro assay and was associated with prolonged ECG conduction indices in control individuals and in patients with BrS.[87]

The noncoding region surrounding *SCN5A* has been more extensively investigated in GWASs that have recently been conducted in the general population. These studies have sought to identify common genetic variation that modulates ECG indices of conduction and repolarization (reviewed by Kolder and colleagues[88] and Marsman and colleagues[89]). Multiple independent genetic variants at the locus of *SCN5A* and neighboring *SCN10A* have been associated with changes in PR interval, QRS duration, and corrected QT (QTc) interval in the general population (summarized in **Table 1**).[90–96] Although there are a few exceptions (eg, association with pacemaker implantation,[91] AF,[92,97–99] and ventricular fibrillation in the setting of acute myocardial infarction[90]), these single-nucleotide polymorphisms (SNPs) have not yet been extensively studied for their potential role in modulating disease expression in the cardiac sodium channelopathies and other (acquired) arrhythmias.

The GWAS approach has recently been applied by our group and international collaborators for the study of genetic factors underlying the BrS. We hypothesized that the inheritance pattern of this disorder is more complex than was previously appreciated and likely entails the inheritance of multiple genetic variants of different effect sizes located in different genes. This hypothesis is based on several observations, including that there is low disease penetrance in families harboring mutations in *SCN5A*, that many patients with BrS are sporadic, and that classical linkage analysis has largely been unsuccessful in identifying new disease genes. Our GWAS effort in the disorder uncovered 3 independent loci, 2 of which (rs10428132 and rs11708996) reside at the *SCN5A/SCN10A* chromosomal locus.[100] These 2 loci had previously been linked to the PR and QRS interval durations in the general population.[90–93,96] For both haplotypes, the PR-prolonging and QRS-prolonging allele was associated with BrS risk, providing support for the concept that the cardiomyocyte depolarization process has an important role in the pathogenesis of BrS.[101] This work not only supports the concept of a more complex inheritance pattern for the BrS but also shows that polymorphisms previously shown to modulate cardiac conduction in GWAS in the general population can also influence susceptibility to a rare primary electrical disorder.

The ENCODE (Encyclopedia Of DNA Elements) project[102] and efforts at individual laboratories[103–106] are rapidly providing insight into the functional regulatory elements such as enhancers in the noncoding part of the genome. These developments are crucial to furthering understanding of the genetic mechanisms associated with GWAS loci located in noncoding regions such as the 2 associated with BrS (and most of the loci

**Table 1**
**Single-nucleotide polymorphisms (SNPs) at the *SCN5A/SCN10A* locus identified by GWAS**

| *SCN5A* SNPs Identified in GWAS | Other Associated Cardiac Traits |
|---|---|
| **SNPs Associated with PR** | |
| rs3922844,[96] rs11708996,[92] rs6599222,[96] rs6795970 or rs6801957[90–92,96] | Altered QT interval,[93–95] QRS interval,[91,93,97] and P-wave duration[90]; AF[92,97–99]; pacemaker implantation[91]; BrS[100]; MI-induced VF[90]; cardiac arrhythmias[97] |
| **SNPs Associated with QRS** | |
| rs6795970 or rs6801957,[91,93,97] rs2051211,[93] rs10865879,[93,97] rs11710077,[93] rs11708996,[93] rs9851724[93] | Altered QT interval,[93–95] QRS interval,[91,93,97] and P-wave duration[90]; AF[92,97–99]; pacemaker implantation[91]; BrS[100]; MI-induced VF[90]; cardiac arrhythmias[97] |
| **SNP Associated with QTc** | |
| rs11129795[94,95] | Altered QRS interval[93,97] |
| **SNPs Associated with the BrS** | |
| rs10428132 and rs11708996[100] | Altered QT interval,[93–95] QRS interval,[91,93,97] and P-wave duration[90]; AF[92,97–99]; pacemaker implantation[91]; MI-induced VF[90]; cardiac arrhythmias[97] |

*Abbreviations:* MI, myocardial infarction; VF, ventricular fibrillation.

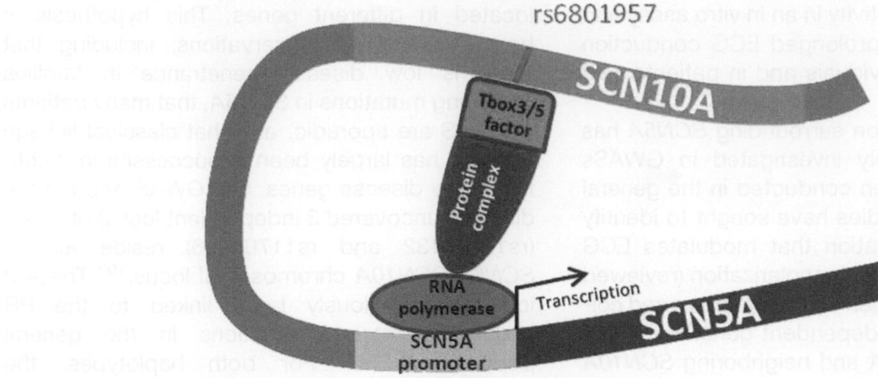


**Fig. 2.** The *SCN10/SCN5A* chromosomal region conformation and the interaction of the enhancer region containing the rs6801957 polymorphism with the *SCN5A* promoter.

uncovered for ECG parameters including cardiac conduction). This insight provides a means to prioritize the potentially causal variants within haplotypes for further downstream functional studies. The potential of this approach has recently been shown by the groups of Christoffels, Nobrega, Barnett, and Moskowitz, who have unraveled the genomic mechanism by which the *SCN10A* haplotype tagged by rs10428132 affects cardiac conduction and BrS.[105,107,108] These investigators showed that the G to A nucleotide change at SNP rs6801957 (located on the haplotype tagged by rs10428132) resides in a consensus T-box transcription factor binding site within a cardiac enhancer. Through a series of in vitro and in vivo studies they showed how the G to A change reduced T-box transcription factor binding to the enhancer; affected the stimulation and repression by TBX5 and TBX3, respectively, of a reporter in in vitro assays; and reduced the activity of the enhancer in vivo.[105,107] Furthermore, the haplotype tagged by rs6801957 was associated with reduced *SCN5A* expression in human heart.[107] In aggregate, these data provide strong evidence that rs6801957 is the causal variant within the rs6801957/rs10428132-tagged haplotype (**Fig. 2**).

Despite the strong evidence for rs6801957 in mediating the pathophysiologic effect of the haplotype on which it occurs through differences in transcription factor binding, SNP rs6795970, which is also on this haplotype (r2 = 0.93 with rs6801957), encodes a nonsynonymous substitution (Ala1073Val) in the *SCN10A*-encoded Nav1.8 sodium channel, which suggests the possibility that the effects of the haplotype on conduction could still arise, at least in part, through effects on the biophysical properties for Nav1.8. However, this seems unlikely because the level of expression of the *SCN10A* transcript in heart seems to be very low.[107]

## SUMMARY

Commensurate with the central role of the cardiac sodium channel in cardiac electrical function, mutations in *SCN5A* have been associated with a broad spectrum of cardiac rhythm disorders associated with sudden cardiac death. Recent work dealing with the effect of noncoding genetic variation at the *SCN5A* locus has now extended insight into *SCN5A* disease mechanisms beyond the coding region of the gene. Work in this regard is expected to grow as insight concerning the regulatory noncoding regions of the genome continues to increase.

## REFERENCES

1. Gellens ME, George AL, Chen LQ, et al. Primary structure and functional expression of the human cardiac tetrodotoxin-insensitive voltage-dependent sodium channel. Proc Natl Acad Sci U S A 1992;89(2): 554–8. Available at: http://www.pubmedcentral.nih.gov/articlerender.fcgi?artid=48277&tool=pmcentrez&rendertype=abstract. Accessed April 15, 2014.
2. George AL, Varkony TA, Drabkin HA, et al. Assignment of the human heart tetrodotoxin-resistant voltage-gated Na+ channel alpha-subunit gene (SCN5A) to band 3p21. Cytogenet Cell Genet 1995; 68(1–2):67–70. Available at: http://www.ncbi.nlm.nih.gov/pubmed/7956363. Accessed April 12, 2014.
3. Wang Q, Shen J, Splawski I, et al. SCN5A mutations associated with an inherited cardiac arrhythmia, long QT syndrome. Cell 1995;80:805–11, 0092-8674 (Print).
4. Remme CA, Bezzina CR. Sodium channel (dys) function and cardiac arrhythmias. Cardiovasc Ther 2010;28(5):287–94. http://dx.doi.org/10.1111/j.1755-5922.2010.00210.x.
5. Jervell A, Lange-Nielsen F. Congenital deaf-mutism, functional heart disease with prolongation

of the Q-T interval and sudden death. Am Heart J 1957;54:59–68, 0002-8703 (Print).

6. Schwartz PJ, Crotti L, Insolia R. Long-QT syndrome: from genetics to management. Circ Arrhythm Electrophysiol 2012;5(4):868–77. http://dx.doi.org/10.1161/CIRCEP.111.962019.
7. Tester DJ, Will ML, Haglund CM, et al. Compendium of cardiac channel mutations in 541 consecutive unrelated patients referred for long QT syndrome genetic testing. Heart Rhythm 2005; 2(5):507–17. http://dx.doi.org/10.1016/j.hrthm.2005.01.020.
8. Splawski I, Shen J, Timothy KW, et al. Spectrum of mutations in long-QT syndrome genes. KVLQT1, HERG, SCN5A, KCNE1, and KCNE2. Circulation 2000;102:1178–85.
9. Zimmer T, Surber R. SCN5A channelopathies–an update on mutations and mechanisms. Prog Biophys Mol Biol 2008;98:120–36, 0079-6107 (Print).
10. Tester DJ, Benton AJ, Train L, et al. Prevalence and spectrum of large deletions or duplications in the major long QT syndrome-susceptibility genes and implications for long QT syndrome genetic testing. Am J Cardiol 2010;106(8):1124–8. http://dx.doi.org/10.1016/j.amjcard.2010.06.022.
11. Barc J, Briec F, Schmitt S, et al. Screening for copy number variation in genes associated with the long QT syndrome: clinical relevance. J Am Coll Cardiol 2011;57:40–7, 1558-3597 (Electronic).
12. Bennett PB, Yazawa K, Makita N, et al. Molecular mechanism for an inherited cardiac arrhythmia. Nature 1995;376:683–5, 0028-0836 (Print).
13. Amin AS, Asghari-Roodsari A, Tan HL. Cardiac sodium channelopathies. Pflugers Arch 2010; 460(2):223–37. http://dx.doi.org/10.1007/s00424-009-0761-0.
14. Schwartz PJ, Priori SG, Spazzolini C, et al. Genotype-phenotype correlation in the long-QT syndrome: gene-specific triggers for life-threatening arrhythmias. Circulation 2001;103:89–95, 1524-4539 (Electronic).
15. Schott JJ, Alshinawi C, Kyndt F, et al. Cardiac conduction defects associate with mutations in SCN5A. Nat Genet 1999;23(1):20–1. http://dx.doi.org/10.1038/12618.
16. Probst V, Kyndt F, Potet F, et al. Haploinsufficiency in combination with aging causes SCN5A-linked hereditary Lenegre disease. J Am Coll Cardiol 2003;41:643–52, 0735-1097 (Print).
17. Kapplinger JD, Tester DJ, Alders M, et al. An international compendium of mutations in the SCN5A-encoded cardiac sodium channel in patients referred for Brugada syndrome genetic testing. Heart Rhythm 2010;7(1):33–46. http://dx.doi.org/10.1016/j.hrthm.2009.09.069.
18. Brugada P, Brugada J. Right bundle branch block, persistent ST segment elevation and sudden cardiac death: a distinct clinical and electrocardiographic syndrome. A multicenter report. J Am Coll Cardiol 1992;20:1391–6, 0735-1097 (Print).
19. Chen Q, Kirsch GE, Zhang D, et al. Genetic basis and molecular mechanism for idiopathic ventricular fibrillation. Nature 1998;392:293–6, 0028-0836 (Print).
20. Crotti L, Marcou CA, Tester DJ, et al. Spectrum and prevalence of mutations involving BrS1- through BrS12-susceptibility genes in a cohort of unrelated patients referred for Brugada syndrome genetic testing: implications for genetic testing. J Am Coll Cardiol 2012;60(15):1410–8. http://dx.doi.org/10.1016/j.jacc.2012.04.037.
21. Smits JP, Eckardt L, Probst V, et al. Genotype-phenotype relationship in Brugada syndrome: electrocardiographic features differentiate SCN5A-related patients from non-SCN5A-related patients. J Am Coll Cardiol 2002;40:350–6, 0735-1097 (Print).
22. Remme CA, Wilde AA, Bezzina CR. Cardiac sodium channel overlap syndromes: different faces of SCN5A mutations. Trends Cardiovasc Med 2008;18(3):78–87. http://dx.doi.org/10.1016/j.tcm.2008.01.002.
23. Kyndt F, Probst V, Potet F, et al. Novel SCN5A mutation leading either to isolated cardiac conduction defect or Brugada syndrome in a large French family. Circulation 2001;104:3081–6, 1524-4539 (Electronic).
24. Eastaugh LJ, James PA, Phelan DG, et al. Brugada syndrome caused by a large deletion in SCN5A only detected by multiplex ligation-dependent probe amplification. J Cardiovasc Electrophysiol 2011;22(9):1073–6. http://dx.doi.org/10.1111/j.1540-8167.2010.02003.x.
25. Meregalli PG, Tan HL, Probst V, et al. Type of SCN5A mutation determines clinical severity and degree of conduction slowing in loss-of-function sodium channelopathies. Heart Rhythm 2009;6(3):341–8. http://dx.doi.org/10.1016/j.hrthm.2008.11.009.
26. Smits JP, Koopmann TT, Wilders R, et al. A mutation in the human cardiac sodium channel (E161K) contributes to sick sinus syndrome, conduction disease and Brugada syndrome in two families. J Mol Cell Cardiol 2005;38(6):969–81. http://dx.doi.org/10.1016/j.yjmcc.2005.02.024.
27. Holst AG, Liang B, Jespersen T, et al. Sick sinus syndrome, progressive cardiac conduction disease, atrial flutter and ventricular tachycardia caused by a novel SCN5A mutation. Cardiology 2010;115(4):311–6. http://dx.doi.org/10.1159/000312747.
28. Nakajima S, Makiyama T, Hanazawa K, et al. A novel SCN5A mutation demonstrating a variety of clinical phenotypes in familial sick sinus syndrome. Intern Med 2013;52(16):1805–8. Available at: http://www.ncbi.nlm.nih.gov/pubmed/23955615. Accessed April 6, 2014.

29. Tan BH, Iturralde-Torres P, Medeiros-Domingo A, et al. A novel C-terminal truncation SCN5A mutation from a patient with sick sinus syndrome, conduction disorder and ventricular tachycardia. Cardiovasc Res 2007;76(3):409–17. http://dx.doi.org/10.1016/j.cardiores.2007.08.006.
30. Ziyadeh-Isleem A, Clatot J, Duchatelet S, et al. A truncating SCN5A mutation combined with genetic variability causes sick sinus syndrome and early atrial fibrillation. Heart Rhythm 2014. http://dx.doi.org/10.1016/j.hrthm.2014.02.021.
31. Kodama T, Serio A, Disertori M, et al. Autosomal recessive paediatric sick sinus syndrome associated with novel compound mutations in SCN5A. Int J Cardiol 2013;167(6):3078–80. http://dx.doi.org/10.1016/j.ijcard.2012.11.062.
32. Selly JB, Boumahni B, Edmar A, et al. Cardiac sinus node dysfunction due to a new mutation of the SCN5A gene. Arch Pediatr 2012;19(8):837–41. http://dx.doi.org/10.1016/j.arcped.2012.04.017 [in French].
33. Benson DW, Wang DW, Dyment M, et al. Congenital sick sinus syndrome caused by recessive mutations in the cardiac sodium channel gene (SCN5A). J Clin Invest 2003;112:1019–28, 0021-9738 (Print).
34. Neu A, Eiselt M, Paul M, et al. A homozygous SCN5A mutation in a severe, recessive type of cardiac conduction disease. Hum Mutat 2010;31(8):E1609–21. http://dx.doi.org/10.1002/humu.21302.
35. Otagiri T, Kijima K, Osawa M, et al. Cardiac ion channel gene mutations in sudden infant death syndrome. Pediatr Res 2008;64:482–7, 1530-0447 (Electronic).
36. Turillazzi E, La Rocca G, Anzalone R, et al. Heterozygous nonsense SCN5A mutation W822X explains a simultaneous sudden infant death syndrome. Virchows Arch 2008;453(2):209–16. http://dx.doi.org/10.1007/s00428-008-0632-7.
37. Ackerman MJ, Siu BL, Sturner WQ, et al. Postmortem molecular analysis of SCN5A defects in sudden infant death syndrome. JAMA 2001;286:2264–9, 0098-7484 (Print).
38. Wedekind H, Smits JP, Schulze-Bahr E, et al. De novo mutation in the SCN5A gene associated with early onset of sudden infant death. Circulation 2001;104:1158–64, 1524-4539 (Electronic).
39. Schwartz PJ, Priori SG, Dumaine R, et al. A molecular link between the sudden infant death syndrome and the long-QT syndrome. N Engl J Med 2000;343:262–7, 0028-4793 (Print).
40. Keller DI, Barrane FZ, Gouas L, et al. A novel nonsense mutation in the SCN5A gene leads to Brugada syndrome and a silent gene mutation carrier state. Can J Cardiol 2005;21:925–31, 0828-282X (Print).
41. Andreasen C, Refsgaard L, Nielsen JB, et al. Mutations in genes encoding cardiac ion channels previously associated with sudden infant death syndrome (SIDS) are present with high frequency in new exome data. Can J Cardiol 2013;29(9):1104–9. http://dx.doi.org/10.1016/j.cjca.2012.12.002.
42. Ellinor PT, Nam EG, Shea MA, et al. Cardiac sodium channel mutation in atrial fibrillation. Heart Rhythm 2008;5(1):99–105. http://dx.doi.org/10.1016/j.hrthm.2007.09.015.
43. Makiyama T, Akao M, Shizuta S, et al. A novel SCN5A gain-of-function mutation M1875T associated with familial atrial fibrillation. J Am Coll Cardiol 2008;52:1326–34, 1558-3597 (Electronic).
44. Li Q, Huang H, Liu G, et al. Gain-of-function mutation of Nav1.5 in atrial fibrillation enhances cellular excitability and lowers the threshold for action potential firing. Biochem Biophys Res Commun 2009;380(1):132–7. http://dx.doi.org/10.1016/j.bbrc.2009.01.052.
45. Darbar D, Kannankeril PJ, Donahue BS, et al. Cardiac sodium channel (SCN5A) variants associated with atrial fibrillation. Circulation 2008;117:1927–35, 1524-4539 (Electronic).
46. Olesen MS, Yuan L, Liang B, et al. High prevalence of long QT syndrome-associated SCN5A variants in patients with early-onset lone atrial fibrillation. Circ Cardiovasc Genet 2012;5(4):450–9. http://dx.doi.org/10.1161/CIRCGENETICS.111.962597.
47. McNair WP, Ku L, Taylor MR, et al. SCN5A mutation associated with dilated cardiomyopathy, conduction disorder, and arrhythmia. Circulation 2004;110:2163–7, 1524-4539 (Electronic).
48. Olson TM, Michels VV, Ballew JD, et al. Sodium channel mutations and susceptibility to heart failure and atrial fibrillation. JAMA 2005;293(4):447–54. http://dx.doi.org/10.1001/jama.293.4.447.
49. Greenlee PR, Anderson JL, Lutz JR, et al. Familial automaticity-conduction disorder with associated cardiomyopathy. West J Med 1986;144(1):33–41. Available at: http://www.pubmedcentral.nih.gov/articlerender.fcgi?artid=1306503&tool=pmcentrez&rendertype=abstract. Accessed April 13, 2014.
50. Laitinen-Forsblom PJ, Mäkynen P, Mäkynen H, et al. SCN5A mutation associated with cardiac conduction defect and atrial arrhythmias. J Cardiovasc Electrophysiol 2006;17(5):480–5. http://dx.doi.org/10.1111/j.1540-8167.2006.00411.x.
51. Groenewegen WA, Firouzi M, Bezzina CR, et al. A cardiac sodium channel mutation cosegregates with a rare connexin40 genotype in familial atrial standstill. Circ Res 2003;92(1):14–22. Available at: http://www.ncbi.nlm.nih.gov/pubmed/12522116. Accessed April 5, 2014.
52. Frigo G, Rampazzo A, Bauce B, et al. Homozygous SCN5A mutation in Brugada syndrome with monomorphic ventricular tachycardia and structural heart abnormalities. Europace 2007;9:391–7, 1099-5129 (Print).

53. Bezzina CR, Rook MB, Groenewegen WA, et al. Compound heterozygosity for mutations (W156X and R225W) in SCN5A associated with severe cardiac conduction disturbances and degenerative changes in the conduction system. Circ Res 2003;92(2):159–68. Available at: http://www.ncbi.nlm.nih.gov/pubmed/12574143. Accessed March 24, 2014.
54. Ge J, Sun A, Paajanen V, et al. Molecular and clinical characterization of a novel SCN5A mutation associated with atrioventricular block and dilated cardiomyopathy. Circ Arrhythm Electrophysiol 2008;1(2):83–92. http://dx.doi.org/10.1161/CIRCEP.107.750752.
55. Watanabe H, Yang T, Stroud DM, et al. Striking in vivo phenotype of a disease-associated human SCN5A mutation producing minimal changes in vitro. Circulation 2011;124(9):1001–11. http://dx.doi.org/10.1161/CIRCULATIONAHA.110.987248.
56. Laurent G, Saal S, Amarouch MY, et al. Multifocal ectopic Purkinje-related premature contractions: a new SCN5A-related cardiac channelopathy. J Am Coll Cardiol 2012;60(2):144–56. http://dx.doi.org/10.1016/j.jacc.2012.02.052.
57. Nair K, Pekhletski R, Harris L, et al. Escape capture bigeminy: phenotypic marker of cardiac sodium channel voltage sensor mutation R222Q. Heart Rhythm 2012;9(10):1681–8.e1. http://dx.doi.org/10.1016/j.hrthm.2012.06.029.
58. McNair WP, Sinagra G, Taylor MR, et al. SCN5A mutations associate with arrhythmic dilated cardiomyopathy and commonly localize to the voltage-sensing mechanism. J Am Coll Cardiol 2011;57(21):2160–8. http://dx.doi.org/10.1016/j.jacc.2010.09.084.
59. Mann SA, Castro ML, Ohanian M, et al. R222Q SCN5A mutation is associated with reversible ventricular ectopy and dilated cardiomyopathy. J Am Coll Cardiol 2012;60(16):1566–73. http://dx.doi.org/10.1016/j.jacc.2012.05.050.
60. Makita N. Phenotypic overlap of cardiac sodium channelopathies. Circ J 2009;73:810–7, 1346-9843 (Print).
61. Veldkamp MW, Wilders R, Baartscheer A, et al. Contribution of sodium channel mutations to bradycardia and sinus node dysfunction in LQT3 families. Circ Res 2003;92:976–83, 1524-4571 (Electronic).
62. Remme CA, Verkerk AO, Nuyens D, et al. Overlap syndrome of cardiac sodium channel disease in mice carrying the equivalent mutation of human SCN5A-1795insD. Circulation 2006;114:2584–94. http://dx.doi.org/10.1161/CIRCULATIONAHA.106.653949, 1524-4539 (Electronic).
63. Grant AO, Carboni MP, Neplioueva V, et al. Long QT syndrome, Brugada syndrome, and conduction system disease are linked to a single sodium channel mutation. J Clin Invest 2002;110:1201–9, 0021-9738 (Print).
64. Makita N, Behr E, Shimizu W, et al. The E1784K mutation in SCN5A is associated with mixed clinical phenotype of type 3 long QT syndrome. J Clin Invest 2008;118:2219–29, 0021-9738 (Print).
65. Abecasis GR, Auton A, Brooks LD, et al. An integrated map of genetic variation from 1,092 human genomes. Nature 2012;491(7422):56–65. http://dx.doi.org/10.1038/nature11632.
66. Tennessen JA, Bigham AW, O'Connor TD, et al. Evolution and functional impact of rare coding variation from deep sequencing of human exomes. Science 2012;337(6090):64–9. http://dx.doi.org/10.1126/science.1219240.
67. Fu W, O'Connor TD, Jun G, et al. Analysis of 6,515 exomes reveals the recent origin of most human protein-coding variants. Nature 2013;493(7431):216–20. http://dx.doi.org/10.1038/nature11690.
68. NHLBI GO exome sequencing project. Available at: http://evs.gs.washington.edu/EVS/. Accessed January, 2014.
69. Risgaard B, Jabbari R, Refsgaard L, et al. High prevalence of genetic variants previously associated with Brugada syndrome in new exome data. Clin Genet 2013;84(5):489–95. http://dx.doi.org/10.1111/cge.12126.
70. Cooper GM, Shendure J. Needles in stacks of needles: finding disease-causal variants in a wealth of genomic data. Nat Rev Genet 2011;12(9):628–40. http://dx.doi.org/10.1038/nrg3046.
71. Scicluna BP, Wilde AA, Bezzina CR. The primary arrhythmia syndromes: same mutation, different manifestations. Are we starting to understand why? J Cardiovasc Electrophysiol 2008;19:445–52, 1540-8167 (Electronic).
72. Postema PG, Van den Berg M, van Tintelen JP, et al. Founder mutations in the Netherlands: SCN5a 1795insD, the first described arrhythmia overlap syndrome and one of the largest and best characterised families worldwide. Neth Heart J 2009;17:422–8, 1876-6250 (Electronic).
73. Probst V, Wilde AA, Barc J, et al. SCN5A mutations and the role of genetic background in the pathophysiology of Brugada syndrome. Circ Cardiovasc Genet 2009;2:552–7, 1942-3268 (Electronic).
74. Ackerman MJ, Splawski I, Makielski JC, et al. Spectrum and prevalence of cardiac sodium channel variants among black, white, Asian, and Hispanic individuals: implications for arrhythmogenic susceptibility and Brugada/long QT syndrome genetic testing. Heart Rhythm 2004;1:600–7, 1547-5271 (Print).
75. Viswanathan PC, Benson DW, Balser JR. A common SCN5A polymorphism modulates the biophysical effects of an SCN5A mutation. J Clin Invest 2003;111:341–6, 0021-9738 (Print).
76. Ye B, Valdivia CR, Ackerman MJ, et al. A common human SCN5A polymorphism modifies expression

of an arrhythmia causing mutation. Physiol Genomics 2003;12:187–93, 1531-2267 (Electronic).
77. Poelzing S, Forleo C, Samodell M, et al. SCN5A polymorphism restores trafficking of a Brugada syndrome mutation on a separate gene. Circulation 2006;114:368–76, 1524-4539 (Electronic).
78. Splawski I, Timothy KW, Tateyama M, et al. Variant of SCN5A sodium channel implicated in risk of cardiac arrhythmia. Science 2002;297:1333–6, 1095-9203 (Electronic).
79. Burke A, Creighton W, Mont E, et al. Role of SCN5A Y1102 polymorphism in sudden cardiac death in blacks. Circulation 2005;112:798–802, 1524-4539 (Electronic).
80. Plant LD, Bowers PN, Liu Q, et al. A common cardiac sodium channel variant associated with sudden infant death in African Americans, SCN5A S1103Y. J Clin Invest 2006;116(2):430–5. http://dx.doi.org/10.1172/JCI25618.
81. Van Norstrand DW, Tester DJ, Ackerman MJ. Overrepresentation of the proarrhythmic, sudden death predisposing sodium channel polymorphism S1103Y in a population-based cohort of African-American sudden infant death syndrome. Heart Rhythm 2008;5(5):712–5. http://dx.doi.org/10.1016/j.hrthm.2008.02.012.
82. Cheng J, Tester DJ, Tan BH, et al. The common African American polymorphism SCN5A-S1103Y interacts with mutation SCN5A-R680H to increase late Na current. Physiol Genomics 2011;43(9):461–6. http://dx.doi.org/10.1152/physiolgenomics.00198.2010.
83. Tan BH, Valdivia CR, Rok BA, et al. Common human SCN5A polymorphisms have altered electrophysiology when expressed in Q1077 splice variants. Heart Rhythm 2005;2(7):741–7. http://dx.doi.org/10.1016/j.hrthm.2005.04.021.
84. Vatta M, Dumaine R, Varghese G, et al. Genetic and biophysical basis of sudden unexplained nocturnal death syndrome (SUNDS), a disease allelic to Brugada syndrome. Hum Mol Genet 2002;11:337–45, 0964-6906 (Print).
85. Wang Q, Chen S, Chen Q, et al. The common SCN5A mutation R1193Q causes LQTS-type electrophysiological alterations of the cardiac sodium channel. J Med Genet 2004;41:e66, 1468-6244 (Electronic).
86. Makielski JC, Ye B, Valdivia CR, et al. A ubiquitous splice variant and a common polymorphism affect heterologous expression of recombinant human SCN5A heart sodium channels. Circ Res 2003;93(9):821–8. http://dx.doi.org/10.1161/01.RES.0000096652.14509.96.
87. Bezzina CR, Shimizu W, Yang P, et al. Common sodium channel promoter haplotype in Asian subjects underlies variability in cardiac conduction. Circulation 2006;113:338–44, 1524-4539 (Electronic).
88. Kolder IC, Tanck MW, Bezzina CR. Common genetic variation modulating cardiac ECG parameters and susceptibility to sudden cardiac death. J Mol Cell Cardiol 2012;52:620–9, 1095-8584 (Electronic).
89. Marsman RF, Tan HL, Bezzina CR. Genetics of sudden cardiac death caused by ventricular arrhythmias. Nat Rev Cardiol 2014;11(2):96–111. http://dx.doi.org/10.1038/nrcardio.2013.186.
90. Chambers JC, Zhao J, Terracciano CM, et al. Genetic variation in SCN10A influences cardiac conduction. Nat Genet 2010;42:149–52, 1546-1718 (Electronic).
91. Holm H, Gudbjartsson DF, Arnar DO, et al. Several common variants modulate heart rate, PR interval and QRS duration. Nat Genet 2010;42:117–22, 1546-1718 (Electronic).
92. Pfeufer A, van Noord C, Marciante KD, et al. Genome-wide association study of PR interval. Nat Genet 2010;42(2):153–9. http://dx.doi.org/10.1038/ng.517.
93. Sotoodehnia N, Isaacs A, de Bakker PI, et al. Common variants in 22 loci are associated with QRS duration and cardiac ventricular conduction. Nat Genet 2010;42:1068–76, 1546-1718 (Electronic).
94. Pfeufer A, Sanna S, Arking DE, et al. Common variants at ten loci modulate the QT interval duration in the QTSCD Study. Nat Genet 2009;41:407–14, 1546-1718 (Electronic).
95. Newton-Cheh C, Eijgelsheim M, Rice KM, et al. Common variants at ten loci influence QT interval duration in the QTGEN Study. Nat Genet 2009;41:399–406, 1546-1718 (Electronic).
96. Smith JG, Magnani JW, Palmer C, et al. Genome-wide association studies of the PR interval in African Americans. PLoS Genet 2011;7(2):e1001304. http://dx.doi.org/10.1371/journal.pgen.1001304.
97. Ritchie MD, Denny JC, Zuvich RL, et al. Genome- and phenome-wide analyses of cardiac conduction identifies markers of arrhythmia risk. Circulation 2013;127(13):1377–85. http://dx.doi.org/10.1161/CIRCULATIONAHA.112.000604.
98. Andreasen L, Nielsen JB, Darkner S, et al. Brugada syndrome risk loci seem protective against atrial fibrillation. Eur J Hum Genet 2014. http://dx.doi.org/10.1038/ejhg.2014.46.
99. Delaney JT, Muhammad R, Shi Y, et al. Common SCN10A variants modulate PR interval and heart rate response during atrial fibrillation. Europace 2014;16(4):485–90. http://dx.doi.org/10.1093/europace/eut278.
100. Bezzina CR, Barc J, Mizusawa Y, et al. Common variants at SCN5A-SCN10A and HEY2 are associated with Brugada syndrome, a rare disease with high risk of sudden cardiac death. Nat Genet 2013;45(9):1044–9. http://dx.doi.org/10.1038/ng.2712.

101. Wilde AA, Postema PG, Di JM, et al. The pathophysiological mechanism underlying Brugada syndrome: depolarization versus repolarization. J Mol Cell Cardiol 2010;49(4):543–53. http://dx.doi.org/10.1016/j.yjmcc.2010.07.012.
102. Bernstein BE, Birney E, Dunham I, et al. An integrated encyclopedia of DNA elements in the human genome. Nature 2012;489:57–74, 1476-4687 (Electronic).
103. May D, Blow MJ, Kaplan T, et al. Large-scale discovery of enhancers from human heart tissue. Nat Genet 2012;44:89–93, 1546-1718 (Electronic).
104. He A, Kong SW, Ma Q, et al. Co-occupancy by multiple cardiac transcription factors identifies transcriptional enhancers active in heart. Proc Natl Acad Sci U S A 2011;108:5632–7, 1091-6490 (Electronic).
105. van den Boogaard M, Wong LY, Tessadori F, et al. Genetic variation in T-box binding element functionally affects SCN5A/SCN10A enhancer. J Clin Invest 2012;23–8. http://dx.doi.org/10.1172/JCI62613DS1.
106. Visel A, Blow MJ, Li Z, et al. ChIP-seq accurately predicts tissue-specific activity of enhancers. Nature 2009;457(7231):854–8. http://dx.doi.org/10.1038/nature07730.
107. van den Boogaard M, Smemo S, Burnicka-turek O, et al. A common genetic variant within SCN10A modulates cardiac SCN5A expression. J Clin Invest 2014;124(4). http://dx.doi.org/10.1172/JCI73140.1844.
108. Arnolds DE, Liu F, Fahrenbach JP, et al. TBX5 drives Scn5a expression to regulate cardiac conduction system function. J Clin Invest 2012;122(7):2509–18. http://dx.doi.org/10.1172/JCI62617.

# Na$_V$1.5 and Regulatory β Subunits in Cardiac Sodium Channelopathies

Yangyang Bao, BS, Lori L. Isom, PhD*

**KEYWORDS**

• Arrhythmia • β Subunit • Voltage-gated sodium channel • Animal model

**KEY POINTS**

- Voltage-gated sodium channel (VGSC) β subunits are not auxiliary.
- β Subunits signal through multiple pathways on multiple time scales.
- β Subunits modulate tetrodotoxin-sensitive (TTX-S) and tetrodotoxin-resistant (TTX-R) $Na^+$ channel expression, localization, and function.
- β Subunits associate with $K^+$ channels.
- β Subunits are immunoglobulin superfamily cell adhesion molecules (CAMs) that associate homophilically and heterophilically with other CAMs.
- β Subunits associate with cytoskeletal, scaffolding, and extracellular matrix proteins.
- β Subunits are substrates for sequential cleavage by β and γ secretases. The cleaved intracellular domain translocates to the nucleus to modulate transcription. The cleaved extracellular domain may function as a CAM ligand.
- *SCN1B* encodes 2 splice variants: a transmembrane β1 and a secreted β1B subunit.
- β Subunit expression alters VGSC pharmacology.
- Mutations in β subunit genes result in neurologic and cardiac disease.

## TOPOLOGY OF VOLTAGE-GATED SODIUM CHANNEL α AND β SUBUNITS

Voltage-gated sodium channels (VGSCs) are responsible for the upstroke of the cardiac action potential (AP) and are required for impulse propagation in the heart.[1] Three different structural subunits are required to assemble the VGSC complex in brain: 1 pore-forming α subunit that is both covalently and noncovalently linked to 2 different β subunits.[2] Because cardiac VGSCs have not been purified, it is assumed, but not proven, that they are also heterotrimers. Five β subunit proteins have been identified in mammals: β1, β1B, β2, β3, and β4. They are encoded by 4 genes: *SCN1B* to *SCN4B*.[3–7] Although the pore-forming VGSC α subunit is sufficient for ion conduction, at least in heterologous systems, β subunits regulate sodium current ($I_{Na}$) density, kinetics, voltage dependence of activation and inactivation, as well as surface expression. In addition to $I_{Na}$ modification, β subunits also function as cell adhesion molecules (CAMs),[8] mediating cellular aggregation, neuronal migration, pathfinding, and axonal fasciculation in brain.[9] Although knowledge of β subunit–mediated cell-cell adhesion in heart is not as extensive, we propose that β subunits contribute to cell-cell coupling at the intercalated disk (ID).[10] With the exception of β1B, all of the VGSC β subunits share similar topologies, containing a single, heavily glycosylated immunoglobulin fold in the extracellular region, a single transmembrane domain, and an

Disclosure: The authors have nothing to disclose.
Department of Pharmacology, University of Michigan Medical School, 1301 MSRB III, 1150 West Medical Center Drive, Ann Arbor, MI 48109, USA
* Corresponding author. Department of Pharmacology, University of Michigan Medical School, 3422 Med Sci I, SPC 5632, Ann Arbor, MI 48109-5632.
*E-mail address:* lisom@umich.edu

Card Electrophysiol Clin 6 (2014) 679–694
http://dx.doi.org/10.1016/j.ccep.2014.07.002
1877-9182/14/$ – see front matter 

intracellular C terminus.[7] β1B (originally called β1A[4]), a *SCN1B* splice variant formed through retention of intron 3, contains an immunoglobulin loop that is identical to that of β1, but lacks a transmembrane domain and is thus a secreted protein.[11] β1B functions as a soluble CAM ligand in addition to a modulator of $I_{Na}$.[11] Of the 5 β subunits, β1B, β1, and β3 are noncovalently linked to VGSC α subunits, whereas β2 and β4 are covalently linked through disulfide bonds. The residue responsible for the covalent interaction between β2 and α subunits was recently identified as cysteine-26.[12] It is postulated that β4, which shares several similar cysteine sites with β2, links to VGSC α subunits through cysteine-28.[5]

## LOCALIZATION OF VOLTAGE-GATED SODIUM CHANNEL α AND β SUBUNITS IN THE HEART

### *Tissue Distribution*

Similar to cardiac potassium channels,[13,14] VGSC α and β subunits show gradients of expression throughout the heart. All β subunits, except for β1B, are expressed in mouse sinoatrial (SA) node.[15] The predominant cardiac VGSC α subunit, $Na_V1.5$, is absent from the central region of the SA node but its expression increases in a gradient fashion toward the peripheral SA nodal region.[16] This arrangement is proposed to play a key role in controlling impulse exit from the node.[17] The tetrodotoxin-sensitive (TTX-S) VGSCs $Na_V1.1$ and $Na_V1.3$ are expressed in the central SA node, with $Na_V1.1$ as the predominant VGSC in this region. In mouse heart, the SA and atrioventricular (AV) nodal regions have higher expression levels of *SCN1B* (encoding β1/β1B) and *SCN3B* (encoding β3) compared with the atrium.[18] *SCN1A* (encoding $Na_V1.1$) and *SCN9A* (encoding $Na_V1.7$) are also highly expressed in AV node.[18] Profiling of ion channel genes in nondiseased human heart revealed that *SCN5A* (encoding $Na_V1.5$) and *SCN9A* transcript levels are higher in left atrium than left ventricle, whereas *SCN1B* is expressed at a higher level in both left and right atria compared with the two ventricles.[19] *SCN3A* (encoding $Na_V1.3$) is expressed at lower levels in right atrium than right ventricle. The TTX-S VGSC *SCN9A*, which is more often expressed in neurons, is more highly expressed in neuronal-like Purkinje fibers compared with right ventricle. Both *SCN5A* and *SCN1B* transcript levels are higher in endocardium than in epicardium.[19] Nevertheless, *SCN2B* (encoding β2) and *SCN3B* seem to be homogeneously distributed throughout the heart.[19] In contrast with findings in human heart, *SCN3B* is highly expressed in the ventricles and Purkinje fibers but not in atrium in sheep heart.[20] Expression of β1 is higher in the trabeculated myocardium and the bundle branches in postnatal mouse.[21] Taken together, a detailed understanding of VGSC subunit localization is critical to understanding the mechanisms of cardiac physiology and pathophysiology.

### *Subcellular Localization*

Both TTX-S and tetrodotoxin-resistant (TTX-R) VGSCs are expressed in cardiac myocytes. TTX-R $Na_V1.5$ colocalizes with tyrosine-phosphorylated β1, β2, and β4 at the ID, whereas nonphosphorylated β1, β2, and β3 colocalize with TTX-S $Na_V1.1$, $Na_V1.3$, and $Na_V1.6$ at the transverse tubules (T tubules) in rodent ventricular myocytes.[10,22,23] A recent study also revealed low-level cell surface expression of $Na_V1.4$ and $Na_V1.6$ in mouse ventricular myocytes.[24] In human atrial myocytes, $Na_V1.2$ is colocalized at IDs with β1 and β3. $Na_V1.4$ and the predominant $Na_V1.5$ channels are colocalized with β2 in a striated pattern. $Na_V1.1$, $Na_V1.3$, and $Na_V1.6$ are located in scattered puncta on the cell surface in a pattern similar to β3 and β4.[25] Because the subcellular distributions of VGSC α and β subunits in human heart seem to be different than in mouse and rat, a more complete study using reliable antibodies will be an important next step in the pursuit of novel therapeutic agents to treat cardiac disease in human patients.

## VOLTAGE-GATED SODIUM CHANNELS EXIST AS MACROMOLECULAR COMPLEXES IN HEART

Mammalian VGSCs exist as macromolecular complexes in vivo. Immunoprecipitation studies show that $Na_V1.5$, β1, and β2 associate in solubilized rat heart membranes.[22] Phosphorylated β1 (at residue tyrosine-181) colocalizes with connexin-43, N-cadherin, and $Na_V1.5$ at rodent IDs but is not detected at the T tubules.[10] Coimmunoprecipitation shows that N-cadherin, an adherens junction protein, interacts with phosphorylated β1 in rodent heart membranes as well as in a heterologous system via the β1 extracellular domain. Connexin-43, a gap junction protein that is critical for impulse propagation, associates with the $Na_V1.5$ complex in heart membranes.[10] The cytoskeletal adaptor protein, ankyrin, is a member of the VGSC signaling complex in heart.[26] $Ankyrin_G$ (AnkG), which interacts directly with $Na_V1.5$ at the ID, is required for $Na_V1.5$ targeting, expression, and biophysical function.[27] Disruption of AnkG-$Na_V1.5$ interactions is associated with Brugada syndrome (BrS).[28] Plakophilin-2 (a desmosomal protein) interacts with connexin-43, and AnkG at the ID.[29] Thus, desmosomes, gap junctions, and VGSC α and β subunits constitute an interacting network, or "connexome," at the ID, controlling excitability, electrical coupling, and intercellular adhesion in the heart.[30] At T tubules, another ankyrin isoform, ankyrin$_B$ (AnkB) coassembles with TTX-S VGSCs by binding to the nonphosphorylated C-terminal region of β1.[10] Mutations in *ANK2*, encoding AnkB, result in ankyrin-B syndrome (formerly long QT type 4 [LQT4]) with a wide spectrum of phenotypes.[31,32] Interactions between β1 and ankyrin are abolished in a heterologous system by expression of a β1 construct that mimics phosphorylated β1 (β1Y181E), suggesting that β1 tyrosine phosphorylation is important for ankyrin recruitment and thus VGSC complex formation in heart.[33] These interactions are summarized in **Fig. 1**.

## HOW ARE CARDIAC VOLTAGE-GATED SODIUM CHANNELS MODULATED IN VITRO?

A conventional method to study ion channels and mutant channels linked to channelopathies is functional expression in heterologous systems. Although different from the native environment, in vitro studies are a convenient first approach to gain structure-function information. Coexpression of β subunits with the predominant cardiac VGSC Na$_V$1.5 in heterologous systems has yielded valuable, but also confusing, information. Effects on Na$_V$1.5 mediated by β1 are inconsistent between laboratories. Some groups report no effect of β1 on Na$_V$1.5 function.[34,35] Others report that β1 increases Na$_V$1.5 I$_{Na}$ density without affecting the gating properties,[36] that β1 shifts the voltage dependence of inactivation,[22,37,38] or that β1 alters the rate of recovery from inactivation.[20,38] This variety of results may stem from differences in cell background, endogenous β subunits, or differential expression of channel interacting proteins.[39–42] We found that Na$_V$1.5 retains β1B, the secreted splice variant of *SCN1B*, at the cell surface in heterologous cells.[11] Coexpression of β1B results in increased Na$_V$1.5-mediated I$_{Na}$ density and a hyperpolarized shift in the voltage dependence of gating.[43] In contrast, β2 coexpression consistently seems to have no effect on Na$_V$1.5-mediated I$_{Na}$ density, kinetics, or gating properties in vitro.[12,22,44] In *Xenopus* oocytes, a system in

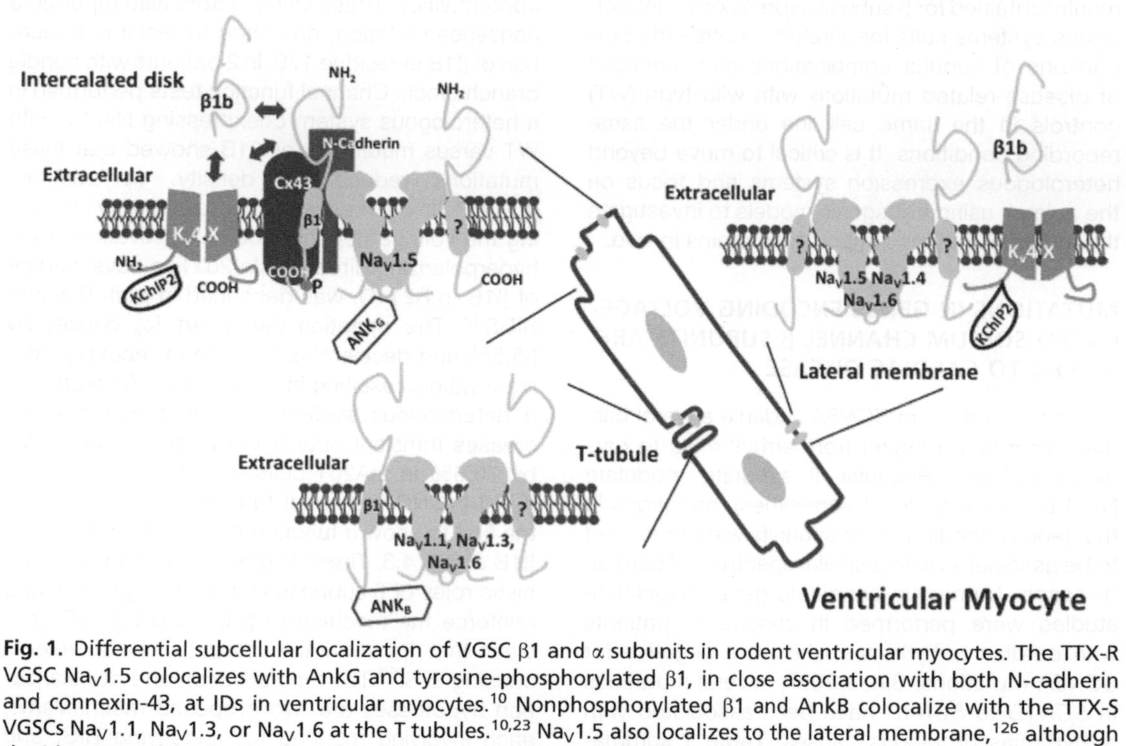


**Fig. 1.** Differential subcellular localization of VGSC β1 and α subunits in rodent ventricular myocytes. The TTX-R VGSC Na$_V$1.5 colocalizes with AnkG and tyrosine-phosphorylated β1, in close association with both N-cadherin and connexin-43, at IDs in ventricular myocytes.[10] Nonphosphorylated β1 and AnkB colocalize with the TTX-S VGSCs Na$_V$1.1, Na$_V$1.3, or Na$_V$1.6 at the T tubules.[10,23] Na$_V$1.5 also localizes to the lateral membrane,[126] although the identities of β subunits there are unknown. In addition, low levels of Na$_V$1.4 and Na$_V$1.6 are detected at the myocyte surface.[24] Although both β1 and β1B have been shown to modulate I$_{to}$, their spatial relationship to the K$_V$4.x/KChIP2 complex is unknown.[55,93,107] Thus, K$_V$4.x/KChIP2, β1, and β1B are drawn at both the ID and lateral membrane. As shown by coimmunoprecipitation,[22] β2 associates with Nav1.5 in heart and has been detected at both IDs[23] and T tubules[22] separately by different groups using immunofluorescence. In addition, β3 and β4 immunofluorescence shows preferential expression at T tubules and IDs, respectively.[23] Thus, heterotrimeric VGSCs composed of many different permutations of α and β subunits may exist in heart. Because of this, we have inserted a question mark on at least one β subunit structure in each domain.

which $I_{Na}$ is considered to be nonphysiologic, β3 increases $Na_V1.5$ $I_{Na}$ density, shifts the voltage dependence of inactivation in the depolarizing direction, and increases the rate of recovery from inactivation.[20] In Chinese hamster ovary (CHO) K1 (CHOK1) cells, β3 has no effect on $Na_V1.5$ peak $I_{Na}$ but reduces persistent $I_{Na}$, shifts the voltage dependence of inactivation in the hyperpolarizing direction, and decelerates the rate of recovery from inactivation.[38] Because of its capability of resurgent $I_{Na}$ generation,[45] β4, which contains a sequence in its intracellular domain (ICD) that causes open channel block, is unique among VGSC β subunits (although *Scn1b* null mice show reduced resurgent $I_{Na}$ current in the cerebellum, also implicating β1/β1B in this mechanism[46]). Resurgent $I_{Na}$ mediated by β4 can be recapitulated with $Na_V1.5$ in vitro.[47] Compared with $Na_V1.5$ alone, β4 coexpression decreases the slope of both the voltage dependence of activation and inactivation[48] with a hyperpolarizing shift in inactivation,[49] and accelerates recovery from inactivation in HEK293 cells.[48]

Taken together, the large variability in functional results obtained for β subunit expression in heterologous systems calls for carefully controlled comparisons of subunit combinations and functions of disease-related mutations with wild-type (WT) controls in the same cell line under the same recording conditions. It is critical to move beyond heterologous expression systems and focus on the animal, using transgenic models to investigate the functions of these important proteins in vivo.

## MUTATIONS IN GENES ENCODING VOLTAGE-GATED SODIUM CHANNEL β SUBUNITS ARE LINKED TO CARDIAC DISEASE

Human mutations in *SCN5A* underlie several cardiac disorders, ranging from arrhythmias to cardiomyopathies. Because β subunits modulate $Na_V1.5$ in vitro (at least sometimes), mutations in the genes encoding these subunits were predicted to be associated with a similar spectrum of cardiac diseases. Numerous candidate gene association studies were performed in cohorts of patients with cardiac arrhythmias who were negative for *SCN5A* mutations. Since 2007, several mutations in *SCN1B* to *SCN4B* have been associated with arrhythmias of various causes. **Table 1** summarizes these results. These mutations can generally be characterized either as resulting in $Na_V1.5$ gain or loss of function. The β subunit gene mutations resulting in $Na_V1.5$ gain of function are linked to long QT syndrome (LQTS)[48] and sudden infant death syndrome (SIDS).[49] The β subunit gene mutations resulting in $Na_V1.5$ loss of function are linked to BrS,[43] progressive cardiac conduction disease (CCD),[43] atrial fibrillation (AF),[44] and idiopathic ventricular fibrillation (IVF).[50] In addition, homozygous *SCN1B* loss-of-function mutations are linked to Dravet syndrome (DS), a severe pediatric epileptic encephalopathy with a high risk of sudden unexpected death in epilepsy (SUDEP).[51,52] We and others have proposed that the expression of *SCN1B* mutations in brain and heart may result in epilepsy and cardiac arrhythmias, with sometimes fatal results.[53,54]

## *SCN1B*

### *Ventricular arrhythmias and cardiac conduction system defects*

The first cardiac disease mutations identified in *SCN1B* were associated with BrS (BRGDA5 OMIM 612838) and cardiac conduction defects (OMIM 612838).[43] In this study, 282 patients with BrS and 44 patients with CCD were screened. A missense mutation in *SCN1B*, p.Glu87Gln, predicted to affect both β1 and β1B, was reported in a patient with BrS who also manifested conduction abnormalities. These investigators also reported a nonsense mutation, predicted to result in truncation of β1B at residue 179, in 2 patients with bundle branch block. Channel function tests performed in a heterologous system coexpressing $Na_V1.5$ with WT versus mutant β1 or β1B showed that these mutations reduce $I_{Na}$ density. In addition, p.Glu87Gln decreases channel availability by shifting the voltage dependence of inactivation in the hyperpolarizing direction. In 2011, a novel variant of β1B, p.R214Q, was described in both BrS and SIDS.[55] This mutation decreases $I_{Na}$ density by 56.5% and decelerates the rate of recovery from inactivation, resulting in loss of $Na_V1.5$ function in a heterologous system. This mutation also increases transient outward potassium current ($I_{to}$) by 70.6% in tsA201 cells, resulting in a gain of $K_v4.3$ (*KCND3*) channel function. This study was the first to show a functional association between β1B and $K_v4.3$. These findings extend the mechanistic roles of β subunits in arrhythmogenesis and reinforce the mechanism proposed for BrS. It is clear that $I_{Na}$ reduction plays a pivotal role in causing BrS.[56] The repolarization and depolarization hypotheses are two proposed mechanisms, each involving reduced $I_{Na}$ underlying BrS, and are supported by experimental and clinical data.[57] In brief, in the repolarizing hypothesis, AP durations are shorter in the epicardium, attributed to the more prominent expression of repolarizing $I_{to}$. Reduction in opposing or depolarizing $I_{Na}$ would further shorten epicardial AP durations, resulting in higher heterogeneity of transmural

**Table 1**
**Human cardiac arrhythmia-associated VGSC β subunit mutations**

| Gene | Affected Isoform | Model | Location | Affected AA | Mutation | MAF (%)[a] | Disease | Functional Alteration(Ref) |
|---|---|---|---|---|---|---|---|---|
| *SCN1B* | β1, β1b | Human | ECD | R85H | c.254G>A | NA | AF or GEFS+ | Reduced $I_{Na}$, and altered gating (CHO)[44] |
| | β1, β1b | | ECD | E87Q | c.259G>C | NA | CCD | Reduced $I_{Na}$, altered gating (CHO)[43] |
| | β1, β1b | | ECD | D153N | c.457G>A | NA | AF | Reduced $I_{Na}$, (CHO)[44] |
| | β1, β1b | | ECD | V138I | c.412G>A | 0.0231 | SUNDS | NA[60] |
| | β1 | | TMD | T189M | c.583G>A | NA | SUNDS | NA[60] |
| | β1b | | — | W179X | c.537G>A | NA | CCD | Reduced $I_{Na}$ and altered gating (CHO)[43] |
| | | | | | c.536G>A | | BrS and CCD | |
| | β1b | | — | R214Q | c.641G>A | 0.3306 | BrS, SIDS, AF | Reduced $I_{Na}$, slower recovery from inactivation; increased $I_{to}$ decelerated $I_{to}$ decay (tsA 201)[55,58] |
| | β1b | | — | H162P | c.641G>A | NA | BrS | Reduced $I_{Na}$ altered gating; slower recovery from inactivation (CHO-K1)[127] |
| | β1, β1b | Mouse | — | Null | — | — | LQT | Increased $I_{Na,peak}$ and $I_{Na,persistent}$, increased APD[54] |
| *SCN2B* | β2 | Human | SP | R28W | c.82C>T | 0.0077 | AF | Reduced $I_{Na}$, and altered gating (CHO)[44] |
| | | | SP | R28Q | c.83G>A | NA | AF | Reduced $I_{Na}$ and altered gating (CHO)[44] |
| | | | ICD | D211G | c.632A>G | NA | BrS | Reduced $I_{Na}$ (CHO), decreased surface expression[67] |
| *SCN3B* | β3 | Human | SP | R6K | c.17G>A | NA | AF | Altered gating of $I_{Na}$ (CHO-Pro5)[77] |
| | | | SP | L10P | c.29T>C | 0.0077 | BrS, AF | Reduced $I_{Na}$, altered gating, and trafficking defect (tsA201, CHO-Pro5)[70,77] |
| | | | ECD | V36M | c.106G>A | NA | SIDS | Reduced $I_{Na,peak}$, increased $I_{Na,persistent}$ (HEK293)[49] |
| | | | ECD | V54G | c.161A>C | NA | SIDS, IVF | Reduced $I_{Na}$, altered gating, and trafficking defect (CHO, HEK293)[49,50] |
| | | | ECG | A130V | c.389C>T | NA | AF | Reduced $I_{Na}$ (HEK293)[76] |
| | | | TMD | M161T | c.482T>C | NA | AF | Reduced $I_{Na}$ (CHO-Pro5)[77] |
| | | | ECM | V110I | c.328G>A | 0.0385 | BrS | Reduced $I_{Na}$, trafficking defect (tsA201)[71] |
| | | | ICD | A195T | c.583G>A | 0.0077 | SUNDS | NA[60] |
| | | Mouse | — | Null | — | — | BrS and sinus dysfunction | Reduced $I_{Na}$ and altered gating[78,79] |
| *SCN4B* | β4 | Human | TMD | L179F | c.535C>T | NA | LQT and AVB | Altered gating of $I_{Na}$, increased $I_{Na,persistent}$ (HEK293)[48] |
| | | | ICD | S206L | c.617G>A | 0.0154 | SIDS | Increased $I_{Na,persistent}$ (HEK293 and myocytes), increased APD (myocytes)[49] |
| | | | TMD | V162G | c.485T>G | NA | AF | NA[83] |
| | | | TMD | I166L | c.496A>C | NA | AF | NA[83] |

*Abbreviations:* AA, affected amino acid; AF, atrial fibrillation; AVB, atrial-ventricular block; BrS, Brugada syndrome; CCD, cardiac conduction disease; CHO, chinese hamster ovary; ECD, extracellular domain; ECG, electrocardiogram; GEFS+, genetic epilepsy with febrile seizure plus; HEK, human embryonic kidney 293 cells; ICD, intracellular domain; LQT, long QT syndrome; MAF, minor allele frequency; NA, not available; SIDS, sudden infant death syndrome; SP, signal peptide; SUNDS, sudden unexpected nocturnal death syndrome; TMD, transmembrane domain; tsA201, SV40 transformed human embryonic kidney cells.

[a] Listed frequency is the frequency in all populations including European American and African American, based on NHLBI GO Exome Sequencing Project (http://evs.gs.washington.edu/EVS/).

voltage gradients between the right ventricular epicardium and endocardium. Thus, reentrant excitation waves (phase 2 reentry) between depolarized endocardium and prematurely repolarized epicardium may be facilitated. In the depolarization hypothesis, right ventricular outflow tract activation delay caused by preferential conduction slowing is aggravated by $I_{Na}$ reduction, which could trigger the occurrence of epicardial reentry. In addition to $I_{Na}$ reduction, β1B p.R214Q may cause further augmentation of the transmural voltage gradient because of increased $I_{to}$. Because both β1 and β1B transcript expression levels are higher in the right versus left ventricle,[43] *SCN1B* tissue distribution may confer preferential conduction slowing in the right ventricle when defects occur. Thus, the pathogenesis proposed to be associated with β1B p.R214Q fits both hypotheses underlying BrS. This same mutation was later identified in 1 patient with BrS and 2 patients with early-onset lone AF from a different cohort collected in Denmark.[58] Both patients with AF presented with incomplete right bundle branch block and a downslope ST segment, suggesting a phenotypic overlap between this *SCN1B* mutation and *SCN5A* loss-of-function mutation–related arrhythmias. To discriminate true monogenetic disease-causing variants from low-frequency genetic variants, the β subunit genes *SCN1B* to *SCN4B* were screened for variations in a population of *SCN5A* mutation–negative Danish and Iranian patients with BrS. This group also reinvestigated prior associations using newly released exome sequencing data. They identified a new *SCN1B* mutation in β1B, p.H162, which was not present in controls or public databases. However, they also identified p.R214Q in the general population with 0.4% minor allele frequency (MAF), thus raising doubts about p.R214Q as a causative mutation.[59] After these studies, *SCN1B* p.V138I and p.T189M were found to be linked to sudden unexplained nocturnal death syndrome (SUNDS).[60] SUNDS and BrS are considered by some investigators to be phenotypically similar.[61]

### *Atrial arrhythmias*

Defects in *SCN5A* leading to loss of $I_{Na}$ are involved in the pathogenesis of familial AF,[62,63] and the same is true for *SCN1B*. In addition to *SCN1B* p.R214Q as described earlier, *SCN1B* p.R85H and p.D153N are associated with familial AF (ATFB 13 OMIM 615377). *SCN1B* p.R85H, located in the immunoglobulin loop region, affects both β1 and β1B. In contrast, p.D153N is located in exon 4 of *SCN1B* and thus can only affect β1. Both mutations result in $I_{Na}$ reduction in heterologous expression systems. In addition, p.R85H, which has also been described in a patient with epilepsy,[64] shifts both the voltage dependence of activation and inactivation positively. Decreased $I_{Na}$ density may shorten the refractory period and reduce conduction velocity, creating a substrate for reentry initiation and perpetuation and thereby contributing to AF susceptibility.[65]

### *Animal models of SCN1B mutations*

All of the human patients thus far described with *SCN1B*-linked cardiac disease are heterozygotes. In contrast, patients with epilepsy have been identified with both heterozygous and homozygous mutations,[51,52] suggesting that patients homozygous for *SCN1B* with cardiac disease may also be identified. Most of these mutations are located in the extracellular immunoglobulin domain, emphasizing the importance of this domain in current modulation and supporting the hypothesis that *SCN1B*-mediated cell-cell adhesion is clinically relevant.[66] To study the physiologic roles of *SCN1B* in the heart, we generated *Scn1b* null mice and studied their cardiac phenotype.[53,54] *Scn1b* null mice are models of DS and show severe seizures and SUDEP.[53,66] Consistent with patients with *SCN1B* mutations that affect the heart, we observed both bradycardia and a prolonged QT interval, suggesting VGSC gain of function. We found a 1.6-fold increase in both peak and persistent $I_{Na}$ density as well as increased AP duration in ventricular cardiac myocytes. These electrophysiologic changes could be explained by increases in transcript and protein levels of *Scn5a* and $Na_V1.5$, respectively. Although *Scn1b*$^{+/-}$ mice are closer to the situation in human patients with heterozygous loss-of-function *SCN1B* mutations, the cardiac phenotype of these mice is unremarkable. The reason why the *Scn1b*$^{+/-}$ model fails to recapitulate clinical findings in humans is unknown, although genetic background differences may play a role. Moreover, the atrial phenotype of *Scn1b* null mice has not yet been described. To further separate the role of β1 from β1B in the heart, reintroduction of 1 splice variant at a time into the *Scn1b* null mice remains under investigation.

## SCN2B

Only 3 missense mutations have been identified in *SCN2B* to date, 2 of which result in amino acid substitution at residue 28 in the β2 signal peptide domain, p.R28W and R28Q, as reported in 2009. Both result in loss of function in a heterologous system and are linked to paroxysmal AF in human patients. Both patients with AF, who were heterozygous for these mutations, showed saddleback-type ST segment elevation in the right precordial leads and 1 patient had PR interval prolongation

(220 milliseconds).[44] Thus, a BrS-like phenotype and conduction abnormalities may be concomitant with an atrial phenotype in a single patient with AF. The β2 p.D211G mutation, located in the ICD, was discovered in 2013 associated with BrS. This mutation results in reduced $Na_V1.5$ cell surface expression, without affecting single channel conductance, in heterologous cells.[67] Similar to amyloid precursor protein, β2 can be sequentially cleaved by β and γ secretases.[68] The cleaved ICD of β2 translocates to the nucleus to modulate *Scn1a* transcription in neurons.[69] Although it is not known whether the β2 ICD also exerts transcriptional modulation on *SCN5A* in cardiomyocytes, this might be an alternative explanation for reduced surface expression.

## *SCN3B*

### *Ventricular arrhythmia*

The first mutation found in *SCN3B*, p.L10P, was linked to BrS (BRGDA7 OMIM 613120).[70] Heterologous expression showed an 82.6% decrease in peak $I_{Na}$ density, an accelerated rate of inactivation, a slowed recovery from inactivation, and a negative 9.6-mV shift in the voltage dependence of inactivation. Immunofluorescence revealed that $Na_V1.5$ remained trapped in intracellular organelles when coexpressed with WT *SCN1B* and mutant *SCN3B* p.L10P. Another trafficking mutation, β3 p.V110I, was similarly found in 3 Japanese patients with BrS from a cohort of 181 individuals.[71] Because of the high prevalence of β3 p.V110I in *SCN5A* mutation–negative Japanese patients with BrS (10.5% familial cases and 0.6% sporadic cases), a recommendation was made to begin testing for *SCN3B* mutations in the *SCN5A*-negative Japanese BrS patients.[72] β3 trafficking mutation, p.V54G, was identified in IVF[50] and SIDS.[49] This mutation did not disrupt the association between α and mutant β subunits, but shifted the voltage dependence of channel gating toward more positive potentials. In the case of IVF, the patient was a 20-year-old man whose positive baseline electrocardiogram (ECG) finding was limited only to epsilon waves, which is often a characteristic manifestation of arrhythmogenic right ventricular dysplasia (ARVD).[73] However, the T waves were not inverted in the right precordial leads, and there was no other evidence to suggest ARVD. Although neither *SCN5A* nor β subunit genes have been implicated in ARVD, a disease more likely caused by defects in desmosomal genes,[74,75] VGSCs have been implicated in the connexome and their dysfunction may harm the integrity of this multimolecular complex. Therefore, VGSC subunit mutations may share some clinical features of ARVD.[30] Thus, if a patient presents with ARVD-like symptoms but without mutations in the usual ARVD-linked desmosomal genes, VGSC genes might be good candidates for screening. In addition, β3 p.A195T was detected in a 31-year-old patient with SUNDS, although functional studies were not reported.

### *Atrial arrhythmias*

In 2010, a candidate gene association study in a cohort of 477 Chinese patients with AF reported β3 p.A130V. This mutation results in decreased $I_{Na}$ density and acts as a dominant negative in the presence of WT β3. However, surface biotinylation experiments revealed no changes in cell surface expression level of $Na_V1.5$.[76] Single channel recording of unitary conductance would have been helpful to further elucidate the $I_{Na}$ reduction mechanism. Later, to increase the probability of screen hits, a cohort was tested with more restricted inclusion criteria in which only patients with early-onset (<40 years of age) lone AF were included.[77] Three mutations, β3 p.R6K, p.L10P, and p.M161T, were identified. Coexpression of β3 p.L10P with $Na_V1.5$ and WT β1 results in a 45% decrease in peak $I_{Na}$ and a 3.8-mV negative shift of voltage dependence of inactivation compared with $Na_V1.5$ coexpressed with WT β1 and β3. p.M161T causes a 57% decrease in peak $I_{Na}$ without observable changes in the voltage dependence of gating. In contrast, p.R6K only shifts the voltage dependence of inactivation by 5 mV in the hyperpolarizing direction. Both p.R6K and p.L10P are located in the signal peptide region of β3, whereas p.M161T is at the border of the transmembrane domain. p.L10P was previously identified in BrS[70] and was shown to interrupt protein trafficking. Overall, additional in vivo work is required to understand the mechanisms of these mutations.

### *Animal models of SCN3B*

Monomorphic VT can be induced in *Scn3b* null mice using programmed electrical stimulation that degenerates to polymorphic VT, suggesting that the ventricles in these animals are prone to arrhythmia.[78] This idea is supported by additional findings, including conduction abnormalities, shorter ventricular effective refractory periods, and a reduction in $I_{Na}$ despite an increase in the expression levels of *Scn5a* mRNA in the right ventricle. The similarity of these electrophysiologic features to clinical BrS suggests that *Scn3b* null mice may serve as a BrS model.[78] Soon after their initial publication, the same group also reported bradycardia, increased P-wave duration, prolonged PR interval, and complete AV block in *Scn3b* null mice, showing electrical abnormalities in the cardiac conduction system and atria. In addition, they found increased SA node recovery times and inducibility of atrial tachycardia and AF by burst pacing, extending the potential use of these animals as models for sick sinus syndrome (SSS) or AF.[79] In contrast to *Scn1b* null mice, no neurologic phenotypes were reported, suggesting that the most important functional roles of *Scn3b* may be in the heart. A recent study resolved the crystal structure of the β3 immunoglobulin domain, revealing that it assembles as a trimer in the crystal asymmetric unit. Using fluorescence photoactivated localization microscopy, these investigators detected full-length β3 trimers on the plasma membrane of transfected HEK293 cells.[80] In addition, β3 subunits bind to more than 1 site on $Na_V1.5$ and induce the formation of α subunit oligomers including trimers. Thus, these results suggest that β3 may participate in cell adhesion via *cis*-homophilic interactions, despite a controversy in the literature regarding the ability of β3 to mediate *trans*-homophilic cell adhesion.[81,82] Furthermore, mutations that perturb the formation of channel trimers are proposed to contribute to arrhythmia.[80]

## *SCN4B*

So far, of the 4 VGSC β subunit genes, only *SCN4B* is linked to LQTS (LQT10, OMIM 611819).[48] In addition, *SCN4B* is the only β subunit gene with a mutation that shows complete penetrance in a family affected by AF.[83] Similar to *SCN3B*, *SCN4B* is linked to SIDS.[49] The β4 p.L179F mutation, identified in a patient with LQTS, does not alter $I_{Na}$ density or channel kinetics. Instead, it increases window current through a positive shift in the voltage dependence of inactivation, widening the voltage range in which $I_{Na}$ may reactivate.[84] More importantly, β4 p.L179F causes a dramatic 8-fold increase in persistent $I_{Na}$ at −60 mV. Increased persistent $I_{Na}$ prolongs the AP duration. The resulting delay in repolarization triggers early afterdepolarizations, which are proposed to induce torsades de pointes.[85] This patient with LQTS also showed asymptomatic bradycardia and 2:1 AV block. Intermittent functional 2:1 AV block in the setting of LQTS is usually an isolated disorder[86] with poor prognosis.[87] Based on these data, direct and independent pathologic roles of β4 in 2:1 AV block in patients with LQTS were suspected.[48] Although *SCN4B* is not yet associated with conduction disease in humans, *Scn4b* is a genetic modifier of disease severity of cardiac conduction defects in mice.[88] *SCN4B* variants may accordingly be considered in risk stratification in patients with LQTS. Similar to β4 p.L179F, another gain-of-function mutation, β4 p.S206L identified in SIDS does not affect peak $I_{Na}$, but shifts inactivation positively by 7 mV, and increases both window current and persistent $I_{Na}$. To more closely mimic the native environment, functional assays were performed in rat cardiomyocytes infected with adenovirus.[49] Because of the close proximity of p.S206 to the β4 open channel blocking sequence, it was postulated that the mutation may enhance the degree of resurgent current. Resurgent $I_{Na}$-specific protocols in whole-cell patch clamp recordings are necessary to test this hypothesis. In 2013, 2 transmembrane domain mutations in β4, p.V162G and p.I166L, were detected in 2 Chinese families affected by AF.[83] Linkage analysis revealed complete penetrance in both pedigrees, although $I_{Na}$ modulation was not tested. In one family member with p.V162G, LQTS was also diagnosed, implying gain of function. No mutations related to arrhythmia have yet been found in the extracellular domain of β4, suggesting that, rather than the extracellular immunoglobulin loop domain functions being clinically relevant as in β1, malfunction in β4 may be more associated with the transmembrane domain and ICD. However, the recent crystallization of the β4 extracellular domain may provide new data on the pathophysiologic relevance of this region.[89]

### *Summary*

The penetrance of VGSC β subunit gene mutations in human patients is variable. Not all carriers develop arrhythmia and individuals with the same mutation may develop different clinical phenotypes that include epilepsy in addition to cardiac disease.[64] Low penetrance and variable expressivity may stem from epigenetic factors, age, gender, or genetic modifiers. Sporadic occurrence without familial cosegregation and the rarity of these genetic diseases add complexity to understanding the role of mutant VGSC β subunits in arrhythmogenesis. Conclusions of causality have become more difficult to draw, in contrast with the rapid growth of genetic information from cohorts of cardiac patients. A practical process of determining potential disease-causing mutations, proposed by Møller and colleagues,[90] is recommended here. Regardless of the genetic information, there is no substitute for expression studies, especially the generation of transgenic animal models. However, the cost in time and resources required to perform these experiments necessitates the careful selection of variants to be studied.

# β SUBUNITS AS ACCOMPLICES OF ABERRANT $Na_V1.5$

β Subunits are not innocent bystanders in *SCN5A*-linked cardiac disease. Instead, they can modify disease severity and, in some cases, their expression is required for pathogenesis. For example, the *SCN5A* LQT mutation, p.D1790G, results in abolishment of α-β1 association and subsequent loss of channel modulation by β1.[37] Functional defects of the BrS-related *SCN5A* mutation p.T1620M are aggravated by coexpression of β1.[91] In another example, reduced expression of β4 in hearts of transgenic mice carrying the BrS-related and CCD-related *Scn5a*-1798insD mutation correlates with more severe conduction abnormalities.[88] In a study investigating the mechanism of a BrS-associated trafficking defective mutation, *SCN5A* p.R1432G, a dominant negative effect of the mutant α subunit on WT channels could be achieved only in the presence of β1,[92] suggesting that β1 is required for mutant-WT $Na_V1.5$ association. In sum, β subunits are actively involved in modulating the severity of *SCN5A*-linked cardiac diseases.

## ADDITIONAL ARRHYTHMOGENIC ROLES OF β SUBUNIT GENE MUTATIONS

Thus far this article has characterized cardiac β subunit gene mutations relative to their effects on $Na_V1.5$ function. However, these mutations may not contribute to cardiac pathogenesis solely through modulation of $Na_V1.5$. In addition, β subunits associate with and modulate TTX-S VGSCs and $K^+$ channels in heart.[10,93] As CAMs, β subunits, especially β1, function in cell-cell coupling and serve as adaptor proteins that link cytoskeletal, signaling, and other adhesion molecules to macromolecular ion channel complexes.[10] Thus, β subunit gene mutations can disrupt more than $Na_V1.5$ function to cause cardiac disease.

### *Voltage-gated Sodium Channel α Subunits Other than $Na_V1.5$ Are Modulated by β Subunits in Heart*

Besides $Na_V1.5$, other VGSCs are expressed in the heart and are modulated by β subunits, contributing to the maintenance of normal cardiac function. TTX-S VGSCs in SA node are important contributors to cardiac automaticity. In isolated SA node cells, TTX-S $I_{Na}$ initiates during the late phase of the pacemaker potential. Blockade of TTX-S $I_{Na}$ results in slowed pacemaking in both intact SA node preparations and isolated SA node cells.[16] On perfusion of nanomolar concentrations of TTX into the intact isolated mouse heart, a significant reduction in spontaneous heart rate and markedly greater heart rate variability are observed, similar to SSS in humans.[15] In a volume-overloaded heart failure (HF) rat model, downregulation of TTX-S $Na_V1.1$ and $Na_V1.6$ expression contributes to HF-induced SA node dysfunction.[94] TTX-S VGSCs in T tubules of ventricular myocytes play an important role in coupling depolarization of the cell membrane to contraction. Low TTX concentrations reduce left ventricular function.[95] This important role was also confirmed in the rabbit.[96] To understand the role of one of the TTX-S VGSCs in heart, the cardiac phenotype of global *Scn8a* null mice was characterized. Both the PR and QRS intervals were prolonged in this model and $Ca^{2+}$ transients were longer in isolated null myocytes compared with controls. Optical mapping showed that hyperkalemia exaggerates the slowing of conduction velocity in *Scn8a* null mouse hearts, implying that $Na_V1.6$ may serve as a protective functional reserve in maintaining the integrity of AP propagation at depolarized potentials. Thus, $Na_V1.6$, and possibly other TTX-S VGSCs, may contribute to the maintenance of propagation in the myocardium and to excitation-contraction coupling.[97] Another TTX-S VGSC, $Na_V1.3$, which is elevated as a result of *Scn1b* deletion, contributes to arrhythmogenesis by disrupting intracellular calcium homeostasis via functional coupling at T tubules.[98]

It has been well established using heterologous systems that TTX-S VGSCs are modulated by β subunits.[3,6,7,11,99] This modulation also occurs in vivo, although the magnitude and direction of the changes vary with cell type. *Scn1b* null ventricular myocytes have increased transient and persistent $I_{Na}$ and a fraction of this is TTX-S.[54] *Scn1b* null hippocampal neurons isolated from the CA3 region express decreased levels of $Na_V1.1$ and increased levels of $Na_V1.3$ without changes in somal $I_{Na}$ density compared with WT.[53] *Scn1b* null cerebellar granule neurons have altered VGSC localization in the axon initial segment and reduced resurgent $I_{Na}$.[46] In the peripheral nervous system, the voltage dependence of TTX-S $I_{Na}$ inactivation is shifted in a depolarizing direction in *Scn1b* null small dorsal root ganglion (DRG) neurons.[100] In *Scn2b* null mice, the loss of β2 results in negative shifts in the voltage dependence of TTX-S $I_{Na}$ inactivation as well as significant decreases in $I_{Na}$ density in acutely dissociated hippocampal neurons. The integral of the compound AP in optic nerve is significantly reduced, and the threshold for AP generation is increased, indicating a reduction in the level of functional plasma membrane VGSCs.[101] In acutely isolated small-fast DRG neurons, *Scn2b* null mice show significant decreases in TTX-S $I_{Na}$ with no detectable changes in the voltage dependence of activation or inactivation. Activation and inactivation kinetics of TTX-S, but not TTX-R, $I_{Na}$ are slower because of *Scn2b* deletion. This selective regulation of TTX-S $I_{Na}$ is supported by reductions in transcript and protein levels of TTX-S *Scn1a*/$Na_V1.1$

and *Scn9a*/$Na_V1.7$.[102] Therefore, β subunits may also contribute to pathogenesis in cardiac disease by disturbing the regulation of TTX-S $I_{Na}$ in heart as well as in the cardiac innervation.

VGSC β subunits may also contribute to cardiac arrhythmia via neuronal mechanisms that include modulation of *SCN10A*, encoding the TTX-R VGSC $Na_V1.8$, whose association with cardiac conduction was identified by genome-wide association study (GWAS).[103] This VGSC, originally identified in nociceptors and known to associate with β subunits,[104] is also localized to intracardiac neurons, where its blockade markedly reduces AP firing frequency.[105] $Na_V1.8$ current characteristics vary in heterologous systems depending on the type of β subunit expressed.[104,106] In *Scn10a* null mice, the cardiac PR interval is shorter than in WT littermates, with no differences in other ECG parameters or echocardiographic cardiac dimensions and function.[103] In addition to $Na_V1.8$, β subunits associate with several peripheral nerve TTX-S VGSCs, including $Na_V1.1$, $Na_V1.2$, and $Na_V1.6$. Thus, through disruptions of some or all of these interactions, β-subunit gene mutations may generate arrhythmias via neural mechanisms.

### *Voltage-gated Sodium Channel β Subunits Modulate $K^+$ Channels*

The β1 subunit is a multifunctional molecule that is not specific to VGSC complexes. β1 coassembles with and modulates the properties of the $K_V4.x$ subfamily of channels that underlie $I_{to}$ in heart and $I_A$ in brain.[93,107,108] $I_{to}$ is an important contributor to AP repolarization in heart.[109] β1 associates with $K_V4.3$, increases the amplitude of the $K_V4.3$ current, and modifies $K_V4.3$ gating.[93,107] The *SCN1B* mutation p.R214Q, which selectively affects β1B and not β1, is proposed to contribute to the arrhythmogenesis of BrS by concomitantly decreasing $I_{Na}$ and increasing $I_{to}$.[55]

## ROLES OF β SUBUNITS IN CARDIOVASCULAR PHARMACOLOGY AND TREATMENT

Expression of β1 modulates cardiac VGSC sensitivity to lidocaine block with subtle changes in channel kinetics and gating properties.[110] Flecainide is a class Ic agent that is used in provocation tests to unmask the BrS phenotype[111] and that reduces arrhythmogenesis in patients with LQT3.[112] Quinidine is a class Ia agent that reduces arrhythmogenesis in patients with BrS[113] and is reasonable for the treatment of electrical storm in BrS.[114] Flecainide and quinidine are proarrhythmic and antiarrhythmic, respectively, in the *Scn5a*$^{+/-}$ BrS mouse model.[115] In contrast, both flecainide and quinidine exert antiarrhythmic effects in *Scn3b* null hearts through modifying the ventricular effective refractory period rather than changes in AP duration.[116] Although both transgenically engineered mouse lines are VGSC loss-of-function BrS models, their responses to flecainide seem to be different. This genetically specific response to drug was also confirmed in our *Scn1b* null mice, in which carbamazepine, but not lacosamide, failed to block high-frequency firing in nerves.[117] The β subunits not only modify the response of $Na_V1.5$ to drug administration but are also putative drug targets. Late $I_{Na}$ contributes to HF mechanisms. Suppression of late $I_{Na}$ but not transient $I_{Na}$ in failing cardiomyocytes is beneficial.[118] Posttranscriptional silencing of *Scn1b* in an HF canine model results in decreased late $I_{Na}$ without affecting transient $I_{Na}$.[119] Based on these results, *SCN1B* may prove to be a plausible drug target in HF.

## FUTURE DIRECTIONS

Common polymorphisms in VGSC α and/or β subunit genes may influence the severity of disease-causing mutations. For example, common *SCN5A* polymorphisms differentially modulate the biophysical effects and expression levels of disease-causing *SCN5A* mutations.[120,121] Expression levels of *Scn4b* modify the conduction defect severity caused by an *Scn5a* mutation in mice.[88] Deleterious effects of mutations can be additive. Longer corrected QT intervals, a higher incidence of arrhythmia, and more severe symptoms are observed in patients with LQTS carrying 2 different mutations.[122] Thus, an understanding of a patient's genetic background is required to correctly interpret a disease-causing mutation. GWAS and patient-specific induced pluripotent stem cell (iPSC) models will allow clinicians to discover new disease-related genes[123] and perform functional studies in cellular models that recapitulate patients' unique genetic backgrounds.[124] A better knowledge of genotype-to-phenotype correlations will necessarily become the basis for more precise risk stratification and prognosis estimation. In addition, patient-specific iPSC models will be invaluable tools for drug screening[125] and the development of individualized therapies.

## REFERENCES

1. Veeraraghavan R, Gourdie R, Poelzing S. Mechanisms of cardiac conduction: a history of revisions. Am J Physiol Heart Circ Physiol 2014;306:H619–27. http://dx.doi.org/10.1152/ajpheart.00760.2013.
2. Catterall WA. Voltage-gated sodium channels at 60: structure, function and pathophysiology.

J Physiol 2012;590(Pt 11):2577–89. http://dx.doi.org/10.1113/jphysiol.2011.224204.

3. Morgan K, Stevens EB, Shah B, et al. β3: an additional auxiliary subunit of the voltage-sensitive sodium channel that modulates channel gating with distinct kinetics. Proc Natl Acad Sci U S A 2000;97(5):2308–13. http://dx.doi.org/10.1073/pnas.030362197.
4. Kazen-Gillespie KA, Ragsdale DS, D'Andrea MR, et al. Cloning, localization, and functional expression of sodium channel β1A subunits. J Biol Chem 2000;275(2):1079–88. http://dx.doi.org/10.1074/jbc.275.2.1079.
5. Yu FH, Westenbroek RE, Silos-Santiago I, et al. Sodium channel β4, a new disulfide-linked auxiliary subunit with similarity to β2. J Neurosci 2003;23(20):7577–85. Available at: http://www.jneurosci.org/content/23/20/7577.abstract.
6. Isom LL, De Jongh KS, Patton DE, et al. Primary structure and functional expression of the beta 1 subunit of the rat brain sodium channel. Science 1992;256(5058):839–42. Available at: http://www.jstor.org/stable/2877043. Accessed February 23, 2014.
7. Isom LL, Ragsdale DS, De Jongh KS, et al. Structure and function of the β2 subunit of brain sodium channels, a transmembrane glycoprotein with a CAM motif. Cell 1995;83(3):433–42. http://dx.doi.org/10.1016/0092-8674(95)90121-3.
8. Isom LL. The role of sodium channels in cell adhesion. Front Biosci 2002;7:12–23.
9. Brackenbury WJ, Isom LL. Na channel β subunits: overachievers of the ion channel family. Front Pharmacol 2011;2:53. http://dx.doi.org/10.3389/fphar.2011.00053.
10. Malhotra JD, Thyagarajan V, Chen C, et al. Tyrosine-phosphorylated and nonphosphorylated sodium channel beta1 subunits are differentially localized in cardiac myocytes. J Biol Chem 2004;279(39):40748–54. http://dx.doi.org/10.1074/jbc.M407243200.
11. Patino GA, Brackenbury WJ, Bao Y, et al. Voltage-gated Na+ channel β1B: a secreted cell adhesion molecule involved in human epilepsy. J Neurosci 2011;31(41):14577–91. http://dx.doi.org/10.1523/jneurosci.0361-11.2011.
12. Chen C, Calhoun JD, Zhang Y, et al. Identification of the cysteine residue responsible for disulfide linkage of Na+ channel α and β2 subunits. J Biol Chem 2012;287(46):39061–9. http://dx.doi.org/10.1074/jbc.M112.397646.
13. Rosati B, Pan Z, Lypen S, et al. Regulation of KChIP2 potassium channel beta subunit gene expression underlies the gradient of transient outward current in canine and human ventricle. J Physiol 2001;533(Pt 1):119–25. Available at: http://www.pubmedcentral.nih.gov/articlerender.fcgi?artid=2278594&tool=pmcentrez&rendertype=abstract. Accessed February 27, 2014.
14. Dixon JE, McKinnon D. Quantitative analysis of potassium channel mRNA expression in atrial and ventricular muscle of rats. Circ Res 1994;75(2):252–60. Available at: http://www.ncbi.nlm.nih.gov/pubmed/8033339. Accessed February 27, 2014.
15. Maier SK, Westenbroek RE, Yamanushi TT, et al. An unexpected requirement for brain-type sodium channels for control of heart rate in the mouse sinoatrial node. Proc Natl Acad Sci U S A 2003;100(6):3507–12. http://dx.doi.org/10.1073/pnas.2627986100.
16. Lei M, Jones SA, Liu J, et al. Requirement of neuronal- and cardiac-type sodium channels for murine sinoatrial node pacemaking. J Physiol 2004;559(3):835–48. http://dx.doi.org/10.1113/jphysiol.2004.068643.
17. Lei M, Goddard C, Liu J, et al. Sinus node dysfunction following targeted disruption of the murine cardiac sodium channel gene Scn5a. J Physiol 2005;567(2):387–400. http://dx.doi.org/10.1113/jphysiol.2005.083188.
18. Marionneau C, Couette B, Liu J, et al. Specific pattern of ionic channel gene expression associated with pacemaker activity in the mouse heart. J Physiol 2005;562(Pt 1):223–34. http://dx.doi.org/10.1113/jphysiol.2004.074047.
19. Gaborit N, Le Bouter S, Szuts V, et al. Regional and tissue specific transcript signatures of ion channel genes in the non-diseased human heart. J Physiol 2007;582(Pt 2):675–93. http://dx.doi.org/10.1113/jphysiol.2006.126714.
20. Fahmi AI, Patel M, Stevens EB, et al. The sodium channel beta-subunit SCN3b modulates the kinetics of SCN5a and is expressed heterogeneously in sheep heart. J Physiol 2001;537(Pt 3):693–700. Available at: http://www.pubmedcentral.nih.gov/articlerender.fcgi?artid=2278985&tool=pmcentrez&rendertype=abstract. Accessed February 20, 2014.
21. Dominguez JN, Navarro F, Franco D, et al. Temporal and spatial expression pattern of beta1 sodium channel subunit during heart development. Cardiovasc Res 2005;65(4):842–50. http://dx.doi.org/10.1016/j.cardiores.2004.11.028.
22. Malhotra JD, Chen C, Rivolta I, et al. Characterization of sodium channel α- and β-subunits in rat and mouse cardiac myocytes. Circulation 2001;103(9):1303–10. http://dx.doi.org/10.1161/01.cir.103.9.1303.
23. Maier SK, Westenbroek RE, McCormick KA, et al. Distinct subcellular localization of different sodium channel alpha and beta subunits in single ventricular myocytes from mouse heart. Circulation 2004;109(11):1421–7. http://dx.doi.org/10.1161/01.CIR.0000121421.61896.24.
24. Westenbroek RE, Bischoff S, Fu Y, et al. Localization of sodium channel subtypes in mouse ventricular myocytes using quantitative immunocytochemistry.

J Mol Cell Cardiol 2013;64:69–78. http://dx.doi.org/10.1016/j.yjmcc.2013.08.004.

25. Kaufmann SG, Westenbroek RE, Maass AH, et al. Distribution and function of sodium channel subtypes in human atrial myocardium. J Mol Cell Cardiol 2013;61:133–41. http://dx.doi.org/10.1016/j.yjmcc.2013.05.006.
26. Hashemi SM, Hund TJ, Mohler PJ. Cardiac ankyrins in health and disease. J Mol Cell Cardiol 2009;47(2):203–9. http://dx.doi.org/10.1016/j.yjmcc.2009.04.010.
27. Lowe JS, Palygin O, Bhasin N, et al. Voltage-gated Nav channel targeting in the heart requires an ankyrin-G dependent cellular pathway. J Cell Biol 2008;180(1):173–86. http://dx.doi.org/10.1083/jcb.200710107.
28. Mohler PJ, Rivolta I, Napolitano C, et al. Nav1.5 E1053K mutation causing Brugada syndrome blocks binding to ankyrin-G and expression of Nav1.5 on the surface of cardiomyocytes. Proc Natl Acad Sci U S A 2004;101(50):17533–8. http://dx.doi.org/10.1073/pnas.0403711101.
29. Sato PY, Coombs W, Lin X, et al. Interactions between ankyrin-G, Plakophilin-2, and Connexin43 at the cardiac intercalated disc. Circ Res 2011;109(2):193–201. http://dx.doi.org/10.1161/CIRCRESAHA.111.247023.
30. Agullo-Pascual E, Cerrone M, Delmar M. Arrhythmogenic cardiomyopathy and Brugada syndrome: diseases of the connexome. FEBS Lett 2014. http://dx.doi.org/10.1016/j.febslet.2014.02.008.
31. Mohler PJ, Schott JJ, Gramolini AO, et al. Ankyrin-B mutation causes type 4 long-QT cardiac arrhythmia and sudden cardiac death. Nature 2003;421(6923):634–9. http://dx.doi.org/10.1038/nature01335.
32. Le Scouarnec S, Bhasin N, Vieyres C, et al. Dysfunction in ankyrin-B-dependent ion channel and transporter targeting causes human sinus node disease. Proc Natl Acad Sci U S A 2008;105(40):15617–22. http://dx.doi.org/10.1073/pnas.0805500105.
33. Malhotra JD, Koopmann MC, Kazen-Gillespie KA, et al. Structural requirements for interaction of sodium channel beta 1 subunits with ankyrin. J Biol Chem 2002;277(29):26681–8. http://dx.doi.org/10.1074/jbc.M202354200.
34. Yang JS, Bennett PB, Makita N, et al. Expression of the sodium channel β1 subunit in rat skeletal muscle is selectively associated with the tetrodotoxin-sensitive α subunit isoform. Neuron 1993;11(5):915–22. http://dx.doi.org/10.1016/0896-6273(93)90121-7.
35. Makita N, Bennett PB, George AL. Voltage-gated Na+ channel beta 1 subunit mRNA expressed in adult human skeletal muscle, heart, and brain is encoded by a single gene. J Biol Chem 1994;269(10):7571–8. Available at: http://www.jbc.org/content/269/10/7571.abstract.
36. Qu Y, Isom LL, Westenbroek RE, et al. Modulation of cardiac Na+ channel expression in *Xenopus* oocytes by β1 subunits. J Biol Chem 1995;270(43):25696–701. http://dx.doi.org/10.1074/jbc.270.43.25696.
37. An RH, Wang XL, Kerem B, et al. Novel LQT-3 mutation affects Na+ channel activity through interactions between alpha- and beta1-subunits. Circ Res 1998;83(2):141–6. Available at: http://www.ncbi.nlm.nih.gov/pubmed/9686753. Accessed February 23, 2014.
38. Ko SH, Lenkowski PW, Lee HC, et al. Modulation of Na(v)1.5 by beta1- and beta3-subunit co-expression in mammalian cells. Pflugers Arch 2005;449(4):403–12. http://dx.doi.org/10.1007/s00424-004-1348-4.
39. Moran O, Nizzari M, Conti F. Endogenous expression of the β1A sodium channel subunit in HEK-293 cells. FEBS Lett 2000;473(2):132–4. http://dx.doi.org/10.1016/s0014-5793(00)01518-0.
40. Moran O, Conti F, Tammaro P. Sodium channel heterologous expression in mammalian cells and the role of the endogenous β1-subunits. Neurosci Lett 2003;336(3):175–9. http://dx.doi.org/10.1016/s0304-3940(02)01284-3.
41. Moran O, Tammaro P, Nizzari M, et al. Functional properties of sodium channels do not depend on the cytoskeleton integrity. Biochem Biophys Res Commun 2000;276(1):204–9. http://dx.doi.org/10.1006/bbrc.2000.3463.
42. Meadows LS, Isom LL. Sodium channels as macromolecular complexes: implications for inherited arrhythmia syndromes. Cardiovasc Res 2005;67(3):448–58. http://dx.doi.org/10.1016/j.cardiores.2005.04.003.
43. Watanabe H, Koopmann TT, Le Scouarnec S, et al. Sodium channel beta1 subunit mutations associated with Brugada syndrome and cardiac conduction disease in humans. J Clin Invest 2008;118(6):2260–8. http://dx.doi.org/10.1172/JCI33891.
44. Watanabe H, Darbar D, Kaiser DW, et al. Mutations in sodium channel beta1- and beta2-subunits associated with atrial fibrillation. Circ Arrhythm Electrophysiol 2009;2(3):268–75. http://dx.doi.org/10.1161/CIRCEP.108.779181.
45. Grieco TM, Malhotra JD, Chen C, et al. Open-channel block by the cytoplasmic tail of sodium channel β4 as a mechanism for resurgent sodium current. Neuron 2005;45(2):233–44. http://dx.doi.org/10.1016/j.neuron.2004.12.035.
46. Brackenbury WJ, Calhoun JD, Chen C, et al. Functional reciprocity between Na+ channel Nav1.6 and beta1 subunits in the coordinated regulation of excitability and neurite outgrowth. Proc Natl Acad Sci U S A 2010;107(5):2283–8. http://dx.doi.org/10.1073/pnas.0909434107.
47. Wang GK, Edrich T, Wang SY. Time-dependent block and resurgent tail currents induced by

mouse β4154–167 peptide in cardiac Na+ channels. J Gen Physiol 2006;127(3):277–89. http://dx.doi.org/10.1085/jgp.200509399.
48. Medeiros-Domingo A, Kaku T, Tester DJ, et al. SCN4B-encoded sodium channel β4 subunit in congenital long-QT syndrome. Circulation 2007;116(2):134–42. http://dx.doi.org/10.1161/circulationaha.106.659086.
49. Tan BH, Pundi KN, Van Norstrand DW, et al. Sudden infant death syndrome–associated mutations in the sodium channel beta subunits. Heart Rhythm 2010;7(6):771–8. http://dx.doi.org/10.1016/j.hrthm.2010.01.032.
50. Valdivia CR, Medeiros-Domingo A, Ye B, et al. Loss-of-function mutation of the SCN3B-encoded sodium channel β3 subunit associated with a case of idiopathic ventricular fibrillation. Cardiovasc Res 2010;86(3):392–400. http://dx.doi.org/10.1093/cvr/cvp417.
51. Patino GA, Claes LR, Lopez-Santiago LF, et al. A functional null mutation of SCN1B in a patient with Dravet syndrome. J Neurosci 2009;29(34):10764–78. http://dx.doi.org/10.1523/JNEUROSCI.2475-09.2009.
52. Ogiwara I, Nakayama T, Yamagata T, et al. A homozygous mutation of voltage-gated sodium channel β(I) gene SCN1B in a patient with Dravet syndrome. Epilepsia 2012;53(12):e200–3. http://dx.doi.org/10.1111/epi.12040.
53. Chen C, Westenbroek RE, Xu X, et al. Mice lacking sodium channel β1 subunits display defects in neuronal excitability, sodium channel expression, and nodal architecture. J Neurosci 2004;24(16):4030–42. http://dx.doi.org/10.1523/jneurosci.4139-03.2004.
54. Lopez-Santiago LF, Meadows LS, Ernst SJ, et al. Sodium channel Scn1b null mice exhibit prolonged QT and RR intervals. J Mol Cell Cardiol 2007;43(5):636–47. http://dx.doi.org/10.1016/j.yjmcc.2007.07.062.
55. Hu D, Barajas-Martínez H, Medeiros-Domingo A, et al. A novel rare variant in SCN1Bb linked to Brugada syndrome and SIDS by combined modulation of Nav1.5 and Kv4.3 channel currents. Heart Rhythm 2012. http://dx.doi.org/10.1016/j.hrthm.2011.12.006.
56. Li A, Behr ER. Brugada syndrome: an update. Future Cardiol 2013;9(2):253–71. http://dx.doi.org/10.2217/fca.12.82.
57. Meregalli PG, Wilde AM, Tan HL. Pathophysiological mechanisms of Brugada syndrome: depolarization disorder, repolarization disorder, or more? Cardiovasc Res 2005;67(3):367–78. http://dx.doi.org/10.1016/j.cardiores.2005.03.005.
58. Olesen MS, Holst AG, Svendsen JH, et al. SCN1Bb R214Q found in 3 patients: 1 with Brugada syndrome and 2 with lone atrial fibrillation. Heart Rhythm 2012;9(5):770–3. http://dx.doi.org/10.1016/j.hrthm.2011.12.005.
59. Holst AG, Saber S, Houshmand M, et al. Sodium current and potassium transient outward current genes in Brugada syndrome: screening and bioinformatics. Can J Cardiol 2012. http://dx.doi.org/10.1016/j.cjca.2011.11.011.
60. Liu C, Tester DJ, Hou Y, et al. Is sudden unexplained nocturnal death syndrome in southern China a cardiac sodium channel dysfunction disorder? Forensic Sci Int 2014;236C:38–45. http://dx.doi.org/10.1016/j.forsciint.2013.12.033.
61. Vatta M, Dumaine R, Varghese G, et al. Genetic and biophysical basis of sudden unexplained nocturnal death syndrome (SUNDS), a disease allelic to Brugada syndrome. Hum Mol Genet 2002;11(3):337–45. Available at: http://www.ncbi.nlm.nih.gov/pubmed/11823453. Accessed February 18, 2014.
62. Ellinor PT, Nam EG, Shea MA, et al. Cardiac sodium channel mutation in atrial fibrillation. Heart Rhythm 2008;5(1):99–105. http://dx.doi.org/10.1016/j.hrthm.2007.09.015.
63. Remme CA. Cardiac sodium channelopathy associated with SCN5A mutations: electrophysiological, molecular and genetic aspects. J Physiol 2013. http://dx.doi.org/10.1113/jphysiol.2013.256461.
64. Scheffer IE, Harkin LA, Grinton BE, et al. Temporal lobe epilepsy and GEFS+ phenotypes associated with SCN1B mutations. Brain 2007;130(Pt 1):100–9. http://dx.doi.org/10.1093/brain/awl272.
65. Nattel S. New ideas about atrial fibrillation 50 years on. Nature 2002;415(6868):219–26. http://dx.doi.org/10.1038/415219a.
66. Brackenbury WJ, Yuan Y, O'Malley HA, et al. Abnormal neuronal patterning occurs during early postnatal brain development of Scn1b-null mice and precedes hyperexcitability. Proc Natl Acad Sci U S A 2013;110(3):1089–94. http://dx.doi.org/10.1073/pnas.1208767110.
67. Riuró H, Beltran-Alvarez P, Tarradas A, et al. A missense mutation in the sodium channel β2 subunit reveals SCN2B as a new candidate gene for Brugada syndrome. Hum Mutat 2013;34(7):961–6. http://dx.doi.org/10.1002/humu.22328.
68. Wong HK, Sakurai T, Oyama F, et al. β Subunits of voltage-gated sodium channels are novel substrates of β-site amyloid precursor protein-cleaving enzyme ($BACE_1$) and γ-secretase. J Biol Chem 2005;280(24):23009–17. http://dx.doi.org/10.1074/jbc.M414648200.
69. Kim DY, Carey BW, Wang H, et al. BACE1 regulates voltage-gated sodium channels and neuronal activity. Nat Cell Biol 2007;9(7):755–64. Available at: http://www.nature.com/ncb/journal/v9/n7/suppinfo/ncb1602_S1.html.
70. Hu D, Barajas-Martinez H, Burashnikov E, et al. A mutation in the β3 subunit of the cardiac sodium channel associated with Brugada ECG phenotype/clinical perspective. Circ Cardiovasc Genet 2009;

2(3):270–8. http://dx.doi.org/10.1161/circgenetics.108.829192.

71. Ishikawa T, Takahashi N, Ohno S, et al. Novel SCN3B mutation associated with Brugada syndrome affects intracellular trafficking and function of Nav1.5. Circ J 2013;77(4):959–67. http://dx.doi.org/10.1253/circj.CJ-12-0995.
72. Kurakami K, Ishii K. Is a novel SCN3B mutation commonly found in SCN5A-negative Brugada syndrome patients? Circ J 2013;77(4):900–1. http://dx.doi.org/10.1253/circj.CJ-13-0242.
73. Marcus FI, Zareba W. The electrocardiogram in right ventricular cardiomyopathy/dysplasia. How can the electrocardiogram assist in understanding the pathologic and functional changes of the heart in this disease? J Electrocardiol 2009;42(2):136.e1–5. http://dx.doi.org/10.1016/j.jelectrocard.2008.12.011.
74. Cox MG, van der Zwaag PA, van der Werf C, et al. Arrhythmogenic right ventricular dysplasia/cardiomyopathy: pathogenic desmosome mutations in index-patients predict outcome of family screening: Dutch arrhythmogenic right ventricular dysplasia/cardiomyopathy genotype-phenotype follow-up study. Circulation 2011;123(23):2690–700. http://dx.doi.org/10.1161/CIRCULATIONAHA.110.988287.
75. Marcus FI, Zareba W, Calkins H, et al. Arrhythmogenic right ventricular cardiomyopathy/dysplasia clinical presentation and diagnostic evaluation: results from the North American Multidisciplinary Study. Heart Rhythm 2009;6(7):984–92. http://dx.doi.org/10.1016/j.hrthm.2009.03.013.
76. Wang P, Yang Q, Wu X, et al. Functional dominant-negative mutation of sodium channel subunit gene SCN3B associated with atrial fibrillation in a Chinese GeneID population. Biochem Biophys Res Commun 2010;398(1):98–104. http://dx.doi.org/10.1016/j.bbrc.2010.06.042.
77. Olesen MS, Jespersen T, Nielsen JB, et al. Mutations in sodium channel β-subunit SCN3B are associated with early-onset lone atrial fibrillation. Cardiovasc Res 2011;89(4):786–93. http://dx.doi.org/10.1093/cvr/cvq348.
78. Hakim P, Gurung IS, Pedersen TH, et al. Scn3b knockout mice exhibit abnormal ventricular electrophysiological properties. Prog Biophys Mol Biol 2008;98(2–3):251–66. http://dx.doi.org/10.1016/j.pbiomolbio.2009.01.005.
79. Hakim P, Brice N, Thresher R, et al. Scn3b knockout mice exhibit abnormal sino-atrial and cardiac conduction properties. Acta Physiol (Oxf) 2010;198(1):47–59. http://dx.doi.org/10.1111/j.1748-1716.2009.02048.x.
80. Namadurai S, Balasuriya D, Rajappa R, et al. Crystal structure and molecular imaging of the Nav channel β3 subunit indicates a trimeric assembly. J Biol Chem 2014. http://dx.doi.org/10.1074/jbc.M113.527994.
81. McEwen DP, Chen C, Meadows LS, et al. The voltage-gated Na+ channel β3 subunit does not mediate trans homophilic cell adhesion or associate with the cell adhesion molecule contactin. Neurosci Lett 2009;462(3):272–5. http://dx.doi.org/10.1016/j.neulet.2009.07.020.
82. Yereddi NR, Cusdin FS, Namadurai S, et al. The immunoglobulin domain of the sodium channel β3 subunit contains a surface-localized disulfide bond that is required for homophilic binding. FASEB J 2013;27(2):568–80. http://dx.doi.org/10.1096/fj.12-209445.
83. Li RG, Wang Q, Xu YJ, et al. Mutations of the SCN4B-encoded sodium channel β4 subunit in familial atrial fibrillation. Int J Mol Med 2013;32(1):144–50. http://dx.doi.org/10.3892/ijmm.2013.1355.
84. Wang DW, Yazawa K, George AL, et al. Characterization of human cardiac Na+ channel mutations in the congenital long QT syndrome. Proc Natl Acad Sci U S A 1996;93(23):13200–5. Available at: http://www.pubmedcentral.nih.gov/articlerender.fcgi?artid=24070&tool=pmcentrez&rendertype=abstract. Accessed February 21, 2014.
85. Yan GX, Wu Y, Liu T, et al. Phase 2 early afterdepolarization as a trigger of polymorphic ventricular tachycardia in acquired long-QT syndrome: direct evidence from intracellular recordings in the intact left ventricular wall. Circulation 2001;103(23):2851–6. Available at: http://www.ncbi.nlm.nih.gov/pubmed/11401944. Accessed February 15, 2014.
86. Trippel DL, Parsons MK, Gillette PC. Infants with long-QT syndrome and 2:1 atrioventricular block. Am Heart J 1995;130(5):1130–4. Available at: http://www.ncbi.nlm.nih.gov/pubmed/7484750. Accessed February 21, 2014.
87. Gorgels AP, Al Fadley F, Zaman L, et al. The long QT syndrome with impaired atrioventricular conduction: a malignant variant in infants. J Cardiovasc Electrophysiol 1998;9(11):1225–32. Available at: http://www.ncbi.nlm.nih.gov/pubmed/9835268. Accessed February 21, 2014.
88. Remme CA, Scicluna BP, Verkerk AO, et al. Genetically determined differences in sodium current characteristics modulate conduction disease severity in mice with cardiac sodium channelopathy. Circ Res 2009;104(11):1283–92. http://dx.doi.org/10.1161/circresaha.109.194423.
89. Gilchrist J, Das S, Van Petegem F, et al. Crystallographic insights into sodium-channel modulation by the β4 subunit. Proc Natl Acad Sci U S A 2013;110(51):E5016–24. http://dx.doi.org/10.1073/pnas.1314557110.
90. Møller DV, Andersen PS, Hedley P, et al. The role of sarcomere gene mutations in patients with idiopathic dilated cardiomyopathy. Eur J Hum Genet 2009;17(10):1241–9. http://dx.doi.org/10.1038/ejhg.2009.34.

91. Makita N, Shirai N, Wang DW, et al. Cardiac Na+ channel dysfunction in Brugada syndrome is aggravated by 1-subunit. Circulation 2000;101(1): 54–60. http://dx.doi.org/10.1161/01.CIR.101.1.54.
92. Mercier A, Clément R, Harnois T, et al. The β1-subunit of Na(v)1.5 cardiac sodium channel is required for a dominant negative effect through α-α interaction. PLoS One 2012;7(11):e48690. http://dx.doi.org/10.1371/journal.pone.0048690.
93. Deschênes I, Armoundas AA, Jones SP, et al. Post-transcriptional gene silencing of KChIP2 and Navbeta1 in neonatal rat cardiac myocytes reveals a functional association between Na and Ito currents. J Mol Cell Cardiol 2008;45(3):336–46. http://dx.doi.org/10.1016/j.yjmcc.2008.05.001.
94. Du Y, Huang X, Wang T, et al. Downregulation of neuronal sodium channel subunits Nav1.1 and Nav1.6 in the sinoatrial node from volume-overloaded heart failure rat. Pflugers Arch 2007; 454(3):451–9. http://dx.doi.org/10.1007/s00424-007-0216-4.
95. Maier SK, Westenbroek RE, Schenkman KA, et al. An unexpected role for brain-type sodium channels in coupling of cell surface depolarization to contraction in the heart. Proc Natl Acad Sci U S A 2002;99(6):4073–8. http://dx.doi.org/10.1073/pnas.261705699.
96. Torres NS, Larbig R, Rock A, et al. Na+ currents are required for efficient excitation-contraction coupling in rabbit ventricular myocytes: a possible contribution of neuronal Na+ channels. J Physiol 2010;588(Pt 21):4249–60. http://dx.doi.org/10.1113/jphysiol.2010.194688.
97. Noujaim SF, Kaur K, Milstein M, et al. A null mutation of the neuronal sodium channel NaV1.6 disrupts action potential propagation and excitation-contraction coupling in the mouse heart. FASEB J 2012;26(1):63–72. http://dx.doi.org/10.1096/fj.10-179770.
98. Lin X, O'Malley H, Chen C, et al. Scn1b deletion leads to increased tetrodotoxin-sensitive sodium current, altered intracellular calcium homeostasis, and arrhythmias in murine hearts. J Physiol 2014. [Epub ahead of print].
99. Aman TK, Grieco-Calub TM, Chen C, et al. Regulation of persistent Na current by interactions between β subunits of voltage-gated Na channels. J Neurosci 2009;29(7):2027–42. http://dx.doi.org/10.1523/jneurosci.4531-08.2009.
100. Lopez-Santiago LF, Brackenbury WJ, Chen C, et al. Na+ channel Scn1b gene regulates dorsal root ganglion nociceptor excitability in vivo. J Biol Chem 2011;286(26):22913–23. http://dx.doi.org/10.1074/jbc.M111.242370.
101. Chen C, Bharucha V, Chen Y, et al. Reduced sodium channel density, altered voltage dependence of inactivation, and increased susceptibility to seizures in mice lacking sodium channel beta 2-subunits. Proc Natl Acad Sci U S A 2002;99(26):17072–7. http://dx.doi.org/10.1073/pnas.212638099.
102. Lopez-Santiago LF, Pertin M, Morisod X, et al. Sodium channel β2 subunits regulate tetrodotoxin-sensitive sodium channels in small dorsal root ganglion neurons and modulate the response to pain. J Neurosci 2006;26(30):7984–94. http://dx.doi.org/10.1523/jneurosci.2211-06.2006.
103. Chambers JC, Zhao J, Terracciano CM, et al. Genetic variation in SCN10A influences cardiac conduction. Nat Genet 2010;42(2):149–52. http://dx.doi.org/10.1038/ng.516.
104. Zhao J, O'Leary ME, Chahine M. Regulation of Nav1.6 and Nav1.8 peripheral nerve Na+ channels by auxiliary β-subunits. J Neurophysiol 2011;106(2): 608–19. http://dx.doi.org/10.1152/jn.00107.2011.
105. Verkerk AO, Remme CA, Schumacher CA, et al. Functional Nav1.8 channels in intracardiac neurons: the link between SCN10A and cardiac electrophysiology. Circ Res 2012;111(3):333–43. http://dx.doi.org/10.1161/CIRCRESAHA.112.274035.
106. Vijayaragavan K, Powell AJ, Kinghorn IJ, et al. Role of auxiliary beta1-, beta2-, and beta3-subunits and their interaction with Na(v)1.8 voltage-gated sodium channel. Biochem Biophys Res Commun 2004; 319(2):531–40. http://dx.doi.org/10.1016/j.bbrc.2004.05.026.
107. Deschênes I, Tomaselli GF. Modulation of Kv4.3 current by accessory subunits. FEBS Lett 2002; 528(1–3):183–8. Available at: http://www.ncbi.nlm.nih.gov/pubmed/12297301.
108. Marionneau C, Carrasquillo Y, Norris AJ, et al. The sodium channel accessory subunit Navβ1 regulates neuronal excitability through modulation of repolarizing voltage-gated K+ channels. J Neurosci 2012;32(17):5716–27. http://dx.doi.org/10.1523/jneurosci.6450-11.2012.
109. Nerbonne JM, Kass RS. Molecular physiology of cardiac repolarization. Physiol Rev 2005;85(4): 1205–53. http://dx.doi.org/10.1152/physrev.00002.2005.
110. Makielski JC, Limberis JT, Chang SY, et al. Coexpression of beta 1 with cardiac sodium channel alpha subunits in oocytes decreases lidocaine block. Mol Pharmacol 1996;49(1):30–9. Available at: http://www.ncbi.nlm.nih.gov/pubmed/8569709. Accessed February 9, 2014.
111. Brugada R, Brugada J, Antzelevitch C, et al. Sodium channel blockers identify risk for sudden death in patients with ST-segment elevation and right bundle branch block but structurally normal hearts. Circulation 2000;101(5):510–5. Available at: http://www.ncbi.nlm.nih.gov/pubmed/10662748. Accessed February 19, 2014.
112. Windle JR, Geletka RC, Moss AJ, et al. Normalization of ventricular repolarization with flecainide in long

QT syndrome patients with SCN5A: DeltaKPQ mutation. Ann Noninvasive Electrocardiol 2001;6(2):153–8. Available at: http://www.ncbi.nlm.nih.gov/pubmed/11333173. Accessed February 19, 2014.

113. Belhassen B, Glick A, Viskin S. Efficacy of quinidine in high-risk patients with Brugada syndrome. Circulation 2004;110(13):1731–7. http://dx.doi.org/10.1161/01.CIR.0000143159.30585.90.

114. Zipes DP, Camm AJ, Borggrefe M, et al. ACC/AHA/ESC 2006 guidelines for management of patients with ventricular arrhythmias and the prevention of sudden cardiac death: a report of the American College of Cardiology/American Heart Association Task Force and the European Society of Cardiology Committee for Practice Guidelines (Writing Committee to Develop Guidelines for Management of Patients With Ventricular Arrhythmias and the Prevention of Sudden Cardiac Death): developed in collaboration with the European Heart Rhythm Association and the Heart Rhythm Society. Circulation 2006;114:e385–484. http://dx.doi.org/10.1161/CIRCULATIONAHA.106.178233.

115. Stokoe KS, Balasubramaniam R, Goddard CA, et al. Effects of flecainide and quinidine on arrhythmogenic properties of Scn5a+/- murine hearts modelling the Brugada syndrome. J Physiol 2007;581(Pt 1):255–75. http://dx.doi.org/10.1113/jphysiol.2007.128785.

116. Hakim P, Thresher R, Grace AA, et al. Effects of flecainide and quinidine on action potential and ventricular arrhythmogenic properties in Scn3b knockout mice. Clin Exp Pharmacol Physiol 2010;37(8):782–9. http://dx.doi.org/10.1111/j.1440-1681.2010.05369.x.

117. Uebachs M, Albus C, Opitz T, et al. Loss of β1 accessory Na+ channel subunits causes failure of carbamazepine, but not of lacosamide, in blocking high-frequency firing via differential effects on persistent Na+ currents. Epilepsia 2012;53(11):1959–67. http://dx.doi.org/10.1111/j.1528-1167.2012.03675.x.

118. Undrovinas AI, Belardinelli L, Undrovinas NA, et al. Ranolazine improves abnormal repolarization and contraction in left ventricular myocytes of dogs with heart failure by inhibiting late sodium current. J Cardiovasc Electrophysiol 2006;17(Suppl 1):S169–77. http://dx.doi.org/10.1111/j.1540-8167.2006.00401.x.

119. Mishra S, Undrovinas NA, Maltsev VA, et al. Post-transcriptional silencing of SCN1B and SCN2B genes modulates late sodium current in cardiac myocytes from normal dogs and dogs with chronic heart failure. Am J Physiol Heart Circ Physiol 2011;301(4):H1596–605. http://dx.doi.org/10.1152/ajpheart.00948.2009.

120. Viswanathan PC, Benson DW, Balser JR. A common SCN5A polymorphism modulates the biophysical effects of an SCN5A mutation. J Clin Invest 2003;111(3):341–6. http://dx.doi.org/10.1172/JCI16879.

121. Ye B, Valdivia CR, Ackerman MJ, et al. A common human SCN5A polymorphism modifies expression of an arrhythmia causing mutation. Physiol Genomics 2003;12(3):187–93. http://dx.doi.org/10.1152/physiolgenomics.00117.2002.

122. Schwartz PJ, Priori SG, Napolitano C. How really rare are rare diseases?: The intriguing case of independent compound mutations in the long QT syndrome. J Cardiovasc Electrophysiol 2003;14(10):1120–1. Available at: http://www.ncbi.nlm.nih.gov/pubmed/14521668. Accessed February 21, 2014.

123. Olesen MS, Nielsen MW, Haunsø S, et al. Atrial fibrillation: the role of common and rare genetic variants. Eur J Hum Genet 2014;22(3):297–306. http://dx.doi.org/10.1038/ejhg.2013.139.

124. Moretti A, Laugwitz KL, Dorn T, et al. Pluripotent stem cell models of human heart disease. Cold Spring Harb Perspect Med 2013;5(11). http://dx.doi.org/10.1101/cshperspect.a014027.

125. Sarić T, Halbach M, Khalil M, et al. Induced pluripotent stem cells as cardiac arrhythmic in vitro models and the impact for drug discovery. Expert Opin Drug Discov 2014;9(1):55–76. http://dx.doi.org/10.1517/17460441.2014.863275.

126. Shy D, Gillet L, Abriel H. Cardiac sodium channel Na(V)1.5 distribution in myocytes via interacting proteins: the multiple pool model. Biochim Biophys Acta 2012. http://dx.doi.org/10.1016/j.bbamcr.2012.10.026.

127. Yuan L, Koivumaki J, Liang B, et al. Investigations of the Navβ1b sodium channel subunit in human ventricle; functional characterization of the H162P Brugada syndrome mutant. Am J Physiol Heart Circ Physiol 2014. http://dx.doi.org/10.1152/ajpheart.00405.2013.

# Pharmacology and Toxicology of $Na_V1.5$-Class 1 Antiarrhythmic Drugs

Dan M. Roden, MD[a,b,*]

**KEYWORDS**

• Sodium channel • Drugs • Proarrhythmia

**KEY POINTS**

- Sodium channel blocking drugs carry proarrhythmic potential. Despite this risk, however, the drugs continue to be used, notably in the treatment of atrial fibrillation with the caveat that they should be avoided in patients with structural heart disease or in patients in whom the Brugada ECG is present or emerges during treatment.
- Modeling studies have suggested that drugs with appropriate combinations of potassium channel inhibition and specific frequency and/or voltage-dependent sodium channel block could be antiarrhythmic with minimal proarrhythmic potential.
- It is possible that with a deeper understanding of the structure function of the cardiac sodium channel will come opportunities to target entirely new regions of the channel or its function-modifying protein partners to modulate its activity to suppress arrhythmias without proarrhythmia.

## LEARNING FROM HISTORY

It is said that the mid-eighteenth century French physician Jean-Baptiste de Sénac was the first to document an antiarrhythmic effect of the bark of the cinchona plant. Almost exactly a century ago, Wenckebach encountered a patient with atrial fibrillation who reported he could abort his attacks by using quinine, extracted from cinchona plant bark. Quinidine, an isomer of quinine, was subsequently developed as an antiarrhythmic and widely used for decades. Quinidine is a mixed antiarrhythmic, with prominent sodium channel blocking (as well as potassium channel blocking) properties. Quinidine is not widely used for many reasons: treatment carries a risk of potentially fatally adverse effects, including thrombocytopenia and torsades de pointes; most patients will develop gastrointestinal side effects, which can become intolerable; and the drug is no longer under patent and so not commercially promoted. The first few decades of the twentieth century saw the introduction of other antiarrhythmic agents, most developed from initial drug structures identified as depressors of conduction or contractile function in nerve or cardiac muscle preparations. These included lidocaine, which because of near-complete first pass metabolism can only be used intravenously, and procainamide and disopyramide, drugs that, like quinidine, can be antiarrhythmic but are poorly tolerated because of the

Supported in part by grants from the US Public Health Service (R01 HL49989, U19 HL65962).
Conflicts of Interest: None.
[a] Department of Medicine, Vanderbilt University School of Medicine, 2215 Garland Avenue, Nashville, TN 37232, USA; [b] Department of Pharmacology, Vanderbilt University School of Medicine, 2215 Garland Avenue, Nashville, TN 37232, USA
* Vanderbilt University School of Medicine, 2215B Garland Avenue, Room 1285, Nashville, TN 37232-0575.
*E-mail address:* dan.roden@vanderbilt.edu

Card Electrophysiol Clin 6 (2014) 695–704
http://dx.doi.org/10.1016/j.ccep.2014.07.003
1877-9182/14/$ – see front matter 

high incidence of proarrhythmia and other adverse effects.

## *The Arrival of Better Tolerated Drugs*

The 1970s brought the recognition that frequent ventricular ectopic beats, particularly in patients with known structural heart disease such as myocardial scarring, constitute a risk factor for sudden cardiac death (SCD) and, therefore, an interest in suppressing these ectopic beats. New antiarrhythmic drugs that were better tolerated than available drugs became available and they virtually all share the property that they inhibit cardiac sodium current.

One avenue to development of these new drugs was manipulation of the lidocaine structure to result in congeners with similar electrophysiologic properties but pharmacokinetic profiles that allowed chronic oral dosing. Mexiletine is one such congener that continues to be used, whereas others, such as tocainide, have been withdrawn because of a risk for noncardiovascular toxicities.

Another group of sodium channel blockers that became available for clinical investigation in the late 1970s was the class Ic subgroup (see later discussion). The first two members of this class to be introduced into clinical investigation and subsequently marketed were encainide and flecainide. Initial clinical trials of these agents highlighted several unusual properties, some of which seemed to make them desirable as antiarrhythmic agents.[1–4] The most prominent property was that the drugs could suppress ventricular ectopic beats without producing any of the noncardiovascular toxicities (eg, gastrointestinal symptoms, drug-induced lupus syndrome) that characterized drugs available at the time. In patients with preexcitation, the drugs could produce prompt disappearance of a delta wave, an initial clue to potential antiarrhythmic activity in this setting.

Encainide did have unusual pharmacokinetic properties: its antiarrhythmic effects seem to be mediated by biotransformation to active metabolites. This metabolism is accomplished by the cytochrome P450 *CYP2D6*; 5% to 10% of white and African subjects lack *CYP2D6* activity and, therefore, when exposed to encainide do not generate the active metabolites and display little or no antiarrhythmic effect.[5] On the other hand, flecainide seemed to lack this pharmacokinetic drawback and, unlike most other antiarrhythmics available at the time, could be administered twice daily. In fact, flecainide is a *CYP2D6* substrate but is also cleared by renal excretion of unchanged drug; therefore, the *CYP2D6* polymorphism does not affect flecainide dosing except in rare individuals who are poor metabolizers and who have renal dysfunction.

Thus, the development of encainide and flecainide seemed to herald a new era in which arrhythmias could be readily suppressed by drugs that were well tolerated. One feature of treatment with these agents was that arrhythmia suppression was routinely accompanied by obvious and striking prolongation of P wave, PR interval, and QRS durations, evidence of marked conduction slowing across the heart. Such ECG changes had been seen with the aggressive use of a high dose of quinidine to convert atrial fibrillation.[6] They were considered a sign of drug toxicity, occasionally preceding the development of ventricular tachycardia (VT). Even during the early development of encainide and flecainide, case reports emerged that occasional patients seemed to develop paradoxic worsening of ventricular arrhythmias, including patients who developed incessant sustained monomorphic or polymorphic VT, some of whom who could not be resuscitated.[7] This seemed to occur primarily in patients in whom the presenting arrhythmia was sustained monomorphic VT.

## *The Cardiac Arrhythmia Suppression Trial*

The conventional wisdom in the 1980s was that ventricular ectopic activity represented a marker identifying individuals at increased risk for SCD. A commonly adopted therapeutic approach in the cardiovascular community was to attempt to suppress ventricular ectopic beats to reduce the risk for SCD. Accordingly, the National Hearth Lung and Blood Institute (NHBLI) launched a series of studies in the 1980s designed to rigorously test the concept that suppressing ventricular ectopic activity using newly introduced and well-tolerated agents, such as encainide and flecainide, could affect the important public health problem of SCD. The Cardiac Arrhythmia Pilot Study (CAPS) showed that such a trial was feasible and identified no major safety concerns.[8] In follow-up, NHLBI launched the Cardiac Arrhythmia Suppression Trial (CAST) in 1987. CAST was a double-blind, placebo-controlled, randomized trial in patients with ventricular ectopic activity 6 days to 2 years following a myocardial infarction. Because the proarrhythmia risk had been recognized, only patients with ejection fractions greater than 30% were eligible. The trial was halted prematurely in the spring of 1989 when a planned interim data analysis revealed a striking excess of death among patients treated with encainide or flecainide, compared with those randomized to placebo.[9] A third drug, moricizine, continued to be tested in CAST-II but this also did not reduce SCD and may have increased it.[10,11]

CAST was a landmark clinical trial for many reasons. First, it showed the power of the randomized clinical trial to unambiguously determine drug actions in a complex clinical setting compared with placebo. Second, it had the obvious effect of bringing all sodium channel blocker–related antiarrhythmic drug development to a screeching halt. The drug development world then turned to action potential prolongation, largely accomplished by block of $I_{Kr}$, and this strategy, in turn, was also plagued by proarrhythmia. Importantly, none of these drugs were developed at a time when the molecular basis for drug-channel interactions was not well-understood and the mechanisms underlying proarrhythmia of various types were just beginning to be defined. Thus, the CAST result raised important questions regarding the fundamental mechanisms whereby sodium channel blocking drugs act at the molecular, cellular, and whole organ levels to promote or suppress arrhythmias.

## IN VITRO MECHANISMS OF SODIUM CHANNEL BLOCKING DRUG ACTION

The initial studies by Hodgkin and Huxley[12,13] in the squid giant axon generated a formal mathematical description of sodium channel transitions from closed to open to inactivated and then recovery to rest states (gating) as a function of voltage. The first sodium channel was cloned from the electric eel electroplax in the early 1980s[14] and the inferred structure showed that the now familiar model, present in all mammalian voltage-gated sodium channels, including the predominant human cardiac isoform *SCN5A*,[15] of four domains each consisting of six membrane spanning segments, with S4 acting as the voltage sensor. Molecular and mathematical models have provided valuable tools with which to dissect the mechanisms whereby drugs inhibit sodium current. The question of how such block translates into antiarrhythmic or proarrhythmic clinical actions is actually less well understood (see later discussion).

### *Subclassifying Drugs*

With the development of multiple sodium channel blocking antiarrhythmics came the hope that classifying drugs by their fundamental electrophysiologic properties might be useful in understanding their basic mechanisms of action, targeting specific drugs to specific patients or arrhythmia mechanisms, and directing new drug development. A first attempt at such a classification divided sodium channel blocking drugs into those that prolong cardiac action potentials (quinidine, procainamide, disopyramide) and those that have little effect on action potentials or, in fact, shortened them slightly (lidocaine and congeners). It is now recognized that drugs of the first type prolong action potentials by inhibiting cardiac potassium currents, whereas drugs of the second type may shorten action potential by inhibiting the persistent or late sodium current (see later discussion).

Initial studies in nerve[16] and, subsequently, in cardiac tissue[17] demonstrated that a striking feature of the interaction between drugs and sodium channels was that drug effects are time-dependent and voltage-dependent. Thus, for example, lidocaine showed little block of cardiac sodium current (assessed as maximum upstroke slope of phase 0 of action potentials in initial experiments) when the preparation was well polarized and driven slowly. By contrast, block was prominent in depolarized preparations or those driven rapidly. These observations led Hille[18] and Hondeghem and Katzung[19] to propose the “modulated receptor hypothesis.” They postulated that blocking drugs bound to and unbound from a specific receptor on cardiac sodium channels and that this binding and unbinding was determined by specific rate constants that were, themselves, state-dependent. Thus, for example, some drugs associate with and dissociate from the inactivated state much more avidly than with the rest or open states.

At roughly the same time, Campbell[20,21] and Campbell and Vaughn-Williams[22] noted that antiarrhythmic drugs exerted strikingly diverse effects on sodium current (again measured as maximum phase 0 upstroke slope) when rapid pacing was initiated in a quiescent guinea pig papillary muscle. For virtually all drugs, the first upstroke slope was near-identical to that recorded in preparations that were not drug-treated. This result indicates that most drugs evaluated had little affinity for the resting state. For lidocaine and mexiletine, the onset of drug block was very rapid, occurring within a beat or two, whereas with encainide the onset was very slow, taking tens of beats; quinidine and disopyramide were intermediate. Recovery from drug block, assessed by recording maximum upstroke slope after trains of rapid pacing were interrupted for variable periods of time, also varied among drugs, fastest for lidocaine and slowest for encainide. These properties define use-dependence. For example, the block develops as the channel is used, becomes more intense as the channel is used more (ie, at faster rates), and resolves when the channel is at rest. Based on these data, they proposed the now widely used terminology of class Ia for quinidine and disopyramide, class Ib for lidocaine and mexiletine, and class Ic for encainide and flecainide.[20,23] Interpreted in the modulated receptor hypothesis framework, drugs such as lidocaine bind rapidly to their receptor in either the open or inactivated state and, similarly, unbind rapidly. By contrast, class Ic drugs bind slowly and dissociate slowly. As a result, drugs such as lidocaine produce little sodium channel block in normal tissues driven at slow rates, whereas encainide and flecainide produce prominent steady state sodium channel block even in normal tissue driven at slow rates. This interpretation, then, explains the striking increases in ECG intervals such as QRS duration observed during the earliest clinical trials of class Ic drugs.

## *Where Is the Receptor?*

The cloning of sodium channels, including the cardiac sodium channel, was followed by studies to identify the molecular determinants of toxin and drug binding to the channel. An elegant series of site-directed mutagenesis studies more than 20 years ago identified a single extracellular residue in domain I as critical for determining sensitivity to the blocking toxin tetrodotoxin (TTX). The presence of a cysteine in the cardiac isoform renders the sodium channel relatively resistant to TTX block, whereas the presence of a tyrosine in the corresponding position in nerve channels (or by site-directed mutagenesis in the cardiac channel) renders the channel TTX-sensitive.[24,25]

Mutagenizing a phenylalanine residue to alanine in the cytoplasmic aspect of the S6 segment of domain IV in nerve channels eliminated local anesthetic block, thus implicating this site as a receptor for blocking drugs.[26] Subsequent studies have also implicated aromatics in the cytoplasmic aspect of S6 in other domains.[27,28] Multiple pathways have been described whereby drugs access such receptor sites: from the cytoplasm, through the pore from the outside, or through side pores on the channel.[29,30] Taken together, the molecular data support the initial view[18,19] that the voltage and use-dependence of block by antiarrhythmics (or for blockers of other sodium channel isoforms such as local anesthetics or anticonvulsants) can be understood as voltage-dependent changes in channel structure that modulate accessibility of the drug-binding site to drug, dissociation of the drug from the binding site, and specific affinity of the drug for the binding site.

Multiple mechanisms have been proposed to explain how drug binding reduces sodium current. One obvious possibility is that drug binding at S6 (which lines the sodium permeation pathway) blocks current flow through the channel pore. Another likely mechanism is that drug binding alters the transitions channels undergo among rest, open, and inactivated states. Support for this allosteric block concept comes from experiments in which inactivation is removed by site-directed mutagenesis in the III-IV linker and drug block is thereby inhibited.[31]

## *Mutant Channels May Display Altered Drug Sensitivity*

With the increasing catalog of disease-related *SCN5A* mutations has come the recognition that some of these mutant channels display unusual drug sensitivity. For example, D1790G and Y1795H channels, both located in domain IV S6, display greater sensitivity to flecainide than wild-type channels.[32] It is reasonable to think that mutations in this region may alter access of the drug to a binding site. Another example is the N406S mutation located in domain I S6.[33] The index subject failed to show an expected response to challenge with a sodium channel blocking agent (pilsicainide, a class Ic drug) and the investigators postulated that this reflected an absence of use-dependent block by the drug, attributable to the mutation. Interestingly, the N406S channel displayed greater than expected use-dependent block by quinidine, which could reflect differences in the physicochemical properties of the two antiarrhythmics.

Another interesting example of the way in which molecular genetics has informed drug therapy is the observation that Brugada syndrome mutations producing their clinical effects by reducing cell surface expression of mutant channels can be rescued by the administration of blocking drugs.[34,35] Nonsodium channel blocking drugs have also produced this effect. For example, the potent $I_{Kr}$ blocker cisapride increased cell surface expression of the L1825P mutant.[36] The usual explanation for this finding is that drug block to the mutant channel stabilizes it in a conformation that is not recognized as misfolded and, therefore, allowed to traffic to the cell surface.[37] Although mistrafficking can be rescued in vitro, translation to clinical usefulness is more problematic, not only because blocking drugs will certainly inhibit current once channels are expressed at the cell surface, but because many mutant *SCN5A* channels display a mixed long QT and Brugada syndrome phenotype. Rescuing the Brugada phenotype would then run the risk of exacerbating the long QT phenotype, as was suggested in the initial cisapride report[38] and others.[39]

## IN VIVO MECHANISMS OF SODIUM CHANNEL BLOCKING DRUG ACTION

Sodium channel blockers can suppress arrhythmia arising through either abnormal automaticity or reentry. Reentry due to an anatomic or functional substrate is critically dependent on heterogeneous electrophysiologic properties and slow conduction specifically enables reentry. Fast conduction in atrium, ventricle, and Purkinje is critically depends on expression of sodium channels at the ends (intercalated disks) of cardiomyocytes. Thus, a widely held view is that if sodium channel blocking drugs interrupt reentry they do so by further depressing conduction and, thus, converting unidirectional to bidirectional block. An exclusive focus on conduction, however, leads to the conclusion that sodium channel block should almost inevitably be proarrhythmic in reentry. This view is supported by clinical observations such as CAST and earlier trials, and subsequent studies in animal models of myocardial infarction that showed that drugs such as flecainide can enable reentry by slowing conduction sufficiently to allow VT to establish itself.[40] A more complex example of proarrhythmia due to conduction slowing by sodium channel blockers (usually class Ic agents but also seen with quinidine and with amiodarone) can occur in atrial flutter. Here, drug-induced conduction slowing in the flutter circuit paradoxically enables 1:1 atrioventricular conduction with an increase in ventricular rate. The use-dependent properties of the culprit drugs then widen the QRS duration so the resultant clinical arrhythmia resembles VT.[41] For this reason, when these drugs are prescribed in patients with atrial fibrillation or flutter, atrioventricular nodal blocking drugs such as beta-blockers are frequently coprescribed.

However, drug block will also persist during and after the action potential and thereby prolong refractoriness, and it may be that it is this effect that is antiarrhythmic.[42] A further wrinkle has been the ability to model the effect of sodium channel block in unstable reentry caused by rotors or multiple wavelets. In this situation, sodium channel block may decrease vulnerability to initiation of fibrillation and, by modulating conduction from the mother rotor, lead to instability of the fibrillatory activity and thereby termination.[43] Other studies have suggested that sodium channel block can terminate reentry by enlarging the inexcitable center of a rotor, decreasing anchoring (thereby increasing meander and extinction), and/or by reducing the number of daughter wavelets.[44]

### *Proarrhythmia in the Structurally Normal Heart*

The recognition that loss of sodium channel function in Brugada syndrome predisposes to ventricular fibrillation, even in the structurally normal or near-normal heart, and that this can be exacerbated by administration of sodium channel blocking drugs, indicates that structural heart disease is not a sine qua non for sodium channel blocking drug proarrhythmia. An *SCN5A* promoter variant common in Asians seems to reduce channel expression and increase both baseline QRS duration and the extent to which class Ic challenge further prolongs QRS.[45] These data suggest the hypothesis that variants, in *SCN5A* regulatory regions or in genes controlling *SCN5A* expression,[46,47] may reduce sodium channel density and predispose to proarrhythmia. This is an appealing scenario in settings such as CAST, or the occasional development of a Brugada syndrome ECG pattern in a patient treated with flecainide for atrial fibrillation, but further work is required to identify such polymorphisms and their potential role in mediating variable drug responses.

Another situation in which sodium channel block even in the normal heart seems to contribute to cardiovascular morbidity and mortality is tricyclic antidepressant overdose. These drugs, notably imipramine and nortriptyline, have been associated with an increased risk of SCD and in overdose typically produce wide complex rhythms which are either VT or drug-induced sinus tachycardia with use-dependent conduction slowing, resulting in wide QRS complexes.[48] Data from human and experimental annals have suggested that increasing extracellular sodium (by sodium bicarbonate or even sodium chloride administration) can shorten QRS duration and potentially exert antiarrhythmic effects.[49–52]

Another intervention that has proven useful in cases of class Ic-related proarrhythmia is administration of beta-blockers. One likely mechanism is that, by slowing sinus rate, beta-blockers decrease the extent of use-dependent block and therefore reduce proarrhythmia.[53] The idea that sodium channel block can confer proarrhythmic effects has generated interest in the regulatory community in the relationship among sodium current blocking potency and QRS prolongation as a function of plasma concentration of drugs. One report suggested that drugs for which the maximum expected plasma concentration was at least thirtyfold lower than the concentration required to block 50% of sodium current was an acceptable safety margin.[54] However, the blocking potency of drug as a function of voltage or rate was not explicitly considered. Furthermore, animal studies have indicated that the relationship between sodium current recorded in a cardiomyocyte and fast conduction may be dissociated with specific mutations in the channel itself[55] or altered function of proteins such as dystrophin and SAP97 that guide its delivery to specific subdomains in the cell.[56]

### *Most Sodium Channel Blockers Exert Other Pharmacologic Effects*

Almost all sodium channel blocking drugs, with the probable exceptions of lidocaine and mexiletine, exert prominent effects on other pharmacologic targets, notably ion channels, and these effects, in turn, complicate interpretation the extent to which sodium channel block contributes to clinical effects observed.

Quinidine, for example, is a very potent blocker of $I_{Kr}$ and a modestly potent blocker of the transient outward current $I_{to}$, and these effects likely contribute to its clinical actions. In particular, quinidine, even at low doses, can frequently produce torsades de pointes, and this likely reflects its $I_{Kr}$-blocking action.[57,58] The effect of quinidine to block $I_{to}$ has been proposed as an antiarrhythmic effect (balancing the loss of sodium current) in Brugada syndrome and this has been demonstrated in both tissue preparations[59] as well as in occasional patients, especially those with VT storm in whom quinidine seems effective.[60,61]

Another example is the unexpected efficacy of flecainide in suppressing arrhythmias and catecholaminergic polymorphic VT (CPVT). CPVT is caused by leaky RYR2 channels, and the initial demonstration of flecainide efficacy in a mouse model of CPVT led to identification of its RYR2-blocking properties and demonstrations of clinical efficacy.[62,63] These are shared with propafenone (and notably the R-enantiomer) but not with other sodium channel blocking agents, and propafenone and flecainide seem unusually effective in CPVT compared with other sodium channel blockers.[64]

Other reports have demonstrated that propafenone is a blocker of cardiac two-pore-domain potassium channels[65] and that the beta blocker propranolol may exert antiarrhythmic effects in certain forms of the long QT syndrome by blocking sodium channels, albeit at relatively high concentrations.[66]

### *The Late Sodium Current*

The macroscopic signature of sodium current during a voltage clamp experiment is rapid activation followed by rapid inactivation back to baseline. Experiments in the 1970s demonstrated that in some tissues (initially the node of Ranvier[67]), fast sodium channel inactivation might be incomplete and, therefore, a persistent current could develop during long voltage clamp steps. Subsequent studies showed that a low concentration of TTX could shorten action potentials in dog Purkinje fibers without affecting maximal phase 0 upstroke slope, supporting the idea of an inward sodium current flowing during the action potential plateau.[68] A body of evidence now supports the view that inhibition of this persistent or late sodium current ($I_{Na-L}$) can suppress arrhythmias without significant proarrhythmic potential.

Two mechanisms underlying $I_{Na-L}$ have been described and both are probably operative in some clinical situations. One is a window mechanism reflecting overlap of the voltage dependence of steady-state activation and inactivation such that at overlap voltages activation and inactivation are nonzero.[68] A second mechanism is a bursting behavior,[69] reflecting instability of the fast inactivation mechanism. The latter is now most commonly associated with type 3 (*SCN5A*-linked) congenital long QT syndrome mutations (the first one described involves the fast inactivation particle in the domain III-IV linker)[70] but is also recognized in normal tissues, notably those with long action potentials such as the Purkinje cells and the midmyocardial (M cell) layer.[71]

The mechanism whereby certain tissues display $I_{Na-L}$ and others do not has not been fully worked out. One possibility is raised by the observation that activation of calmodulin kinase II increases $I_{Na-L}$,[72] suggesting that variable activation of this or other signaling pathways underlies the presence or absence of late sodium current in specific cells. Another candidate pathway is suggested by the observation that hours of exposure to some QT prolonging drugs can inhibit PI3 kinase and this, in turn, increases $I_{Na-L}$.[73] The current is blocked not only by TTX but also by sodium channel blocking drugs such as flecainide[74] or mexiletine.[75] These drugs have been used in LQT3, although they may also provoke the Brugada ECG in this setting.[76]

In addition, $I_{Na-L}$ block is the likely major mechanism of antiarrhythmic action of the antianginal agent ranolazine.[77] The drug seems modestly selective for late sodium current versus peak sodium current.[78] It also blocks $I_{Kr}$ at somewhat higher concentrations than those required to block late sodium current. The clinical effect is to prolong QT interval minimally, if at all, presumably due to late sodium current block. Ranolazine has not been associated with torsades de pointes during clinical use and in animal models the drug's late sodium channel blocking properties seem to inhibit experimental long QT-related arrhythmias.[79] In a large clinical trial in patients with coronary disease, the drug produced no evidence of CAST-like (or other) proarrhythmia.[80] Ranolazine is currently being evaluated as a potential antiarrhythmic in other settings, including atrial fibrillation,[81] and other more selective late cardiac sodium current blockers have been developed.[82,83]

## SUMMARY

Sodium channel blocking drugs carry proarrhythmic potential. This was recognized with the use of high-dose quinidine in the first half of the twentieth century; with the use of encainide and flecainide in patients with advanced heart disease in the 1980s, in CAST, in atrial flutter; and with the recognition that sodium channel block exacerbates the electrocardiographic and arrhythmia susceptibility phenotype in the Brugada syndrome. Despite this risk, the drugs continue to be used, notably in the treatment of atrial fibrillation with the caveat that they should be avoided in patients with structural heart disease or in patients in whom the Brugada ECG is present or emerges during treatment.

Modeling studies have suggested that drugs with appropriate combinations of potassium channel inhibition and specific frequency and/or voltage-dependent sodium channel block could be antiarrhythmic with minimal proarrhythmic potential. One such study suggested that drugs targeting inactivated channels could be atrial fibrillation-selective.[84] The newer agent AZD1305 is highly effective in animal models of atrial fibrillation and seems to induce far greater sodium channel block in atria than in ventricles[85]; this effect is also seen with ranolazine and may reflect differences between atrial and ventricular tissue in the voltage-dependence of fast inactivation.[86] It is also possible that with a deeper understanding of the structure function of the cardiac sodium channel will come opportunities to target entirely new regions of the channel or its function-modifying protein partners to modulate its activity to suppress arrhythmias without proarrhythmia.

## REFERENCES


1. Sami M, Mason JW, Peters F, et al. Clinical electrophysiologic effects of encainide, a newly developed antiarrhythmic agent. Am J Cardiol 1979;44:527–32.
2. Roden DM, Reele SB, Higgins SB, et al. Total suppression of ventricular arrhythmias by encainide. Pharmacokinetic and electrocardiographic characteristics. N Engl J Med 1980;302:877–82.
3. Olsson SB, Edvardsson N. Clinical electrophysiologic study of antiarrhythmic properties of flecainide: acute intraventricular delayed conduction and prolonged repolarization in regular paced and premature beats using intracardiac monophasic action potentials with programmed stimulation. Am Heart J 1981;102:864–71.
4. Duff HJ, Roden DM, Maffucci RJ, et al. Suppression of resistant ventricular arrhythmias by twice daily dosing with flecainide. Am J Cardiol 1981;48:1133–40.
5. Wang T, Roden DM, Wolfenden HT, et al. Influence of genetic polymorphism on the metabolism and disposition of encainide in man. J Pharmacol Exp Ther 1984;228:605–11.
6. Wetherbee DG, Holzman D, Brown MG. Ventricular tachycardia following the administration of quinidine. Am Heart J 1951;42:89–96.
7. Herre JM, Titus C, Oeff M, et al. Inefficacy and proarrhythmic effects of flecainide and encainide for sustained ventricular tachycardia and ventricular fibrillation. Ann Intern Med 1990;113:671–6.
8. CAPS Investigators. Effects of encainide, flecainide, imipramine and moricizine on ventricular arrhythmias during the year after acute myocardial infarction: the CAPS. Am J Cardiol 1988;61:501–9.
9. Cardiac Arrhythmia Suppression Trial Investigators. Increased mortality due to encainide or flecainide in a randomized trial of arrhythmia suppression after myocardial infarction. N Engl J Med 1989;321:406–12.
10. The Cardiac Arrhythmia Suppression Trial-II Investigators. Effect of the antiarrhythmic agent moricizine on survival after myocardial infarction. N Engl J Med 1991;327:227–33.
11. Epstein AE, Hallstrom AP, Rogers WJ, et al. Mortality following ventricular arrhythmia suppression by encainide, flecainide, and moricizine after myocardial infarction. The original design concept of the Cardiac Arrhythmia Suppression Trial (CAST). JAMA 1993;270:2451–5.
12. Hodgkin AL, Huxley AF. Currents carried by sodium and potassium ions through the membrane of the giant axon of Loligo. J Physiol 1952;116:449–72.
13. Hodgkin AL, Huxley AF. A quantitative description of membrane current and its application to conduction and excitation in nerve. J Physiol 1952;117:500–44.
14. Noda M, Shimizu S, Tanabe T, et al. Primary structure of Electrophorus electricus sodium channel deduced from cDNA sequence. Nature 1984;312:121–7.
15. Gellens ME, George AL Jr, Chen LQ, et al. Primary structure and functional expression of the human cardiac tetrodotoxin-insensitive voltage-dependent sodium channel. Proc Natl Acad Sci U S A 1992;89:554–8.
16. Strichartz G. Molecular mechanisms of nerve block by local anesthetics. Anesthesiology 1976;45:421–41.

17. Hondeghem LM, Katzung BG. Time- and voltage-dependent interactions of antiarrhythmic drugs with cardiac sodium channels. Biochim Biophys Acta 1977;472:373–98.
18. Hille B. Local anesthetics: hydrophilic and hydrophobic pathways for the drug-receptor reaction. J Gen Physiol 1977;69:497–515.
19. Hondeghem LM, Katzung BG. Antiarrhythmic agents: the modulated receptor mechanism of action of sodium and calcium channel-blocking drugs. Annu Rev Pharmacol Toxicol 1984;24:387–423.
20. Campbell TJ. Kinetics of onset of rate-dependent effects of Class I antiarrhythmic drugs are important in determining their effects on refractoriness in guinea-pig ventricle, and provide a theoretical basis for their subclassification. Cardiovasc Res 1983;17:344–52.
21. Campbell TJ. Resting and rate-dependent depression of maximum rate of depolarisation (Vmax) in guinea pig ventricular action potentials by mexiletine, disopyramide, and encainide. J Cardiovasc Pharmacol 1983;5:291–6.
22. Campbell TJ, Vaughan Williams EM. Voltage- and time-dependent of maximum rate of depolarization of guinea pig ventricular action potentials by two new antiarrhythmic drugs, flecainide and lorcainide. Cardiovasc Res 1983;17:251–8.
23. Vaughan Williams EM. A classification of antiarrhythmic actions reassessed after a decade of new drugs. J Clin Pharmacol 1984;24:129–47.
24. Backx PH, Yue DT, Lawrence JH, et al. Molecular localization of an ion-binding site within the pore of mammalian sodium channels. Science 1992; 257:248–51.
25. Satin J, Kyle JW, Chen M, et al. A mutant of TTX-resistant cardiac sodium channels with TTX-sensitive properties. Science 1992;256:1202–5.
26. Ragsdale DS, McPhee JC, Scheuer T, et al. Molecular determinants of state-dependent block of Na + channels by local anesthetics. Science 1994;265:1724–8.
27. Yarov-Yarovoy V, Brown J, Sharp EM, et al. Molecular determinants of voltage-dependent gating and binding of pore-blocking drugs in transmembrane segment IIIS6 of the Na(+) channel alpha subunit. J Biol Chem 2001;276:20–7.
28. Yarov-Yarovoy V, McPhee JC, Idsvoog D, et al. Role of amino acid residues in transmembrane segments IS6 and IIS6 of the Na+ channel alpha subunit in voltage-dependent gating and drug block. J Biol Chem 2002;277:35393–401.
29. Payandeh J, Scheuer T, Zheng N, et al. The crystal structure of a voltage-gated sodium channel. Nature 2011;475:353–8.
30. Fozzard HA, Lee PJ, Lipkind GM. Mechanism of local anesthetic drug action on voltage-gated sodium channels. Curr Pharm Des 2005;11:2671–86.
31. Balser JR, Nuss HB, Orias DW, et al. Local anesthetics as effectors of allosteric gating. Lidocaine effects on inactivation-deficient rat skeletal muscle Na channels. J Clin Invest 1996;98:2874–86.
32. Liu H, Clancy C, Cormier J, et al. Mutations in cardiac sodium channels: clinical implications. Am J Pharmacogenomics 2003;3:173–9.
33. Itoh H, Shimizu M, Takata S, et al. A novel missense mutation in the SCN5A gene associated with Brugada syndrome bidirectionally affecting blocking actions of antiarrhythmic drugs. J Cardiovasc Electrophysiol 2005;16:486–93.
34. Valdivia CR, Ackerman MJ, Tester DJ, et al. A novel SCN5A arrhythmia mutation, M1766L, with expression defect rescued by mexiletine. Cardiovasc Res 2002;55:279–89.
35. Valdivia CR, Tester DJ, Rok BA, et al. A trafficking defective, Brugada syndrome-causing SCN5A mutation rescued by drugs. Cardiovasc Res 2004;62:53–62.
36. Liu K, Yang T, Viswanathan PC, et al. New mechanism contributing to drug-induced arrhythmia: rescue of a misprocessed LQT3 mutant. Circulation 2005;112:3239–46.
37. Bezzina CR, Tan HL. Pharmacological rescue of mutant ion channels. Cardiovasc Res 2002;55: 229–32.
38. Makita N, Horie M, Nakamura T, et al. Drug-induced long-QT syndrome associated with a subclinical SCN5A mutation. Circulation 2002;106: 1269–74.
39. Ruan Y, Denegri M, Liu N, et al. Trafficking defects and gating abnormalities of a novel SCN5A mutation question gene-specific therapy in long QT syndrome type 3. Circ Res 2010; 106:1374–83.
40. Coromilas J, Saltman AE, Waldecker B, et al. Electrophysiological effects of flecainide on anisotropic conduction and reentry in infarcted canine hearts. Circulation 1995;91:2245–63.
41. Crijns HJ, van Gelder IS, Lie KI. Supraventricular tachycardia mimicking ventricular tachycardia during flecainide treatment. Am J Cardiol 1988;62:1303–6.
42. Coronel R, Janse MJ, Opthof T, et al. Postrepolarization refractoriness in acute ischemia and after antiarrhythmic drug administration: action potential duration is not always an index of the refractory period. Heart Rhythm 2012;9:977–82.
43. Qu Z, Weiss JN. Effects of Na+ and K+ channel blockade on vulnerability to and termination of fibrillation in simulated normal cardiac tissue. Am J Physiol Heart Circ Physiol 2005;289: H1692–701.
44. Kneller J, Kalifa J, Zou R, et al. Mechanisms of atrial fibrillation termination by pure sodium channel blockade in an ionically-realistic mathematical model. Circ Res 2005;96:e35–47.

45. Bezzina CR, Shimizu W, Yang P, et al. Common sodium channel promoter haplotype in Asian subjects underlies variability in cardiac conduction. Circulation 2006;113:338–44.
46. van den Boogaard M, Smemo S, Burnicka-Turek O, et al. A common genetic variant within SCN10A modulates cardiac SCN5A expression. J Clin Invest 2014;124:1844–52.
47. Bezzina CR, Barc J, Mizusawa Y, et al. Common variants at SCN5A-SCN10A and HEY2 are associated with Brugada syndrome, a rare disease with high risk of sudden cardiac death. Nat Genet 2013;45:1044–9.
48. Bardai A, Amin AS, Blom MT, et al. Sudden cardiac arrest associated with use of a non-cardiac drug that reduces cardiac excitability: evidence from bench, bedside, and community. Eur Heart J 2013;34:1506–16.
49. Bou-Abboud E, Nattel S. Molecular mechanisms of the reversal of imipramine-induced sodium channel blockade by alkalinization in human cardiac myocytes. Cardiovasc Res 1998;38:395–404.
50. Ranger S, Sheldon R, Fermini B, et al. Modulation of flecainide's cardiac sodium channel blocking actions by extracellular sodium: a possible cellular mechanism for the action of sodium salts in flecainide cardiotoxicity. J Pharmacol Exp Ther 1993;264:1160–7.
51. Bou-Abboud E, Nattel S. Relative role of alkalosis and sodium ions in reversal of class I antiarrhythmic drug-induced sodium channel blockade by sodium bicarbonate. Circulation 1996;94:1954–61.
52. Bajaj AK, Woosley RL, Roden DM. Acute electrophysiologic effects of sodium administration in dogs treated with O-desmethyl encainide. Circulation 1989;80:994–1002.
53. Myerburg RJ, Kessler KM, Cox MM, et al. Reversal of proarrhythmic effects of flecainide acetate and encainide hydrochloride by propranolol. Circulation 1989;80:1571–9.
54. Lu HR, Rohrbacher J, Vlaminckx E, et al. Predicting drug-induced slowing of conduction and proarrhythmia: identifying the 'bad' sodium current blockers. Br J Pharmacol 2010;160:60–76.
55. Watanabe H, Yang T, Stroud DM, et al. Striking in vivo phenotype of a disease-associated human SCN5A mutation producing minimal changes in vitro. Circulation 2011;124:1001–11.
56. Petitprez S, Zmoos AF, Ogrodnik J, et al. SAP97 and dystrophin macromolecular complexes determine two pools of cardiac sodium channels Nav1.5 in cardiomyocytes. Circ Res 2011;108:294–304.
57. Roden DM, Woosley RL, Primm RK. Incidence and clinical features of the quinidine-associated long QT syndrome: implications for patient care. Am Heart J 1986;111:1088–93.
58. Yang T, Roden DM. Extracellular potassium modulation of drug block of IKr. Implications for torsade de pointes and reverse use-dependence. Circulation 1996;93:407–11.
59. Yan GX, Antzelevitch C. Cellular basis for the Brugada syndrome and other mechanisms of arrhythmogenesis associated with ST-segment elevation. Circulation 1999;100:1660–6.
60. Alings M, Dekker L, Sadee A, et al. Quinidine induced electrocardiographic normalization in two patients with Brugada syndrome. Pacing Clin Electrophysiol 2001;24:1420–2.
61. Belhassen B, Glick A, Viskin S. Efficacy of quinidine in high-risk patients with Brugada syndrome. Circulation 2004;110:1731–7.
62. Watanabe H, Chopra N, Laver D, et al. Flecainide prevents catecholaminergic polymorphic ventricular tachycardia in mice and humans. Nat Med 2009;15:380–3.
63. van der Werf C, Kannankeril PJ, Sacher F, et al. Flecainide therapy reduces exercise-induced ventricular arrhythmias in patients with catecholaminergic polymorphic ventricular tachycardia. J Am Coll Cardiol 2011;57:2244–54.
64. Hwang HS, Hasdemir C, Laver D, et al. Inhibition of cardiac $Ca2+$ release channels (RyR2) determines efficacy of class I antiarrhythmic drugs in catecholaminergic polymorphic ventricular tachycardia. Circulation 2011;4:128–35.
65. Schmidt C, Wiedmann F, Schweizer PA, et al. Class I antiarrhythmic drugs inhibit human cardiac two-pore-domain $K+$ (K2P) channels. Eur J Pharmacol 2013;721:237–48.
66. Bankston JR, Kass RS. Molecular determinants of local anesthetic action of beta-blocking drugs: implications for therapeutic management of long QT syndrome variant 3. J Mol Cell Cardiol 2010;48:246–53.
67. Dubois JM, Bergman C. Late sodium current in the node of Ranvier. Pflugers Arch 1975;357:145–8.
68. Coraboeuf E, Deroubaix E, Coulombe A. Effect of tetrodotoxin on action potentials of the conducting system in the dog heart. Am J Physiol 1979;236:HV561–7.
69. Kiyosue T, Arita M. Late sodium current and its contribution to action potential configuration in guinea pig ventricular myocytes. Circ Res 1989;64:389–97.
70. Bennett PB, Yazawa K, Makita N, et al. Molecular mechanism for an inherited cardiac arrhythmia. Nature 1995;376:683–5.
71. Zygmunt AC, Eddlestone GT, Thomas GP, et al. Larger late sodium conductance in M cells contributes to electrical heterogeneity in canine ventricle. Am J Physiol Heart Circ Physiol 2001;281:H689–97.
72. Wagner S, Ruff HM, Weber SL, et al. Reactive oxygen species-activated Ca/Calmodulin Kinase IIδ is required for late I(Na) augmentation leading

to cellular Na and Ca overload. Circ Res 2011;108: 555–65.
73. Lu Z, Wu CY, Jiang YP, et al. Suppression of phosphoinositide 3-Kinase signaling and alteration of multiple ion currents in drug-induced long QT syndrome. Sci Transl Med 2012;4:131ra50.
74. Nagatomo T, January CT, Makielski JC. Preferential block of late sodium current in the LQT3 DeltaKPQ mutant by the class I(C) antiarrhythmic flecainide. Mol Pharmacol 2000;57:101–7.
75. Sunami A, Fan Z, Sawanobori T, et al. Use-dependent block of Na+ currents by mexiletine at the single channel level in guinea-pig ventricular myocytes. Br J Pharmacol 1993;110:183–92.
76. Priori SG, Napolitano C, Schwartz PJ, et al. The elusive link between LQT3 and Brugada syndrome: the role of flecainide challenge. Circulation 2000; 102:945–7.
77. Zaza A, Belardinelli L, Shryock JC. Pathophysiology and pharmacology of the cardiac "late sodium current". Pharmacol Ther 2008;119:326–39.
78. Antzelevitch C, Burashnikov A, Sicouri S, et al. Electrophysiologic basis for the antiarrhythmic actions of ranolazine. Heart Rhythm 2011;8:1281–90.
79. Wu L, Shryock JC, Song Y, et al. Antiarrhythmic effects of ranolazine in a guinea pig in vitro model of long-QT syndrome. J Pharmacol Exp Ther 2004; 310:599–605.
80. Morrow DA, Scirica BM, Karwatowska-Prokopczuk E, et al. Effects of ranolazine on recurrent cardiovascular events in patients with non–ST-elevation acute coronary syndromes. JAMA 2007;297:1775–83.
81. Verrier RL, Kumar K, Nieminen T, et al. Mechanisms of ranolazine's dual protection against atrial and ventricular fibrillation. Europace 2013;15:317–24.
82. Belardinelli L, Liu G, Smith-Maxwell C, et al. A novel, potent, and selective inhibitor of cardiac late sodium current suppresses experimental arrhythmias. J Pharmacol Exp Ther 2013;344: 23–32.
83. Pezhouman A, Madahian S, Stepanyan H, et al. Selective inhibition of late sodium current suppresses ventricular tachycardia and fibrillation in intact rat hearts. Heart Rhythm 2014;11: 492–501.
84. Aguilar-Shardonofsky M, Vigmond Edward J, Nattel S, et al. In silico optimization of atrial fibrillation-selective sodium channel blocker pharmacodynamics. Biophys J 2012;102:951–60.
85. Burashnikov A, Zygmunt AC, Di Diego JM, et al. AZD1305 exerts atrial predominant electrophysiological actions and is effective in suppressing atrial fibrillation and preventing its reinduction in the dog. J Cardiovasc Pharmacol 2010;56: 80–90.
86. Burashnikov A, Di Diego JM, Zygmunt AC, et al. Atrium-selective sodium channel block as a strategy for suppression of atrial fibrillation: differences in sodium channel inactivation between atria and ventricles and the role of ranolazine. Circulation 2007;116:1449–57.

# Congenital Long QT Syndrome Type 3

Yanfei Ruan, MD[a], Nian Liu, MD[a], Rong Bai, MD[a], Silvia G. Priori, MD, PhD[b,c,d], Carlo Napolitano, MD, PhD[b,*]

**KEYWORDS**

• Electrophysiology • Genetics • Long QT syndrome • Sodium • Ion channel • Pharmacology

**KEY POINTS**

- Long QT syndrome type 3 (LQT3) is caused by "gain-of-function" SCN5A mutations. Specific ST-T wave patterns, triggers, and risk for cardiac events are associated with LQT3.
- Beta blockers provided some but inadequate protection for LQT3 patients. Based on the "gain-of-function" mechanism, sodium channel blockers are used as gene-specific therapy in LQT3.
- Response to sodium channel blockade among LQT3 patients is mutation-specific. In vitro assessment of the gating properties may help to predict the patient's response.

## INTRODUCTION

Long QT syndrome (LQTS) is a cardiovascular disorder characterized by abnormally prolonged QT interval leading to life-threatening arrhythmia in the presence of a structurally normal heart. The syndrome is caused by mutations of genes encoding cardiac ion channels or their modulators that control cardiac repolarization. The responsible genetic loci have been named in sequence of discovery. The list of LQTS-causing genes is continuously expanding and has reached a count of 13. Although there is remarkable genetic heterogeneity in LQTS, 3 genes, KCNQ1 (LQT1), KCNH2 (LQT2), and SCN5A (LQT3), dominate the picture and account for greater than 90% of LQTS patients with identified mutations. The estimated prevalence of LQTS is approximately 1:2500. However, due to silent mutation carriers, the actual prevalence in the population could be higher. LQT3 makes up 5% to 10% of LQTS cases.[1] The limited prevalence of LQT3 in the largest registry data results in reduced power to detect robust genotype-phenotype correlation and response to therapies. For this reason, although in vitro studies have been very successful in delineating the biophysical consequences of mutations, the progress of our clinical management skills remains less than optimal.

This article provides an overview of the molecular genetics, clinical presentation, and management of LQT3 and discusses the gene-specific and mutation-specific pharmacotherapy in LQT3.

## MOLECULAR GENETICS

In 1994, LQT3 was mapped to 3p21–24[2]; 1 year later *SCN5A*, the gene encoding $\alpha$-subunit of the human cardiac sodium channel hNav1.5 was mapped to chromosome 3p21.[3] Shortly after, Wang and colleagues[4] demonstrated that SCN5A mutations are the cause of this variant and named it LQT3. They identified genetic linkage between *SCN5A* and LQT3 in 3 unrelated families. No recombination was identified between these loci. They also identified intragenic deletions of *SCN5A* in affected members of 2 LQT families. In vitro functional expression demonstrated a

Disclosures: None.

[a] Department of Cardiology, Beijing An Zhen Hospital, Capital Medical University, 2 Anzhen Road, Beijing 100029, China; [b] Molecular Cardiology, IRCCS Fondazione Salvatore Maugeri, Via Maugeri 10, Pavia 27100, Italy; [c] Cardiovascular Genetics, Leon Charney Division of Cardiology, New York University, 522 First Avenue, New York, NY 10016, USA; [d] Department of Molecular Medicine, University of Pavia, Via Maugeri 10, Pavia 27100, Italy

* Corresponding author.

*E-mail address:* carlo.napolitano@fsm.it

Card Electrophysiol Clin 6 (2014) 705–713
http://dx.doi.org/10.1016/j.ccep.2014.07.007
1877-9182/14/$ – see front matter 

gain-of-function effect.[4] The sodium current (INa) activates normally but it does not inactivate properly and a small noninactivating current remains even after hundred of milliseconds after initial fast (and quantitatively predominant) inactivation (**Fig. 1**).[5] This small current defined as "late INa" or "late sustained inward sodium current (Isus)" occurs during the plateau phase of the action potential. During this phase, small currents can cause large membrane voltage perturbations because of the reduced permeability to potassium ions (increased impedance), which explains why even small INa (fraction of percentage of the total peak current) can cause significant QT prolongation.

With the increasing availability of commercial genetic screening, the list of *SCN5A* mutations responsible for LQT3 is expanding and there are more than 100 variants associated with a typical LQTS phenotype (many more SCN5A mutations are associated with Brugada syndrome (BrS) or conduction defect and a loss of function phenotype). However, the growing number of identified genetic variations is creating the need of distinguishing the disease-causing mutation from rare nonpathogenic variants in the attempt of reducing the number of the so-called variant of unknown significance (VUS). This objective is clinically relevant and critically important. There are no specific data for LQT3 but the prevalence of VUS in LQTS genes found upon screening of normal subjects is of 4%, leading to a signal to noise ratio of 19:1[6]; this means that approximately 1 of 20 of the identified variants cannot be definitely labeled as pathogenic. When familial cosegregation analysis is not possible the functional study of the mutant channel can be very helpful to the clinical assessment,[7] particularly when considering that SCN5A mutations may be associated with other phenotypes like BrS of progressive cardiac conduction detect.

## CLINICAL PRESENTATION

The clinical presentation of LQT3 is similar to that of LQTS in general even if it shows distinctive features in terms of incidence of cardiac events and response to therapy. Accordingly, the typical manifestations are syncopal episodes and QT interval prolongation with ST-T wave morphologic abnormalities.

### *Life-threatening Cardiac Events and Genotype-specific Triggers in Long QT Syndrome Type 3*

The syncopal episodes are due to torsades de pointes (TdP), a polymorphic ventricular tachycardia with a characteristic twist of the QRS complex around the isoelectric baseline, often degenerating into ventricular fibrillation. Arrhythmias can arise without changes in heart rate and without specific sequences, even though long pauses increase the probability of TdP. In LQT3 patients, life-threatening arrhythmias occur more frequently during sleep or at rest in sharp contrast with LQT1 patients, for whom most arrhythmias occurred during exercise.[8] The underlying mechanism may be related to the disproportional QT prolongation at long cycle lengths or during nighttime observed in LQT3 patients. LQT3 also differs from the typical LQTS feature of female preponderance of cardiac events. Zareba and colleagues[9] observed a higher lethality of events with no clear gender difference. The authors substantially confirmed the observation and demonstrated that men are at significantly high risk than women when QTc is greater than 500 ms.

Overall, LQT3 is to be considered a severe LQTS variant. When only patients with ascertained causative mutation are included, the annual cardiac arrest/sudden death rate is of 0.59% and 42% of patient experience a cardiac event before age 40 years.[10]

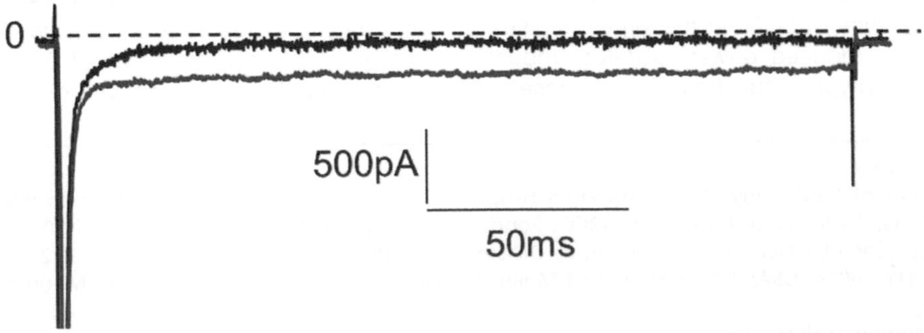


**Fig. 1.** Original current recording from HEK293 cells transiently transfected with wild type (*black line*) or F1473S (*red line*) SCN5A with β1-subunit of cardiac sodium channel. Although the initial gas component is relatively unchanged, the current does not inactivate properly even after 200 ms of depolarizing pulse.

### *Features of Electrocardiogram*

The clinical severity of typical LQT3 is confirmed by the evidence of a longer corrected QT (QTc) duration. The authors showed[11] that QT penetrance (ie, the percentage of patients with QTc greater than the normal limits) is 79%. As a comparison example the penetrance of LQT1 is 55%. So, most of the LQT3 patients have a clinically detectable disease (mean QTc 478 ms). It is clinically useful to measure QT interval at rest or at relatively low rates in LQT3 because the increased adaptation[12] to heart rate (steep QT/RR slope) may reduce the possibility of detecting prolonged QT at fast rates. Moss and colleagues[13] reported that QTonset-c was unusually prolonged in LQT3. LQT3 patients have a distinctive, late-appearing small T wave with straight ST segment that is clearly different from that in LQT1, which shows a broad-based, prolonged T-wave pattern, and in LQT2, which shows a low-amplitude, moderately delayed T wave (**Fig. 2**). This observation was expanded by Zhang and colleagues[14] who reported 2 typical ST-T wave patterns in LQT3 patients: (1) a long ST segment followed by a narrow peaked or biphasic T wave; this pattern type was identified in 53% of LQT3 patients and (2) peaked and asymmetrical T wave with a steep downslope (12% of cases). In other cases, however, a considerable variability existed with overlap of the electrocardiogram (ECG) repolarization patterns among the 3 genotypes. Therefore, although ST-T wave morphology can provide a hint and favor targeted screening, it can not be considered as a surrogate of genetic testing.

Although LQT3 is a high-penetrance variant, approximately 20% of the cases present with normal QT interval.[11,15] Several possibilities have been proposed to explain such incomplete penetrance spanning from QT-modulating single nucleotide polymorphisms[16] to gene-gene interactions.[17] From the clinical standpoint it is important to observe that mutations carriers with normal QT interval retain a marginal risk of events (4%–6%).

## DIAGNOSIS

The diagnosis of LQT3 is generally a 2-step process and it should be approached differently for probands and family members. The first step would be to diagnose LQTS on a clinical basis in the subject who first comes to the medical attention within a given kindred (the proband), who is often also the most severely affected subject. According to the most recent consensus on diagnosis of inherited arrhythmias,[18] the disease can be diagnosed in the presence of a QTc greater than 480 ms or a diagnostic score greater than or equal to 3.5. LQTS is also diagnosed when a pathogenic mutation is identified, independently from QT duration.

Specific consideration to LQT3 includes the need for careful QT interval measurements (see earlier discussion) to avoid heart rate–dependent artifacts. Twelve-lead 24-hour Holter monitoring is very useful to assess QT interval morphology and duration at different heart rates. Secondary causes of QT prolongation (drugs, electrolyte imbalances) should also be excluded before diagnosis.

Genetic testing is critically important to establish diagnosis especially for borderline cases (ie, QTc between 440 ms and 470 ms). Once diagnosis is established a mutation is found; the second step is to expand the analysis to all family members independently from the presence/absence of a prolonged QT interval and symptoms. In the absence of a known disease-causing mutation, first-degree family members should be clinically assessed.

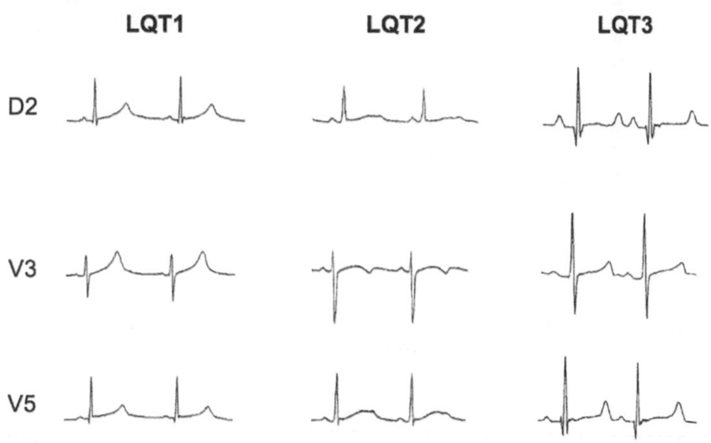


**Fig. 2.** ECG recordings from D2, V3, and V5 in 3 patients from families with LQTS. The typical morphology of LQT3 with straight ST segment and small T wave is shown in the right panel.

## MANAGEMENT OF LONG QT SYNDROME TYPE 3

As for all LQTS patients, the management of LQT3 should start from the estimate of the risk of cardiac events, which is primarily determined by the length of QT interval. It has been confirmed by independent investigators that QTc greater than 500 ms identifies the highest risk subgroup.[10] Genotype and gender modulate the effect of QT interval, and LQT3 is considered a malignant LQTS variant (**Fig. 3**). The risk of becoming symptomatic is also higher among male than female patients in LQT3.[10] Therefore appropriate therapies and close follow-up is required.

### *Lifestyle Modifications*

According to the HRS/EHRA/APHRS expert consensus statement on the diagnosis and management of patients with inherited primary arrhythmia syndromes,[18] lifestyle modifications are recommended in all LQTS patients. These modifications include avoidance of QT-prolonging drugs and prompt correction of electrolyte abnormalities that may occur during diarrhea, vomiting, metabolic conditions, or imbalanced diets for weight loss. Because LQT3 patients tend to experience cardiac events at rest and their QT adapts promptly to heart rate increase, some investigator suggested that sport activity at moderate intensity can be allowed.[19] This is certainly true for low-risk patients with borderline QTc prolongation, no history of syncope. However, less certain is the recommendation for symptomatic patients.

### *Beta-blockers*

Current guidelines do not provide genotype-specific indications for the use of beta-blockers, which are recommended in all patients presenting with QTc greater than or equal to 470 ms. Nevertheless, there has been a long history of debate about the effectiveness of beta-blockers in LQT3. In 1995, Schwartz and colleagues[12] reported that LQT3 patients shortened their QT interval in response to increases in heart rate much more than control subjects. Using an in vitro model, Priori and colleagues[20] reported that LQT3 model shortened action potential duration in response to isoproterenol and rapid pacing. These observations raised the concern that, by reducing heart rate beta-blockers could actually increase the propensity to arrhythmias in LQT3. In 2000, Moss and colleagues[21] reported the lack of effectiveness of beta-blockers among 28 LQT3 patients. In 2001, Schwartz and colleagues[8] reported that among 18 LQT3 patients on beta-blockers, 17% patients experienced cardiac arrest/sudden death versus 7% LQT1 and 4% LQT2. Finally, higher event rate on active beta-blocking therapy was reported in 2004 by Priori and colleagues[22] (**Fig. 4**).

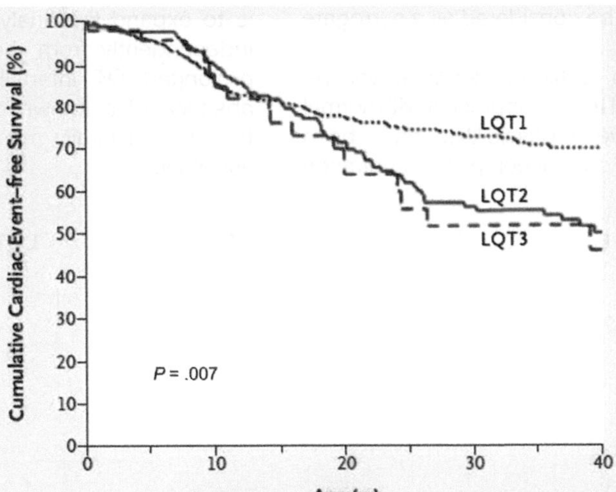


No. at Risk

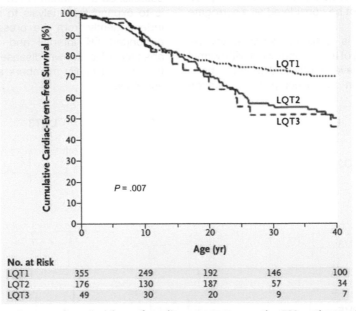

| | | | | | |
|---|---|---|---|---|---|
| LQT1 | 355 | 249 | 192 | 146 | 100 |
| LQT2 | 176 | 130 | 187 | 57 | 34 |
| LQT3 | 49 | 30 | 20 | 9 | 7 |

**Fig. 3.** Kaplan-Meier estimates of survival-free of cardiac events among the 580 patients with LQTS in the risk-stratification analysis, according to the genetic locus of the mutation. The difference among the groups was significant ($P = .007$ by the log-rank test). (*From* Priori SG, Schwartz PJ, Napolitano C, et al. Risk stratification in the long-QT syndrome. N Engl J Med 2003;348:1869; with permission.)

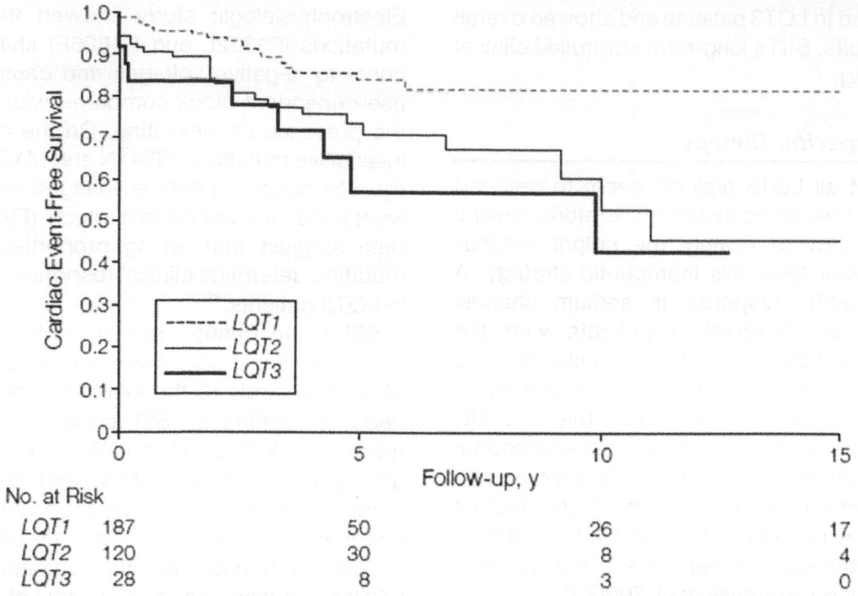


**Fig. 4.** Kaplan-Meier analysis of cumulative cardiac event-free survival in genotyped LQTS patients receiving beta-blockers according to the genetic variant of the disease (log-rank $P<.001$). The definition of events includes syncope, cardiac arrest, and sudden cardiac death. (*From* Priori SG, Napolitano C, Schwartz PJ, et al. Association of long QT syndrome loci and cardiac events among patients treated with beta-blockers. JAMA 2004;292:1341–4; with permission.)

Beta-blockers are likely to be less effective in LQT3 as compared with other LQTS variants, but this does imply they do not reduce the burden of cardiac events. This concept is supported by experimental evidence obtained in ΔKPQ-SCN5A knock-in transgenic mouse model in which propranolol effectively prevents ventricular tachycardia/ventricular fibrillation[23] and by preliminary clinical data showing a reduction of events after therapy in 403 LQT3 patients.[24]

Overall, it is reasonable to recommend the use of beta-blockers among LQT3 unless there is a specific contraindication.

## *Gene-specific Therapy*

Bench studies have elucidated at least 3 major biophysical abnormalities associated with LQT3. First, single-channel reopening behavior induces small Isus,[25] which is the main defect for the most mutant SCN5A associated with LQT3. The second mechanism of mutant SCN5A is called "window current", which results from steady-state channel reopening that occurs over voltage ranges for which steady-state inactivation (SSI) and activation overlap.[26] The third mechanism occurs under nonequilibrium conditions whereby channel reopening result from fast recovery from inactivation at membrane potentials that facilitates activation transition.[27] All the biophysical alterations discussed earlier predispose the sodium channel to a gain of function causing a small increase in net inward current during the plateau phase of action potential. Therefore the use of sodium channel blockers is a rational approach for LQT3.

Interestingly, LQT3 is the only LQTS variant for which a gene-specific therapy is recommended by current guidelines. Indeed, the HRS/EHRA/APHRS expert consensus paper[18] states that "*sodium channel blockers can be useful, as add-on therapy, for LQT3 patients with a QTc >500 ms who shorten their QTc by >40 ms following an acute oral drug test with one of these compounds*" (class IIa). This recommendation is based on a limited number of clinical papers. But experimental findings are consistent and robust. The 40-ms QTc reduction required to indicate the use of these drugs is based on the evidence that not all patients display the same therapeutic response (see later discussion) and it has a practical implication. Indeed, the effect of sodium channel blockers (mexiletine is the most widely used) on QTc should be assessed by acute oral drug testing before chronic administration.

A possible therapeutic effect of mexiletine was first proposed several years ago by the authors in an experimental model[20] and confirmed in a small clinical trial.[12] Other sodium channel blockers such as flecainide[28] and ranolazine[29] were also administrated in LQT3 patients and showed overall positive results. Still a long-term controlled clinical trial is lacking.

## *Mutation-specific Therapy*

Of note, not all LQT3 patients seem to respond favorably to mexiletine therapy. Therefore, several groups attempt to identify the culprit mechanisms to better tailor this therapeutic strategy. A mutation-specific response to sodium channel blockade was observed in patients with the D1790G mutation, who show significant QTc shortening with flecainide but not lidocaine. Electrophysiologic study demonstrated that D1790G markedly increases flecainide use-dependent block of channels, mainly due to the pronounced slow recovery from inactivation of the mutant channel in the presence of flecainide, but not lidocaine; thus the distinct responses are associated with the gating properties of D1790G.[28]

On the basis of these preliminary findings the authors carried out a systematic analysis and identified a set of LQT3 patients with different SCN5A mutations and with variable response to mexiletine.[30] P1332L and R1626P mutation carriers presented QTc shortening by 10% or more after mexiletine administration and were free of cardiac events during follow-up. On the contrary, S941N and M1652R mutation carriers showed negligible or no QTc shortening on mexiletine treatment and died from cardiac events during follow-up. Electrophysiologic study showed that sensitive mutations (P1332L and R1626P) shifted the SSI curve to negative voltages and caused stronger use-dependent block compared with wild type in the presence of mexiletine. On the contrary, the insensitive mutations (S941N and M1652R) shifted the SSI curve to positive voltages and caused a weakened use-dependent block (**Fig. 5**). These data suggest that gating properties of SCN5A mutation determine clinical response to mexiletine in LQT3 patients.[30]

SSI curve defines the proportion of inactive sodium channel at a given membrane potential. Mexiletine binds to the inactive sodium channel; negative shifting of SSI curve would produce more inactive channels and thus increase channel affinity for mexiletine block and better clinical response. Should these data be confirmed in a larger and prospective study, it will be reasonable to use systematic in vitro characterization of SCN5A mutants as a predictor of the clinical response; this could avoid serious side effects as outlined in the following section.

## *Pitfalls for Gene-specific Therapy in LQT3*

The most frequently reported overlap syndrome for SCN5A mutations is LQT3 combined with BrS. Incomplete penetrance raised concerns that sodium channel blocker is used in LQT3 patients with latent BrS. The authors clinically observed Brugada-like ECG changes in LQT3 patients

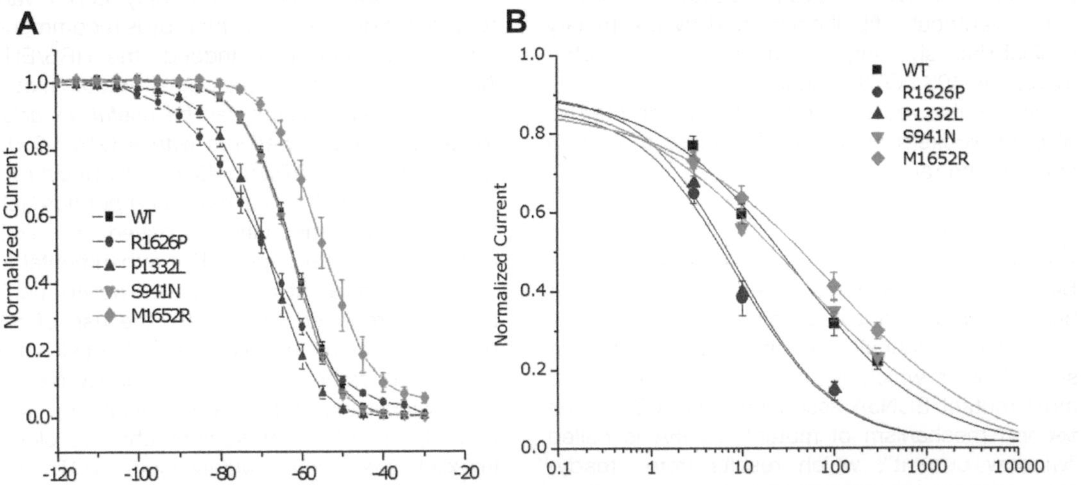


**Fig. 5.** A hyperpolarizing shift of inactivation might be associated with a good clinical response to mexiletine. (*A*) Voltage dependence of inactivation for wild type, R1626P, P1332L, S941N, and M1652R sodium channels. (*B*) Concentration dependence of use-dependent block by mexiletine. EC50 values were 37.99 μmol/L, 8.8 μmol/L, 8.76 μmol/L, 37.57 μmol/L, and 96.14 μmol/L for wild type, R1626P, P1332L, S941N, and M1652R respectively. (*From* Ruan Y, Liu N, Bloise R, et al. Gating properties of SCN5A mutations and the response to mexiletine in long-QT syndrome type 3 patients. Circulation 2007;116:1137–44; with permission.)

treated with flecainide,[31] suggesting that the complex biophysical mechanisms of some SCN5A mutants could result in unexpected clinical responses. More recently they had the opportunity to study in detail one exemplary case of "complex" response to sodium channel blockade. The authors were referred for genetic testing of an LQTS case with an unexpected deleterious effect of mexiletine. The index case was a child treated with beta-blockers and mexiletine at birth due to severe QT prolongation and arrhythmias.[5] After an initial good response, the QT prolonged back to the initial values and the child died for intractable arrhythmias. They identified the F1473S variant and decided to carry out in vitro expression. Data demonstrated a severe gain of function phenotype with very large late sodium current (probably the largest ever reported) and an enhanced window current. Intriguingly, F1473S also caused trafficking defect with an overall reduction of peak sodium current of 80%. The trafficking impairment (loss-of-function phenotype) actually protected patient by the deleterious effects of Isus. Indeed when expressed in vitro therapeutic concentration of mexiletine rescued the trafficking defect and induced further action potential prolongation. This explained why the patient actually worsened the clinical phenotypes after treatment.

These results support the clinical usefulness of in vitro expression of mutants and suggest the need for performing acute oral drug testing before chronic administration of mexiletine in LQT3 patients.[31,32]

### *Implantable Cardioverter-Defibrillator and Left Cardiac Sympathetic Denervation*

Recommendations for implantable cardioverter-defibrillator (ICD) implant and left cardiac sympathetic denervation (LCSD) are not specific for LQT3 and the general LQTS recommendations apply. ICD is recommended to LQT3 patients who are survivors of cardiac arrest (class I) and it could be considered in patients who experience recurrent syncope with beta-blockers (class IIa).

However, the clinical data that suggested higher severity and reduced response to beta-blockers among LQT3 are having a clinical impact on how this genetic variant is approached. Registry data show that ICD implantation is overrepresented among LQT3, with greater proportion of implants in asymptomatic subjects (45% vs 3%–5% among LQT1 and LQT2).[33] However, the worrisome incidence of adverse events in young patients with ICDs discourages a widespread use of devices in low- to medium-risk patients. In this light it should be considered that there is no evidence that ICD implantation in asymptomatic LQT3 improves survival. It would therefore be advisable to enforce the controlled use of mexiletine or the newer specific sodium channel blockers[34] and restrict the ICD use for primary prevention only in the few highest-risk LQT3 subgroup (men with QTc >500 ms).

LCSD can be useful in patients with a diagnosis of LQTS who experience breakthrough events while on therapy with beta-blockers/ICD. LCSD can also be considered in LQTS patients when beta-blocker is contraindicated. However, LCSD cannot be considered as an equally effective alternative to ICD. Recurrence of arrhythmic events is indeed observed in 40% of LQTS patients.[35] Theoretically, the antiadrenergic effect of LCSD without reducing heart rate may be favorable for LQT3 patients but there are no clinical data to support this statement. Therefore LQTS guidelines should be followed.[18]

## SUMMARY

LQT3 is a relatively rare and aggressive LQTS variant. Unfortunately, clinical data and LQT3-specific genotype-phenotype correlation are slowly accumulating due to the limited size of available study cohorts. On the other hand, the robust understanding of the biophysical pathogenesis of SCN5A mutations allows to devise gene- or mutation-specific therapies and to improve the optimization of the available therapeutic armamentarium. The availability of novel and more specific late INa blocker will hopefully allow to further abate the burden of life-threatening events in these patients.

## REFERENCES

1. Schwartz PJ, Crotti L, Insolia R. Long-QT syndrome: from genetics to management. Circ Arrhythm Electrophysiol 2012;5:868–77.
2. Jiang C, Atkinson D, Towbin JA, et al. Two long QT syndrome loci map to chromosomes 3 and 7 with evidence for further heterogeneity. Nat Genet 1994; 8:141–7.
3. George AL Jr, Varkony TA, Drabkin HA, et al. Assignment of the human heart tetrodotoxin-resistant voltage-gated Na+ channel alpha-subunit gene (SCN5A) to band 3p21. Cytogenet Cell Genet 1995;68:67–70.
4. Wang Q, Shen J, Splawski I, et al. SCN5A mutations associated with an inherited cardiac arrhythmia, long qt syndrome. Cell 1995;80:805–11.
5. Ruan Y, Denegri M, Liu N, et al. Trafficking defects and gating abnormalities of a novel SCN5A mutation question gene-specific therapy in long QT syndrome type 3. Circ Res 2010;106:1374–83.
6. Ackerman MJ, Priori SG, Willems S, et al. HRS/EHRA expert consensus statement on the state of genetic

testing for the channelopathies and cardiomyopathies this document was developed as a partnership between the Heart Rhythm Society (HRS) and the European Heart Rhythm Association (EHRA). Heart Rhythm 2011;8:1308–39.
7. Ruan Y, Liu N, Priori SG. Sodium channel mutations and arrhythmias. Nature reviews. Cardiology 2009; 6:337–48.
8. Schwartz PJ, Priori SG, Spazzolini C, et al. Genotype-phenotype correlation in the long-QT syndrome: gene-specific triggers for life-threatening arrhythmias. Circulation 2001;103:89–95.
9. Zareba W, Moss AJ, Schwartz PJ, et al. Influence of genotype on the clinical course of the long-QT syndrome. International long-QT syndrome registry research group. N Engl J Med 1998;339:960–5.
10. Priori SG, Schwartz PJ, Napolitano C, et al. Risk stratification in the long-QT syndrome. N Engl J Med 2003; 348:1866–74.
11. Napolitano C, Priori SG, Schwartz PJ, et al. Genetic testing in the long QT syndrome: development and validation of an efficient approach to genotyping in clinical practice. JAMA 2005;294:2975–80.
12. Schwartz PJ, Priori SG, Locati EH, et al. Long QT syndrome patients with mutations of the SCN5A and HERG genes have differential responses to Na+ channel blockade and to increases in heart rate. Implications for gene-specific therapy. Circulation 1995;92:3381–6.
13. Moss AJ, Zareba W, Benhorin J, et al. ECG T-wave patterns in genetically distinct forms of the hereditary long QT syndrome. Circulation 1995;92:2929–34.
14. Zhang L, Timothy KW, Vincent GM, et al. Spectrum of ST-T-wave patterns and repolarization parameters in congenital long-QT syndrome: ECG findings identify genotypes. Circulation 2000;102:2849–55.
15. Priori SG, Napolitano C, Schwartz PJ. Low penetrance in the long-QT syndrome: clinical impact. Circulation 1999;99:529–33.
16. Tomas M, Napolitano C, De Giuli L, et al. Polymorphisms in the NOS1AP gene modulate QT interval duration and risk of arrhythmias in the long QT syndrome. J Am Coll Cardiol 2010;55:2745–52.
17. van den Boogaard M, Smemo S, Burnicka-Turek O, et al. A common genetic variant within SCN10A modulates cardiac SCN5A expression. J Clin Invest 2014; 124(4):1844–52.
18. Priori SG, Wilde AA, Horie M, et al. HRS/EHRA/APHRS expert consensus statement on the diagnosis and management of patients with inherited primary arrhythmia syndromes: document endorsed by HRS, EHRA, and APHRS in May 2013 and by ACCF, AHA, PACES, and AEPC in June 2013. Heart Rhythm 2013;10:1932–63.
19. Maron BJ, Chaitman BR, Ackerman MJ, et al. Recommendations for physical activity and recreational sports participation for young patients with genetic cardiovascular diseases. Circulation 2004;109:2807–16.
20. Priori SG, Napolitano C, Cantu F, et al. Differential response to Na+ channel blockade, beta-adrenergic stimulation, and rapid pacing in a cellular model mimicking the SCN5A and herg defects present in the long-QT syndrome. Circ Res 1996;78:1009–15.
21. Moss AJ, Zareba W, Hall WJ, et al. Effectiveness and limitations of beta-blocker therapy in congenital long-QT syndrome. Circulation 2000;101:616–23.
22. Priori SG, Napolitano C, Schwartz PJ, et al. Association of long QT syndrome loci and cardiac events among patients treated with beta-blockers. JAMA 2004;292:1341–4.
23. Calvillo L, Spazzolini C, Vullo E, et al. Propranolol prevents life-threatening arrhythmias in LQT3 transgenic mice: implications for the clinical management of LQT3 patients. Heart Rhythm 2014;11:126–32.
24. Wilde AA, kaufman ES, Shimizu W. Sodium channel mutations, risk of cardiac events, and efficacy of beta-blocker therapy in type 3 long QT syndrome. Heart Rhythm 2012;9:S321.
25. Bennett PB, Yazawa K, Makita N, et al. Molecular mechanism for an inherited cardiac arrhythmia. Nature 1995;376:683–5.
26. Wang DW, Yazawa K, George AL Jr, et al. Characterization of human cardiac Na+ channel mutations in the congenital long QT syndrome. Proc Natl Acad Sci U S A 1996;93:13200–5.
27. Clancy CE, Tateyama M, Liu H, et al. Non-equilibrium gating in cardiac Na+ channels: an original mechanism of arrhythmia. Circulation 2003;107:2233–7.
28. Benhorin J, Taub R, Goldmit M, et al. Effects of flecainide in patients with new SCN5A mutation: mutation-specific therapy for long-QT syndrome? Circulation 2000;101:1698–706.
29. Moss AJ, Zareba W, Schwarz KQ, et al. Ranolazine shortens repolarization in patients with sustained inward sodium current due to type-3 long-QT syndrome. J Cardiovasc Electrophysiol 2008;19:1289–93.
30. Ruan Y, Liu N, Bloise R, et al. Gating properties of SCN5A mutations and the response to mexiletine in long-QT syndrome type 3 patients. Circulation 2007;116:1137–44.
31. Priori SG, Napolitano C, Schwartz PJ, et al. The elusive link between LQT3 and Brugada syndrome: the role of flecainide challenge. Circulation 2000;102:945–7.
32. Schwartz PJ, Spazzolini C, Crotti L. All LQT3 patients need an ICD: true or false? Heart Rhythm 2009;6:113–20.
33. Schwartz PJ, Spazzolini C, Priori SG, et al. Who are the long-QT syndrome patients who receive an implantable cardioverter-defibrillator and what happens to them?: data from the european long-QT syndrome implantable cardioverter-defibrillator (LQTS ICD) registry. Circulation 2010;122:1272–82.

34. Sicouri S, Belardinelli L, Antzelevitch C. Antiarrhythmic effects of the highly selective late sodium channel current blocker GS-458967. Heart Rhythm 2013;10:1036–43.

35. Olde Nordkamp LR, Driessen AH, Odero A, et al. Left cardiac sympathetic denervation in the Netherlands for the treatment of inherited arrhythmia syndromes. Neth Heart J 2014;22:160–6.

# Brugada Syndrome and $Na_v1.5$

Vincent Probst, MD, PhD*, Jean-Jacques Schott, PhD, Jean-Baptiste Gourraud, MD, Richard Redon, PhD, Florence Kyndt, PharmD, PhD, Hervé Le Marec, MD, PhD

**KEYWORDS**

• Brugada syndrome • Sodium channel • *SCN5A* gene • $Na_v1.5$

**KEY POINTS**

- The sodium channel and its regulatory subunits play a central role in the pathophysiology of Brugada syndrome (BrS).
- The identification of rare and common variants that modify the sodium current involved in the development of BrS favors the predominant role of conduction abnormalities.
- Even if the sodium current is a key factor in the development of BrS, the relationship between *SCN5A* mutations and BrS is weak and does not allow the use of molecular tests for genetic counseling for families.
- Improved genetic knowledge about this syndrome should help elucidate the pathophysiology and perhaps better define patients at high arrhythmic risk.

## INTRODUCTION

Brugada syndrome (BrS) is characterized by a typical aspect of ST segment elevation in the right precordial leads in patients without gross cardiac morphologic abnormalities and a risk of sudden cardiac death from ventricular fibrillation. The first descriptions of the electrocardiogram aspect were published in 1989,[1] but complete description of the syndrome and identification of a clear relationship between the electrocardiogram aspect and the risk of sudden cardiac death was initially proposed by the Brugada brothers in their famous paper published in 1992.[2] Since then, the role of this syndrome in the occurrence of sudden cardiac death in young, apparently healthy subjects has been progressively better recognized, and after an initial overestimation of the arrhythmic risk, the constitution of large clinical databases has finally allowed a better estimation of the arrhythmic risk and development of better therapeutic strategies in patients affected by the syndrome.[3–5]

Soon after the disease was described, Chen and colleagues[6] used a gene candidate approach to identify 3 different mutations in the *SCN5A* gene, the gene encoding the major sodium channel ($Na_v1.5$) in the heart, leading to the classification of BrS as a channelopathy. Since then, screening of the *SCN5A* gene identified dozens of different mutations in patients with BrS, and genetic research has allowed the identification of several other genes involved in the disease. However, very few linkage analyses are available for this disease, weakening the relation between the genetic defect identified (in the *SCN5A* or in the other genes) and the disease in most cases.

The typical appearance of BrS is shown in **Fig. 1**.

The authors have nothing to disclose.
Reference Centre for Hereditary Arrhythmic Diseases, Cardiologic Department and INSERM U1087, CHU de Nantes, Bd Monod, 44093 Nantes Cedex, France
* Corresponding author.
*E-mail address:* vincent.probst@chu-nantes.fr

Card Electrophysiol Clin 6 (2014) 715–721
http://dx.doi.org/10.1016/j.ccep.2014.08.001
1877-9182/14/$ – see front matter 

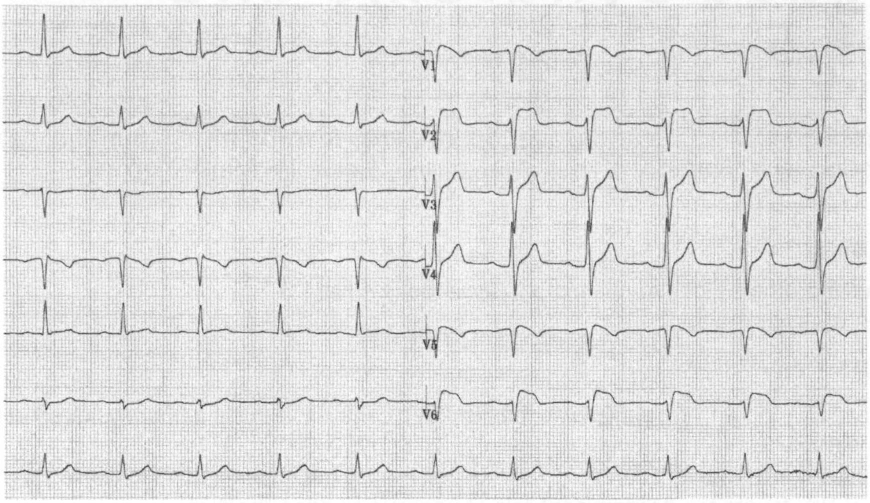

**Fig. 1.** Typical appearance of BrS with a canonical ST-segment elevation in V1 and V2.

## CLINICAL AND PHYSIOPATHOLOGIC CHARACTERISTICS OF THE BRUGADA SYNDROME

The disease exhibits an autosomal dominant pattern of transmission and variable penetrance.

The prevalence of BrS is estimated at approximately 3 to 5 in 10,000 people. The mean age at which the arrhythmic events occur is 40 years but sudden cardiac death can affect individuals of any age. The disease is far more frequent in men than in women, even though the transmission of the disease usually follows an autosomal dominant pattern with variable penetrance.

Even if the main characteristic of the syndrome is the presence of a coved-type ST segment elevation in the right precordial leads, cardiac conduction defects with prolongation of the PR interval and widening of the QRS are frequently found in the patients affected by the disease.[7]

Two hypotheses have been proposed to explain both ST segment elevation and occurrence of arrhythmias. The first, mainly based on experimental data obtained in arterially perfused canine right ventricular wedges, implicates alterations in transmural and regional repolarization gradients leading to localized losses of the subepicardial action potential dome and phase 2 reentries as the arrhythmogenic mechanism. The second, mainly based on clinical studies, implicates abnormal conduction.[8] Today, the debate on this crucial point remains open.

## GENETIC BASIS OF BRUGADA SYNDROME

Today, hundreds of variants in 17 genes have been associated with BrS. Of these, mutations in *SCN5A*, coding for the cardiac voltage-gated sodium channel, account for most (**Table 1**).[9]

Most of these mutations reduce the cardiac sodium current ($I_{Na}$) and are located not only in *SCN5A*[10] but also in its β-subunits *SCN1B* and *SCN3B* or in *GPD1L* and *MOG1*, which are thought to impair trafficking of the cardiac sodium channel to the cell membrane.[11–14] Other mutations associated with BrS reduce the L-type calcium current ($I_{Ca\text{-}L}$) and are located in *CACNA1C*, *CACNB2b*, and *CACNA2D1*, which encode the α1-, β2b-, and α2δ1-subunits of the L-type calcium channel.[15,16]

Other gene mutations that have been associated with BrS occur in *KCNE3* and *KCNE5*, which encode regulatory β-subunits of the $I_{to}/I_{Ks}$ channels; *KCNJ8*, which encodes the ATP-sensitive potassium channel; *TRPM4*, which encodes the transient receptor potential melastatin 4, which is a calcium-activated nonselective cation channel ($NSC_{Ca}$) that mediates transport of monovalent cations across membranes; *SCN2B*, the gene encoding the β2-subunit of the cardiac sodium channel; *SLMAP*, which encodes the sarcolemmal membrane–associated protein, a component of T tubules and sarcoplasmic reticulum; and *HCN4*, a gene encoding a pacemaker channel.[17–22]

However, for most of these gene defects, linkage analyses are missing and, in the National Heart, Lung and Blood Institute "Grand Opportunity" (NHLBI GO) Exome Sequencing Project population, Risgaard and colleagues[23] found a high genotype prevalence of 1:23 genetic variants in 12 genes (*SCN5A*, *GPD1L*, *CACNA1C*, *CACNB2*, *SCN1B*, *KCNE3*, *SCN3B*, *KCNH2*, *CACNA2D1*, *MOG1*, *KCND3*, and *KCNJ8*) previously associated with BrS, thus questioning the true role of these genes in the occurrence of the disease.

**Table 1**
**Mutations in genes associated with Brugada syndrome**

| Brugada Subtype | Locus | Gene | Protein (Function/Ionic Current) | Mutation Effect |
|---|---|---|---|---|
| BrS1 | 3p21 | *SCN5A*[6] | $Na_v1.5$ (sodium channel, α subunit), depolarization/$I_{Na}$ | ↓ $I_{Na}$ |
| BrS2 | 3p22.3[41] | *GPD1L*[13] | Glycerol-3-phosphate dehydrogenase 1–like | ↓ $I_{Na}$ |
| BrS3 | 12p13.3 | *CACNA1C*[15] | $Ca_v1.2$ (calcium channel, α1C subunit), depolarization/$I_{Ca\text{-}L}$ | ↓ $I_{Ca}$ |
| BrS4 | 10p12 | *CACNB2*[15] | $Ca_v\beta_{2b}$ (calcium channel, $\beta_{2b}$ subunit), depolarization/$I_{Ca\text{-}L}$ | ↓ $I_{Ca}$ |
| BrS5 | 19q13.1 | *SCN1B*[11] | $Na_v\beta1$ (sodium channel, β1 subunit), depolarization/$I_{Na}$ | ↓ $I_{Na}$ |
| BrS6 | 11q13-q14 | *KCNE3*[18] | MiRP2 (potassium channel, β subunit), repolarization/$I_{to}$ | ↑ $I_{to}$ |
| BrS7 | 11q23.3 | *SCN3B*[42] | $Na_v\beta3$ (sodium channel, β3 subunit), depolarization/$I_{Na}$ | ↓ $I_{Na}$ |
| BrS8 | 7q36.1 | *KCNH2*[43] | hERG or $K_v11.1$ (potassium channel α), repolarization/$IK_r$ | ↑ $IK_r$ |
| BrS9 | 12p11.23 | *KCNJ8*[44] | Kir6.1 (ATP-dependent potassium channel) | ↑ $IK_{ATP}$ |
| BrS10 | 7q21–q22 | *CACNA2D1*[16] | $Ca_{v2\delta1}$ (calcium channel, δδ1subunit), depolarization/$I_{Ca\text{-}L}$ | Not available |
| BrS11 | Xq22.3 | *KCNE5*[19] | KCNE1L (potassium channel, β subunit), repolarization/$I_{to}$ | ↑ $I_{to}$ |
| BrS12 | 17p13.1 | *MOG1*[14] | Multicopy suppressor of Gsp1 | ↓ $I_{Na}$ |
| BrS13 | 1p13.3 | *KCND3*[45] | Kv4.3 (potassium channel) repolarization/$I_{to}$ | ↑ $I_{to}$ |
| BrS14 | 15q24-q25 | *HCN4*[46,47] | $I_f$ | Not available |
| BrS15 | 3p21.2-p14.3 | *SLMAP*[22] | Sarcolemma-associated protein depolarization/$I_{Na}$ | ↓ $I_{Na}$ |
| BrS16 | 19q13.33 | *TRPM4*[20] | Transient receptor potential cation channel, subfamily M, member 4 (calcium-activated nonselective cation channel) | ↓ or ↑ $NSC_{Ca}$ |
| BrS17 | 11q23 | *SCN2B*[21] | $Na_v\beta2$ (sodium channel, β2 subunit), depolarization/$I_{Na}$ | ↓ $I_{Na}$ |

*Adapted from* Nielsen MW, Holst AG, Olesen SP, et al. The genetic component of Brugada syndrome. Front Physiol 2013;4:179.

Even in a study designed to identify the presence of rare variants in *SCN5A* in control individuals, these variants were particularly identified in the intradomain linker and the *C*-terminus of *SCN5A*.[23]

With this caveat in mind, one should examine cautiously the existing literature and be particularly vigilant before accepting a rare genetic variant as a novel arrhythmia syndrome–susceptibility mutation.

## ROLE OF *SCN5A* MUTATION IN BRUGADA SYNDROME

BrS mutations in the *SCN5A* gene lead to a loss of sodium channel function through several mechanisms, including trafficking defects, generation of truncated proteins, faster channel inactivation, shift of voltage dependence of steady-state activation toward more depolarized membrane potentials, and slower recovery from inactivation. Mutations are identified in the *SCN5A* gene in approximately 25% of patients with BrS, but 2% to 5% of healthy individuals host missense *SCN5A* variants, leading to a potential conundrum in the interpretation of genetic results.[10,24]

In the black population (which is rarely affected by the syndrome), *SCN5A* variations are common and can be related to PR prolongation.[25]

More importantly, Priori and colleagues[26] showed that in families harboring *SCN5A* mutations the penetrance of the disease is low. More surprisingly, the current authors showed that within large families affected by the syndrome and in which the index case of the family is an *SCN5A* mutation carrier, the penetrance of the disease is low (<50% even after sodium channel blocker challenge), the penetrance of cardiac conduction defects is high (>80%), and it is common (in 5 of the 13 families studied) to identify family members who do not carry the familial mutation but are affected by BrS.[27]

The identification of family members who are not carriers of the familial *SCN5A* mutation but are affected by the disease showed that the link between *SCN5A* and the disease is clearly not straightforward and that other factors play a role in the occurrence of the disease.

Recently, Bezzina and colleagues[28] showed, through a genome-wide association study of 312 individuals with BrS and 1115 controls, that the syndrome is not a simple autosomal dominant disease, because 3 common variants can explain 15% of the heritability of the disease. Two of these variants affect the sodium current. The strongest association (rs10428132) resides in intron 14 of the *SCN10A* gene, located adjacent to *SCN5A* on chromosome 3p21-22. The particular haplotype tagged by this single nucleotide polymorphism, which also contains a nonsynonymous variant affecting *SCN10A* (rs6795970, $r^2$ = 0.97 with rs10428132), was previously associated with variability in PR interval and QRS duration in the general population.[29] The other independent association at 3p21-22 (rs11708996) involved another haplotype previously associated with cardiac conduction through its effect on the *SCN5A* gene.[30]

## CLINICAL CHARACTERISTICS OF PATIENTS WITH BRUGADA SYNDROME CARRYING AN *SCN5A* MUTATION

It was constantly demonstrated in the large databases that carriers of an *SCN5A* mutation have more pronounced cardiac conduction defects than patients with BrS who are noncarriers of *SCN5A* mutations.[3–5,31,32]

However, a meta-analysis of the main databases published showed no different risk of life-threatening arrhythmias in carriers of an *SCN5A* mutation.[3–5,31–33]

Meregalli and colleagues[34] published a genotype-phenotype correlation according to the type of *SCN5A* mutation (missense, truncated). Patients and relatives with a truncated protein had a more severe phenotype essentially in term of occurrence of syncope and more severe conduction disorders. However, this study of 147 individuals found no increased risk of sudden cardiac death in the truncated group of patients.

In addition to the mutations that have been identified in the *SCN5A* gene, polymorphisms in the same gene may also alter the electrophysiological property of the sodium channel. Both p.D1690N and p.G1748D produced a marked dominant negative effect when cotransfected with either wild-type or p.H558R channels. Conversely, p.H558R was able to rescue defective trafficking of p.D1690N channels toward the membrane when both the polymorphism and the mutation were in the same construct. Surprisingly, cotransfection with p.D1690N, either alone or together with the polymorphism (p.H558R-D1690N), completely restored the profound gating defects exhibited by p.G1748D channels but only slightly rescued their trafficking.[35]

The common variant H558R can also restore the sodium current in carriers of an R282H *SCN5A* mutation[36] and seems to be a genetic modulator of BrS among carriers of an *SCN5A* mutation, in whom the presence of the less common allele G improves the electrocardiographic characteristics and clinical phenotype.[37]

## GENETIC COUNSELING IN PATIENTS WITH BRUGADA SYNDROME

In the last consensus statement on the state of genetic testing for the channelopathies and cardiomyopathies, comprehensive or BrS1 (*SCN5A*)-targeted BrS genetic testing is considered only a class IIa indication in any patient for whom a cardiologist has established a clinical index of suspicion for BrS based on the patient's clinical history, family history, and expressed electrocardiographic (resting 12-lead electrocardiograms and/or provocative drug challenge testing) phenotype.

Finally, genetic testing is not indicated in the setting of an isolated type 2 or 3 Brugada electrocardiographic pattern, because *SCN5A* has a low frequency of mutation in patients with BrS, and therefore the absence of an *SCN5A* mutation can not rule out the diagnosis.

However, mutation-specific genetic testing is recommended for family members and appropriate relatives after the BrS-causative mutation is identified in an index case class I indication.[38]

Given the complexity of the relationship between the presence of an *SCN5A* mutation and BrS, one must be very cautious during genetic counseling. The presence of the *SNC5A* mutation in a family member does not confirm the presence of the syndrome in this individual, because the penetrance of the disease is less than 50%. Conversely, even in the most favorable case, when the family member is not carrying the mutation, the absence of the mutation cannot rule out the syndrome, and therefore the arrhythmic risk given the frequency of noncarrier but affected family members. It is important to clearly explain to family members that for BrS, the only way to determine who is affected by the disease within the family is to perform an electrocardiogram, and a sodium channel blocker challenge for those with normal electrocardiogram result.

This practice is particularly relevant in young children, in whom the syndrome is infrequent and the identification of the mutation is not enough to determine a specific risk even if the prevalence of the *SCN5A* mutation is higher in this specific population.[39,40]

## SUMMARY

The sodium channel and its regulatory subunits play a central role in the pathophysiology of BrS. The identification of rare and common variants that modify the sodium current involved in the development of BrS favor the predominant role of conduction abnormalities in the development of this condition.

Even if the sodium current is a key player in the development of BrS, however, the relationship between *SCN5A* mutations and BrS is weak and does not allow the use of molecular tests for genetic counseling for families.

In the future, improved genetic knowledge about this syndrome should help elucidate the pathophysiology and perhaps better define patients at high arrhythmic risk.

## REFERENCES


1. Martini B, Nava A, Thiene G, et al. Ventricular fibrillation without apparent heart disease: description of six cases. Am Heart J 1989;118:1203–9.
2. Brugada P, Brugada J. Right bundle branch block, persistent ST segment elevation and sudden cardiac death: a distinct clinical and electrocardiographic syndrome. A multicenter report. J Am Coll Cardiol 1992;20:1391–6.
3. Probst V, Veltmann C, Eckardt L, et al. Long-term prognosis of patients diagnosed with Brugada syndrome: results from the FINGER Brugada syndrome registry. Circulation 2010;121:635–43.
4. Priori SG, Gasparini M, Napolitano C, et al. Risk stratification in Brugada syndrome: results of the PRELUDE (PRogrammed ELectrical stimUlation preDictive valuE) registry. J Am Coll Cardiol 2012;59:37–45.
5. Brugada J, Brugada R, Antzelevitch C, et al. Long-term follow-up of individuals with the electrocardiographic pattern of right bundle-branch block and ST-segment elevation in precordial leads V1 to V3. Circulation 2002;105:73–8.
6. Chen Q, Kirsch GE, Zhang D, et al. Genetic basis and molecular mechanism for idiopathic ventricular fibrillation. Nature 1998;392:293–6.
7. Wilde AA, Antzelevitch C, Borggrefe M, et al. Proposed diagnostic criteria for the Brugada syndrome: consensus report. Circulation 2002;106:2514–9.
8. Hoogendijk MG, Potse M, Linnenbank AC, et al. Mechanism of right precordial ST-segment elevation in structural heart disease: excitation failure by current-to-load mismatch. Heart Rhythm 2010;7:238–48.
9. Nielsen MW, Holst AG, Olesen SP, et al. The genetic component of Brugada syndrome. Front Physiol 2013;4:179.
10. Kapplinger JD, Tester DJ, Alders M, et al. An international compendium of mutations in the SCN5A-encoded cardiac sodium channel in patients referred for Brugada syndrome genetic testing. Heart Rhythm 2010;7:33–46.
11. Watanabe H, Koopmann TT, Le Scouarnec S, et al. Sodium channel beta1 subunit mutations associated with Brugada syndrome and cardiac conduction disease in humans. J Clin Invest 2008;118:2260–8.
12. Valdivia CR, Medeiros-Domingo A, Ye B, et al. Loss-of-function mutation of the SCN3B-encoded sodium channel {beta}3 subunit associated with a case of idiopathic ventricular fibrillation. Cardiovasc Res 2010;86:392–400.
13. London B, Michalec M, Mehdi H, et al. Mutation in glycerol-3-phosphate dehydrogenase 1 like gene (GPD1-L) decreases cardiac Na+ current and causes inherited arrhythmias. Circulation 2007;116:2260–8.
14. Kattygnarath D, Maugenre S, Neyroud N, et al. MOG1: a new susceptibility gene for Brugada syndrome. Circ Cardiovasc Genet 2011;4(3):261–8. Available at: http://www.ncbi.nlm.nih.gov/pubmed/21447824?dopt=Citation.
15. Antzelevitch C, Pollevick GD, Cordeiro JM, et al. Loss-of-function mutations in the cardiac calcium channel underlie a new clinical entity characterized by ST-segment elevation, short QT intervals, and sudden cardiac death. Circulation 2007;115:442–9.
16. Burashnikov E, Pfeiffer R, Barajas-Martinez H, et al. Mutations in the cardiac L-type calcium channel associated with inherited J-wave syndromes and sudden cardiac death. Heart Rhythm 2010;7:1872–82.
17. Barajas-Martínez H, Hu D, Ferrer T, et al. Molecular genetic and functional association of Brugada and early repolarization syndromes with S422L missense mutation in KCNJ8. Heart Rhythm 2012;9:548–55.
18. Delpón E, Cordeiro JM, Nunez L, et al. Functional effects of KCNE3 mutation and its role in the development of Brugada syndrome. Circ Arrhythm Electrophysiol 2008;1:209–18.

19. Ohno S, Zankov DP, Ding W-G, et al. KCNE5 (KCNE1L) variants are novel modulators of Brugada syndrome and idiopathic ventricular fibrillation. Circ Arrhythm Electrophysiol 2011;4:352–61.
20. Liu H, Chatel S, Simard C, et al. Molecular genetics and functional anomalies in a series of 248 Brugada cases with 11 mutations in the TRPM4 channel. PLoS One 2013;8:e54131.
21. Riuró H, Beltran-Alvarez P, Tarradas A, et al. A missense mutation in the sodium channel β2 subunit reveals SCN2B as a new candidate gene for Brugada syndrome. Hum Mutat 2013;34:961–6.
22. Ishikawa T, Sato A, Marcou CA, et al. A novel disease gene for Brugada syndrome: sarcolemmal membrane-associated protein gene mutations impair intracellular trafficking of hNav1.5. Circ Arrhythm Electrophysiol 2012;5:1098–107.
23. Risgaard B, Jabbari R, Refsgaard L, et al. High prevalence of genetic variants previously associated with Brugada syndrome in new exome data. Clin Genet 2013;84:489–95.
24. Ackerman MJ, Splawski I, Makielski JC, et al. Spectrum and prevalence of cardiac sodium channel variants among black, white, Asian, and Hispanic individuals: implications for arrhythmogenic susceptibility and Brugada/long QT syndrome genetic testing. Heart Rhythm 2004;1:600–7.
25. Jeff JM, Brown-Gentry K, Buxbaum SG, et al. SCN5A variation is associated with electrocardiographic traits in the Jackson Heart Study. Circ Cardiovasc Genet 2011;4:139–44.
26. Priori SG, Napolitano C, Gasparini M, et al. Clinical and genetic heterogeneity of right bundle branch block and ST-segment elevation syndrome: a prospective evaluation of 52 families. Circulation 2000;102:2509–15.
27. Probst V, Wilde AA, Barc J, et al. SCN5A mutations and the role of genetic background in the pathophysiology of Brugada syndrome. Circ Cardiovasc Genet 2009;2:552–7.
28. Bezzina CR, Barc J, Mizusawa Y, et al. Common variants at SCN5A-SCN10A and HEY2 are associated with Brugada syndrome, a rare disease with high risk of sudden cardiac death. Nat Genet 2013. http://dx.doi.org/10.1038/ng.2712.
29. Chambers JC, Zhao J, Terracciano CMN, et al. Genetic variation in SCN10A influences cardiac conduction. Nat Genet 2010;42:149–52.
30. Pfeufer A, van Noord C, Marciante KD, et al. Genome-wide association study of PR interval. Nat Genet 2010;42:153–9.
31. Smits JP, Eckardt L, Probst V, et al. Genotype-phenotype relationship in Brugada syndrome: electrocardiographic features differentiate SCN5A-related patients from non-SCN5A-related patients. J Am Coll Cardiol 2002;40:350–6.
32. Eckardt L, Probst V, Smits JPP, et al. Long-term prognosis of individuals with right precordial ST-segment-elevation Brugada syndrome. Circulation 2005;111:257–63.
33. Gehi AK, Duong TD, Metz LD, et al. Risk stratification of individuals with the Brugada electrocardiogram: a meta-analysis. J Cardiovasc Electrophysiol 2006;17:577–83.
34. Meregalli PG, Tan HL, Probst V, et al. Type of SCN5A mutation determines clinical severity and degree of conduction slowing in loss-of-function sodium channelopathies. Heart Rhythm 2009;6:341–8.
35. Núñez L, Barana A, Amoros I, et al. p.D1690N Nav1.5 rescues p.G1748D mutation gating defects in a compound heterozygous Brugada syndrome patient. Heart Rhythm 2013;10:264–72.
36. Poelzing S, Forleo C, Samodell M, et al. SCN5A polymorphism restores trafficking of a Brugada syndrome mutation on a separate gene. Circulation 2006;114:368–76.
37. Lizotte E, Juntilla MJ, Dube MP, et al. Genetic modulation of Brugada syndrome by a common polymorphism. J Cardiovasc Electrophysiol 2009;20:1137–41.
38. Ackerman MJ, Priori SG, Willems S, et al. HRS/EHRA expert consensus statement on the state of genetic testing for the channelopathies and cardiomyopathies: this document was developed as a partnership between the Heart Rhythm Society (HRS) and the European Heart Rhythm Association (EHRA). Europace 2011;13:1077–109.
39. Probst V, Denjoy I, Meregalli PG, et al. Clinical aspects and prognosis of Brugada syndrome in children. Circulation 2007;115:2042–8.
40. Chockalingam P, Clur S-AB, Breur JMPJ, et al. The diagnostic and therapeutic aspects of loss-of-function cardiac sodium channelopathies in children. Heart Rhythm 2012;9:1986–92.
41. Weiss R, Barmada MM, Nguyen T, et al. Clinical and molecular heterogeneity in the Brugada syndrome: a novel gene locus on chromosome 3. Circulation 2002;105:707–13.
42. Hu D, Barajas-Martinez H, Burashnikov E, et al. A mutation in the beta 3 subunit of the cardiac sodium channel associated with Brugada ECG phenotype. Circ Cardiovasc Genet 2009;2:270–8.
43. Verkerk AO, Wilders R, Schulze-Bahr E, et al. Role of sequence variations in the human ether-a-go-go-related gene (HERG, KCNH2) in the Brugada syndrome. Cardiovasc Res 2005;68:441–53.
44. Medeiros-Domingo A, Tan B-H, Crotti L, et al. Gain-of-function mutation S422L in the KCNJ8-encoded cardiac K(ATP) channel Kir6.1 as a pathogenic substrate for J-wave syndromes. Heart Rhythm 2010;7:1466–71.
45. Giudicessi JR, Ye D, Tester DJ, et al. Transient outward current (I(to)) gain-of-function mutations in

the KCND3-encoded Kv4.3 potassium channel and Brugada syndrome. Heart Rhythm 2011;8:1024–32.
46. Ueda K, Nakamura K, Hayashi T, et al. Functional characterization of a trafficking-defective HCN4 mutation, D553N, associated with cardiac arrhythmia. J Biol Chem 2004;279:27194–8.
47. Ueda K, Hirano Y, Higashiuesato Y, et al. Role of HCN4 channel in preventing ventricular arrhythmia. J Hum Genet 2009;54:115–21.

# Conduction Disorders and $Na_v1.5$

Joshua R. Kovach, MD[a], D. Woodrow Benson, MD, PhD[a,b,*]

**KEYWORDS**

- Atrioventricular block • Cardiac conduction disease • Lev/Lenègre disease • SCN5A • $Na_v1.5$
- Channelopathy • Inherited arrhythmia disorder

**KEY POINTS**

- An increasing number of mutations affecting $Na_v1.5$ have been identified that contribute to inherited cardiac conduction disease.
- These mutations can be associated with overlap syndromes, also causing phenotypes consistent with Brugada syndrome, long QT syndrome, or dilated cardiomyopathy.
- Treatment options for inherited cardiac conduction disease remain limited to rate support with pacemaker implantation.

## INTRODUCTION

The atrioventricular (AV) conduction system is comprised of specialized cells that permit synchronized cardiac excitation resulting in contraction of the atria during ventricular filling and rapid depolarization of the ventricles. In the postnatal heart, distinguishable electrophysiologic and anatomic components of the AV conduction system include the sinoatrial node, AV node, and His bundle and left and right bundle branches and Purkinje ramifications.[1–4] Disorders of AV conduction are common clinical problems, and early classification relied on anatomic and electrocardiographic distinctions (electroanatomic classification). Based on family clustering of AV conduction disorders, a genetic cause has long been suspected.[5–10] Nearly 15 years ago, genetic discovery techniques identified heterozygous mutations in SCN5A as a cause of heritable AV conduction disorders.[11–13]

## AV CONDUCTION

### Anatomy

The structure of the AV conduction system was first described by Tawara based on extensive histologic examination.[1] The conduction system comprises the AV node, the penetrating bundle of His, the right and left bundle branches, and distal Purkinje fibers (**Fig. 1**). The AV node is localized to the floor of the right atrium, between the intra-atrial septum and the annulus of the tricuspid valve, within the triangle of Koch.[1,14] This triangle is bound by the septal tricuspid valve annulus, the tendon of Todaro, and the os of the coronary sinus. The His bundle arises from the anterior compact AV node and penetrates the fibrous annulus at the membranous ventricular septum below the aortic root. It divides at the crest of the muscular septum into the right and left fascicles or bundles that descend toward the apex of the heart. The left bundle descends toward the apex in a fanlike distribution, with prominent anterior and posterior fascicles. The right bundle branch descends within the right septal endocardium, then deviates toward the free wall through the moderator band.

### Characteristics of Conduction Tissue

During his initial descriptions, Tawara presented features that distinguished specific conduction

The authors have no disclosures relevant to the content of this article.

[a] Pediatrics, Cardiology, Children's Hospital of Wisconsin, Medical College of Wisconsin, 9000 West Wisconsin Avenue, MS 713, Milwaukee, WI 53226, USA; [b] Pediatrics, Cardiology, Medical College of Wisconsin, 9000 West Wisconsin Avenue, MS 713, Milwaukee, WI 53226, USA

* Corresponding author. Pediatrics, Cardiology, Medical College of Wisconsin, 9000 West Wisconsin Avenue, MS 713, Milwaukee, WI 53226, USA.

*E-mail address:* dbenson@chw.org

Card Electrophysiol Clin 6 (2014) 723–731
http://dx.doi.org/10.1016/j.ccep.2014.07.008
1877-9182/14/$ – see front matter 

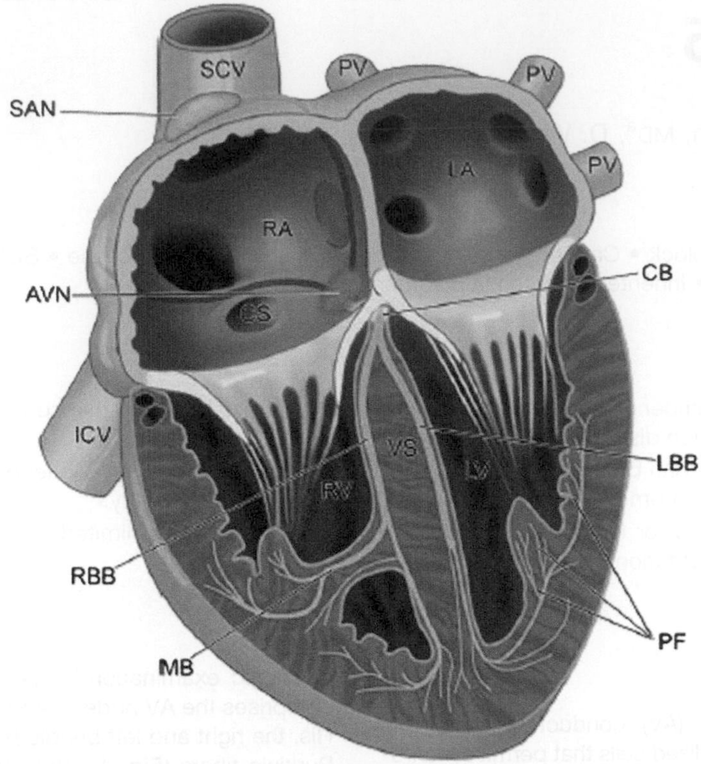


**Fig. 1.** Anatomy of the normal cardiac conduction system. See text for full description. AVN, atrioventricular node; CB, common bundle; CS, coronary sinus; ICV, inferior vena cava; LA, left atrium; LBB, left bundle branch; LV, left ventricle; MB, moderator band; PF, Purkinje fibers; PV, pulmonary vein; RA, right atrium; RBB, right bundle branch; RV, right ventricle; SAN, sinoatrial node; SCV, superior caval vein; VS, ventricular septum. (*From* Jongbloed MR, Steijn RV, Hahurij ND, et al. Normal and abnormal development of the cardiac conduction system; implications for conduction and rhythm disorders in the child and adult. Differentiation 2012;84(1): 131–48; with permission.)

tissue from the rest of the working myocardium.[1,14] These features included (1) continuity from one histologic section to the next; (2) cells are histologically discrete from the working myocardium; and (3) separation from the working myocardium by fibrous tissue. The general features that differentiate conduction tissue from the working myocardium largely revolve around the very rapid conduction and action potential propagation that occurs through this specialized myocardium. Molecular analysis has identified that these features are predominantly attributed to the connections between these specialized myocardial cells, and the specific connexin proteins that inhabit the gap junctions connecting the cells.[15] These specialized connexins facilitate rapid ion transport from myocyte to myocyte, resulting in rapid electrical conduction through the tissue. The propagation of these impulses along the conduction tissue and entrance into the working myocardium ensure coordinated, rapid, and efficient ventricular contraction.

## *Role of $Na_V$1.5 in Atrioventricular Conduction*

During tissue depolarization, $Na_V$1.5 is primarily responsible for phase 0 of the action potential, causing rapid depolarization as the channel opens and sodium ions rapidly enter the myocyte.[16–18] Disruptions in $Na_V$1.5 function result in impaired channel reactivation or expression that may affect the ability to conduct action potentials along and between myocytes. The channel then becomes inactivated by slow- and fast-inactivation conformational changes. Studies evaluating $Na_V$1.5 expression in myocardial tissue demonstrate high concentrations in the atrial and ventricular myocardium, transitional zones around the compact AV node, and distal conduction system, with lesser expression within the compact AV node itself.[19,20] Recent studies have focused on interaction of $Na_V$1.5 with regulatory proteins that are important for correct localization and pooling of $Na_V$1.5 in compartments forming distinct pools of channels (eg, T-tubules; **Fig. 2**; reviewed in Ref.[17]).

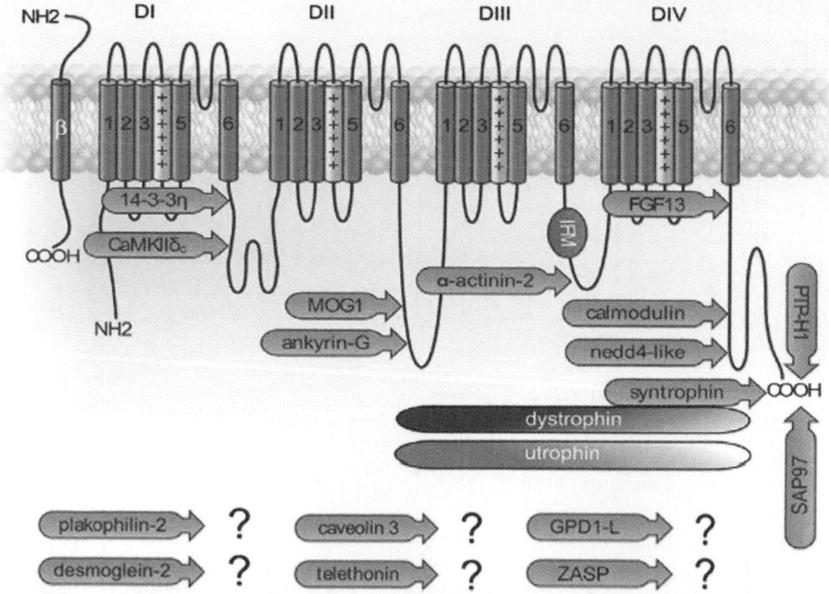


**Fig. 2.** $Na_V1.5$ topology depicting interaction with regulatory proteins. The four homologous domains (DI-DIV) of the pore-forming alpha subunit of $Na_V1.5$ are connected by intracellular and extracellular loops. Several regulatory proteins for $Na_V1.5$ were identified and sites of interaction have been mapped on the channel alpha subunit. Many of these interactions are thought to occur at the intracellular loops or the C-terminus of $Na_V1.5$. However, for some proteins that have been shown to associate with $Na_V1.5$, the sites of interaction on the channel are unknown. (*From* Shy D, Gillet L, Abriel H. Cardiac sodium channel $Na_V1.5$ distribution in myocytes via interacting proteins: the multiple pool model. Biochim Biophys Acta 2013;1833(4):886–94.)

## Clinical Manifestations: Degrees of Atrioventricular Block

The impairment of conduction through the AV conduction system can occur at multiple levels between the atrium, AV node, and bundle of His. The level and degree at which this disruption in conduction occurs determines the clinical effect observed. Three clinical degrees of AV block are typically described, divided into first-, second-, and third-degree block based on the clinical appearance (**Fig. 3**). Second-degree block in turn is divided into two different categories described as Mobitz I or II.

First-degree block is characterized by prolongation of the PR interval, suggestive of a delay of conduction between the atria and the ventricles, but not complete inhibition of conduction. Second-degree block is characterized by conduction of most atrial impulses to the ventricles, but with differences in conduction behavior before the nonconducted beat. In Mobitz I block (Wenckebach), there is evidence of progressive PR prolongation before the nonconducted beat. In contrast, with Mobitz II block, there is no evidence of PR prolongation before the dropped beat. The key differentiation is that Mobitz I block is thought to occur above the level of the His bundle within the compact node, whereas Mobitz II block occurs at the His bundle or below. Although Mobitz I block is often tolerated well, believed to be benign, and frequently encountered in normal people during periods of enhanced vagal tone, Mobitz II block is frequently more concerning for unstable AV conduction that may be progressive. Third-degree AV block represents complete loss of anterograde communication between the atrium and the ventricle. Heart rate in this degree of AV block is primarily determined by whichever endogenous pacemaker is most active to generate an escape rhythm, starting at the level of the AV node with distal progression down the conduction system. This escape rate may be sufficient to support cardiac output and limit symptoms, but may be slow enough to impair perfusion and potentially unstable enough to result in prolonged asystole or Stokes-Adams attacks causing sudden cardiac death.

Although these degrees of block describe conduction impairment through the compact AV node and His bundle, there can be block of the individual bundle branches to each ventricle, with a typical QRS pattern indicative of both (**Fig. 4**). With right bundle-branch block, there is delayed activation of the right ventricle after the left ventricle has depolarized, characterized by an RSR′ pattern

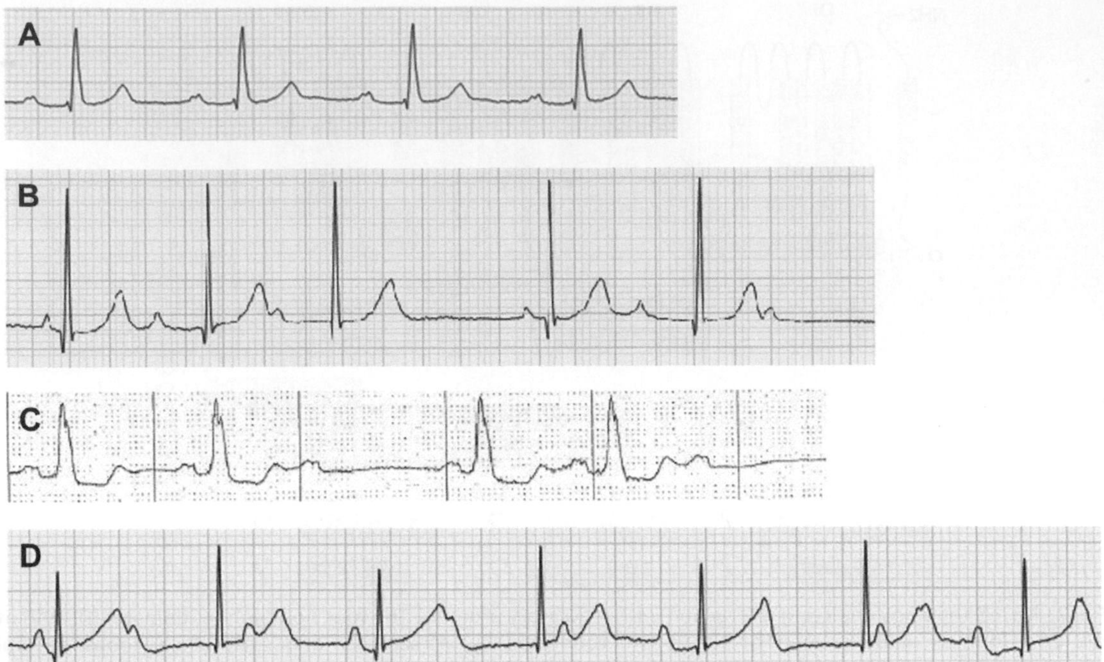


**Fig. 3.** Different clinical degrees of atrioventricular block. (*A*) First-degree AV block. (*B*) Second-degree AV block, Mobitz I (Wenckebach). (*C*) Second-degree AV block, Mobitz II. (*D*) Third-degree (complete) AV block.

in lead V1 and slurred S wave in V6. Left bundle-branch block is typified by a QS pattern in V1, and broad R wave in V6. Also there can be hemiblock of either the left anterior or posterior fascicle, which is characterized by either superior axis or right axis deviation in the limb leads, respectively.

## HISTORY OF FAMILIAL CONDUCTION DISEASE

### *Lev/Lenègre Disease*

A description of inherited heart block was first published by Morquio in 1901.[21] Subsequently, there were multiple reports and publications of familial patterns of inherited conduction disorders.[5–10,22–24] Collectively, these were later classified as either Lev or Lenègre disease based on the age of onset and the type of block encountered. Lenègre disease is typically characterized by multiple family members who develop progressive degrees of AV conduction block. Affected family members often demonstrate variable degrees of first- and second-degree block, and various forms of bundle-branch block, until they eventually develop complete disruption of AV conduction with third-degree AV block (**Fig. 5**). Lev disease has been typically attributed to fibrosis of the left conduction system with aging.[8,10]

Histologic review of the conduction system in affected individuals has frequently demonstrated progressive and variable fibrosis of the conduction tissue specifically that seems to cause the progressive loss of conduction.[10] Interestingly, patients with classic Lev disease demonstrated fibrosis within the proximal His bundle, whereas those diagnosed with Lenègre disease often demonstrated fibrosis within the more distal bundle branches and Purkinje fibers.[25] It was never clear what exactly triggered this fibrosis in affected individuals, and there was no consistent mode of treatment other than providing pacemaker support. Theories regarding development of this fibrosis included an autoimmune reaction, fundamental genetic deficiency in protein structures, and molecular signaling defects causing accelerated aging and degeneration of the conduction tissue.[8,25]

### *Role of SCN5A in Familial Atrioventricular Block*

The role of the SCN5A gene in familial conduction block was first described by Schott and colleagues[11] in 1999. Their report described two families with individuals in multiple generations exhibiting conduction block. In a large French family, affected members demonstrated initial ventricular conduction abnormalities that progressed to complete AV block (see **Fig. 5**). The second was a Dutch family, where affected family members demonstrated various changes in AV conduction, but without progressive disease. Subsequent

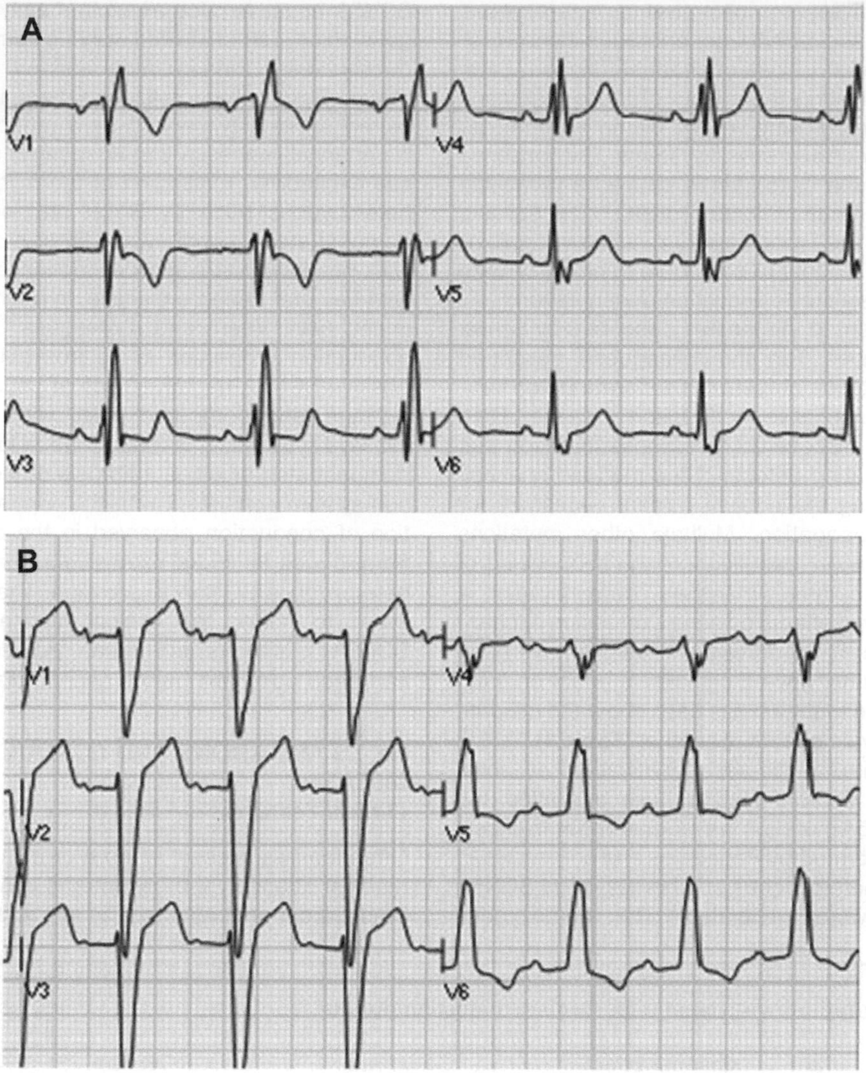


**Fig. 4.** Examples of different forms of bundle-branch block. (*A*) Right bundle-branch block. (*B*) Left bundle-branch block.

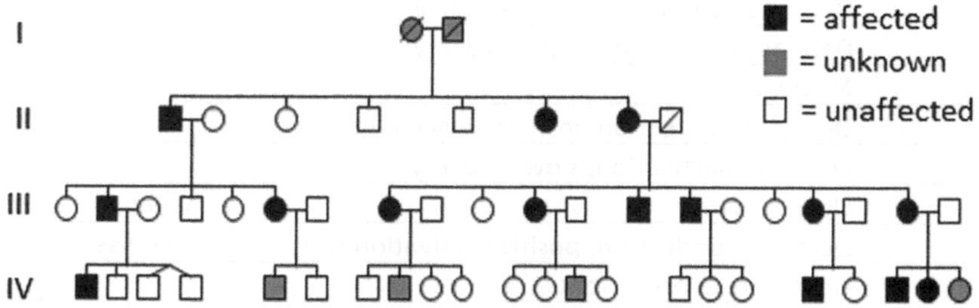


**Fig. 5.** Adaptation of the French family pedigree described by Schott and colleagues in 1999. The pedigree demonstrates an inheritance pattern consistent with autosomal-dominant inheritance. Although the clinical status of two gene-positive family members in generation IV was not known, all other family members carrying the mutation demonstrated some clinical evidence of conduction disease. (*Data from* Schott JJ, Alshinawi C, Kyndt F, et al. Cardiac conduction defects associate with mutations in SCN5A. Nat Genet 1999;23:20–1.)

genetic analysis demonstrated a heterozygous mutation in the SCN5A gene in each family predicted to result in loss of channel function. Later studies evaluating the effects of these mutations were performed using voltage clamp experiments in heterologous expression systems. The nonsense mutation in the Dutch family caused a trafficking defect of a nonfunctional protein.[26] The splicing mutation in the French family resulted in haploinsufficiency, thought to contribute to or exacerbate normal age-related conduction degeneration.[27]

Subsequent to the families described by Schott and colleagues, Tan and colleagues[12] described another mutation present in a separate Dutch family with progressive conduction disease. DNA sequencing discovered a missense mutation that produced gating defects of the mutated channel, thus reducing the sodium current necessary for impulse propagation. Multiple other mutations have since been identified through sequencing of patients and family members, demonstrating a wide variety of effects on gene expression or channel function.[28–30] Additional mutations have been shown to either have a cumulative effect on each other, or one mutation has been shown to mitigate the phenotypic effects of another (**Table 1**).[28,29,31]

Along with continued identification of novel mutations, multiple studies have evaluated the role of SCN5A mutation in a mouse model. In experiments performed by Papadatos and colleagues,[32] mice with heterozygous and homozygous SCN5A deletions were generated. The homozygous SCN5A-negative mice all expired early. Heterozygous mice demonstrated various forms of conduction delay through atrial and AV conduction tissue. Tissue characterization demonstrated impaired excitability caused by a reduced pool of Na channels necessary to adequately recover tissue excitability. Evaluation of the myocardium in heterozygous mice by Royer and colleagues[33] demonstrated conduction fibrosis consistent with previous histologic descriptions of patients with Lev and Lenègre disease. In a further experiment, van Veen and colleagues[34] evaluated conduction properties in heterozygous SCN5A-positive/SCN5A-negative mice at young age and old age, and compared these with young and old wild-type mice. Although old wild-type mice demonstrated significant fibrosis of their conduction system consistent with the normal deterioration of conduction observed in the elderly, this fibrosis was far more extensive in the mice with heterozygous SCN5A expression. These findings seem to mirror the clinical manifestations of SCN5A mutations in human populations that had been observed before genetic diagnoses.

## $Na_v1.5$ MUTATIONS AND CONDUCTION DISEASE

### *Clinical Features*

Often families present when a proband comes to medical attention with symptoms consistent with bradycardia and AV block, such as fatigue with

**Table 1**
**SCN5A mutations associated with cardiac conduction disease**

| Mutation | Channel Effect | Overlap | Reference |
|---|---|---|---|
| S1710 + 75X | No current | | 11,26 |
| IVS22 + 2 T>C | No current | | 11,27 |
| G1406R | Decrease conduction | BrS | 35 |
| G514C | Increase availability, positive activation shift | | 12 |
| delK1500 | Decrease availability, positive activation shift | LQTS, BrS | 39 |
| G298S | Decrease conduction, slow recovery | | 30 |
| D1595N | Decrease conduction, slow recovery | | 30 |
| W156X | No current | | 29 |
| R225W | Decrease conduction, increase availability | | 29 |
| T512I/H558R | Enhance inactivation, slow recovery | | 31 |
| G3823A | Unknown | DCM | 40 |
| E161K | Decrease conduction, positive activation shift | BrS, SSS | 37 |
| W1421X | Unknown, ± no current | | 28 |
| W1440X | Decrease conduction, slow recovery | DCM | 41 |
| T1620K | Decrease availability, negative activation shift | LQTS | 38 |
| A1180V | Unknown | BrS | 42 |

*Abbreviations:* BrS, Brugada syndrome; DCM, dilated cardiomyopathy; LQTS, long QT syndrome; SSS, sick sinus syndrome.

or without exertion, dizziness, or syncope. Patients have classically been characterized by bradycardia and/or dizziness or syncope in the absence of systemic disease, angina, or congestive heart failure.[10] After this initial patient is identified, and family history pursued, then the diagnosis of conduction disease in other family members becomes more apparent. Often affected family members demonstrate a mild degree of impairment in AV conduction with first-degree AV block, left anterior or posterior fascicular block, or complete left or right bundle-branch block (see **Figs. 3** and **4**).[7,9,22,35,36] Subsequently, these family members demonstrate progression in AV conduction severity until they develop complete AV block, which ultimately results in pacemaker implantation at a relatively early age.

Evaluation of probands should include a complete and thorough pedigree. Focus should be given to family members who have had implanted devices, experienced frequent syncope or seizures, or experienced sudden cardiac arrest at an early age. Many younger family members carrying a mutation are likely to demonstrate some degree of abnormal AV conduction. Although these diseases often manifest an autosomal-dominant inheritance pattern, incomplete penetrance or the presence of other moderating genes can create silent mutation carriers.[7,9,22,35,36] Patients often require further investigation into the stability of their AV conduction, including Holter monitoring or exercise stress testing.

### *Overlap Syndromes*

Mutations in $Na_v1.5$ have not only been confirmed in patients with familial cardiac conduction disease, but also in forms of long QT syndrome, Brugada syndrome, and familial dilated cardiomyopathy (see **Table 1**).[35,37–42] The occurrence of overlap syndromes, where a family may demonstrate different familial phenotypes between generations, had been observed before the advent of genetic diagnosis.[43] However, it is becoming increasingly apparent that the same SCN5A mutation may result in different phenotypic expression within families, causing conduction disease in some members, and another $Na_v1.5$-related disease in others. Typically these other diseases, such as Brugada syndrome, also represent a loss of function of the $Na_v1.5$ channel, although there are reports of a long QT syndrome phenotype also being expressed by the same mutation.[38,39] The reasons for this difference in phenotypic expression between these affected individuals remain unclear, and it is suspected that there are certain expression modifiers or other cofactors affecting channel expression or function that are incompletely understood.

### *Treatment and Prognosis*

Currently there are limited treatment options for patients with inherited conduction diseases. Patients require frequent vigilance of their cardiac conduction to monitor for disease progression. The only therapy currently available for symptomatic heart block is a permanent pacemaker, with guidelines for device implant depending on rate, symptoms, and cardiac function.[44] Typically a dual-chamber pacemaker is recommended, even in patients with isolated sinus node dysfunction, because these patients are also at increased risk of developing complete heart block long term.[45] Pacemaker system implantation at an early age commits a patient to long-term device management, including generator changes and lead extractions or revisions, which can bring complications over time. However, pacemaker technology continues to evolve, with advances toward battery longevity and wireless leads possible in the future.

## FUTURE DIRECTIONS

The ability to regenerate cardiac tissue remains limited. However, there is increasing interest in the role stem cell therapy may play in restoring AV conduction in patients who have developed AV block.[46,47] Preliminary studies in canines have demonstrated some regeneration in conduction tissue with stem cell therapy, although these findings are recent and the clinical applicability remains unclear. The use of gene therapy for many genetic disorders continues to be evaluated, although the results of previous efforts have been frustrating. However, the potential for this therapy to treat inherited arrhythmia disorders, and multiple other genetic diseases, remains extremely appealing especially for young patients who face prolonged dependence on a pacing device. Improved genetic diagnosis to screen family members and permit genetic studies to evaluate channel function has provided tremendous insight into the primary dysfunction in familial AV block. However, the exact mechanism behind the progressive fibrosis that is often observed in affected family members remains poorly understood and may represent a target for potential therapy in the future. Also, the effects of other moderating factors in $Na_v1.5$ expression and function continue to require further definition and clarification.

## SUMMARY

The heritable nature of congenital or idiopathic AV block has been recognized for decades. However, only recently have mutations in the SCN5A gene encoding $Na_V1.5$ been identified as the culprits in many of these families. Although knowledge and understanding of the pathogenesis of these mutations continue to improve, it is quickly becoming apparent that there are multiple factors that affect the expressed phenotype of these mutations in particular individuals. A thorough pedigree and electrocardiogram screening of family members remains important, as does the ongoing clinical surveillance of mutation carriers that may be at risk. Certainly the ability to test for mutations has improved the ability to identify carriers and patients at risk for conduction disease, but options for treatment remain limited to implantable pacemaker therapy. As the understanding of these channel mutations and their effects continues to improve, then the ability to target appropriate intervention or innovate new therapies will improve accordingly.

## REFERENCES

1. Anderson RH, Yanni J, Boyett MR, et al. The anatomy of the cardiac conduction system. Clin Anat 2009;22(1):99–113.
2. Jongbloed MR, Steijn RV, Hahurij ND, et al. Normal and abnormal development of the cardiac conduction system: implications for conduction and rhythm disorders in the child and adult. Differentiation 2012; 84(1):131–48.
3. Moorman AF, Christoffels VM. Cardiac chamber formation: development, genes, and evolution. Physiol Rev 2003;83:1223–67.
4. Dobrzynski H, Anderson RH, Atkinson A, et al. Structure, function and clinical relevance of the cardiac conduction system, including the atrioventricular ring and outflow tract tissues. Pharmacol Ther 2013;139(2): 260–88.
5. Lev M. Anatomic basis for atrioventricular block. Am J Med 1964;37:742–8.
6. Greenspahn BR, Denes P, Daniel W, et al. Chronic bifascicular block: evaluation of familial factors. Ann Intern Med 1976;84:521–5.
7. Stephan E. Hereditary bundle branch system defect. Am Heart J 1978;95(1):89–95.
8. Sarachek NS, Leonard JJ. Familial heart block and sinus bradycardia: classification and natural history. Am J Cardiol 1972;29:451–8.
9. Schaal SF, Seidensticker J, Goodman R, et al. Familial RBBB, LAD, CHB, and early death: a heritable disorder of cardiac conduction. Ann Intern Med 1973;79:63–6.
10. Lynch HT, Mohiuddin S, Sketch MH, et al. Hereditary progressive AV conduction defect: a new syndrome. JAMA 1973;225:1465–70.
11. Schott JJ, Alshinawi C, Kyndt F, et al. Cardiac conduction defects associate with mutations in SCN5A. Nat Genet 1999;23:20–1.
12. Tan HL, Bink-Boelkens MT, Bezzina CR, et al. A sodium-channel mutation causes isolated cardiac conduction disease. Nature 2001;409:1043–7.
13. Zimmer T, Surber R. SCN5A channelopathies: an update on mutations and mechanisms. Prog Biophys Mol Biol 2008;98(2–3):120–36.
14. Meijler FL, Janse MJ. Morphology and electrophysiology of the mammalian AV node. Physiol Rev 1988; 68:608–47.
15. Jansen JA, van Veen TA, de Bakker JM, et al. Cardiac connexins and impulse propagation. J Mol Cell Cardiol 2010;48(1):76–82.
16. Marban E, Yamagashi T, Tomaselli GF. Structure and function of voltage-gated sodium channels. J Physiol 1998;508(3):647–57.
17. Shy D, Gillet L, Abriel H. Cardiac sodium channel NaV1.5 distribution in myocytes via interacting proteins: the multiple pool model. Biochim Biophys Acta 2013;1833(4):886–94.
18. Abriel H. Roles and regulation of the cardiac sodium channel Na v 1.5: recent insights from experimental studies. Cardiovasc Res 2007;76(3):381–9.
19. Petrecca K, Amellal F, Laird DW, et al. Sodium channel distribution within the rabbit AV node as analysed by confocal microscopy. J Physiol 1997;501:263–74.
20. Yoo S, Dobrzynski H, Fedorov VV, et al. Localization of Na+ channel isoforms at the atrioventricular junction and atrioventricular node in the rat. Circulation 2006;114(13):1360–71.
21. Morquio L. Sur une maladie infantile et familiale: caracterisee par des modifications permanentes du pouls, des attaques syncopales et epileptiformes et la mort subite. Arch Med Enfants 1901;4:467–75.
22. Myburgh DP, Steenkamp WF. The hereditary nature of adult-onset heart block. S Afr Med J 1973;47:657–8.
23. Gazes PC, Culler RM, Taber E, et al. Congenital familial cardiac conduction defects. Circulation 1965; 32(1):32–4.
24. Morgans CM, Gray KE, Robb GH. A survey of familial heart block. Br Heart J 1974;36:693–6.
25. Stephan E, Aftimos G, Allam C. Familial fascicular block: histologic features of Lev's disease. Am Heart J 1985;109:1399–401.
26. Herfst L, Potet F, Bezzina CR, et al. Na+ channel mutation leading to loss of function and non-progressive cardiac conduction defects. J Mol Cell Cardiol 2003;35(5):549–57.
27. Probst V, Kyndt F, Potet F, et al. Haploinsufficiency in combination with aging causes SCN5A-linked hereditary Lenègre disease. J Am Coll Cardiol 2003; 41(4):643–52.

28. Niu DM, Hwang B, Hwang HW, et al. A common SCN5A polymorphism attenuates a severe cardiac phenotype caused by a nonsense SCN5A mutation in a Chinese family with an inherited cardiac conduction defect. J Med Genet 2006;43(10):817–21.
29. Bezzina CR, Rook MB, Groenewegen WA, et al. Compound heterozygosity for mutations (W156X and R225W) in SCN5A associated with severe cardiac conduction disturbances and degenerative changes in the conduction system. Circ Res 2002; 92(2):159–68.
30. Wang DW, Viswanathan PC, Balser JR, et al. Clinical, genetic, and biophysical characterization of SCN5A mutations associated with atrioventricular conduction block. Circulation 2002;105(3):341–6.
31. Viswanathan PC, Benson DW, Balser JR. A common SCN5A polymorphism modulates the biophysical effects of an SCN5A mutation. J Clin Invest 2003; 111(3):341–6.
32. Papadatos GA, Wallerstein PM, Head CE, et al. Slowed conduction and ventricular tachycardia after targeted disruption of the cardiac sodium channel gene Scn5a. Proc Natl Acad Sci U S A 2002;99(9): 6210–5.
33. Royer A, van Veen TA, Le Bouter S, et al. Mouse model of SCN5A-linked hereditary Lenegre's disease: age-related conduction slowing and myocardial fibrosis. Circulation 2005;111(14):1738–46.
34. van Veen TA, Stein M, Royer A, et al. Impaired impulse propagation in Scn5a-knockout mice: combined contribution of excitability, connexin expression, and tissue architecture in relation to aging. Circulation 2005;112(13):1927–35.
35. Kyndt F, Probst V, Potet F, et al. Novel SCN5A mutation leading either to isolated cardiac conduction defect or Brugada syndrome in a large French family. Circulation 2001;104(25):3081–6.
36. Baruteau AE, Behaghel A, Fouchard S, et al. Parental electrocardiographic screening identifies a high degree of inheritance for congenital and childhood nonimmune isolated atrioventricular block. Circulation 2012;126(12):1469–77.
37. Smits JP, Koopmann TT, Wilders R, et al. A mutation in the human cardiac sodium channel (E161K) contributes to sick sinus syndrome, conduction disease and Brugada syndrome in two families. J Mol Cell Cardiol 2005;38(6):969–81.
38. Surber R, Hensellek S, Prochnau D, et al. Combination of cardiac conduction disease and long QT syndrome caused by mutation T1620K in the cardiac sodium channel. Cardiovasc Res 2008;77(4):740–8.
39. Grant AO, Carboni MP, Neplioueva V, et al. Long QT syndrome, Brugada syndrome, and conduction system disease are linked to a single sodium channel mutation. J Clin Invest 2002;110(8):1201–9.
40. McNair WP, Ku L, Taylor MR, et al. SCN5A mutation associated with dilated cardiomyopathy, conduction disorder, and arrhythmia. Circulation 2004;110(15): 2163–7.
41. Ge J, Sun A, Paajanen V, et al. Molecular and clinical characterization of a novel SCN5A mutation associated with atrioventricular block and dilated cardiomyopathy. Circ Arrhythm Electrophysiol 2008;1(2): 83–92.
42. Vorobiof G, Kroening D, Hall B, et al. Brugada syndrome with marked conduction disease: dual implications of a SCN5A mutation. Pacing Clin Electrophysiol 2008;31:630–4.
43. Greenlee PR, Anderson JL, Lutz JR, et al. Familial automaticity-conduction disorder with associated cardiomyopathy. West J Med 1986;144:33–41.
44. Epstein AE, DiMarco JP, Ellenbogen KA, et al. ACC/AHA/HRS 2008 guidelines for device-based therapy of cardiac rhythm abnormalities. Heart Rhythm 2008;5(6):e1–62.
45. Gillis AM, Russo AM, Ellenbogen KA, et al. HRS/ACCF expert consensus statement on pacemaker device and mode selection. Developed in partnership between the Heart Rhythm Society (HRS) and the American College of Cardiology Foundation (ACCF) and in collaboration with the Society of Thoracic Surgeons. Heart Rhythm 2012;9(8):1344–65.
46. Cho HC, Marban E. Biological therapies for cardiac arrhythmias: can genes and cells replace drugs and devices? Circ Res 2010;106(4):674–85.
47. Xiao YF. Cell and gene therapy for arrhythmias: repair of cardiac conduction damage. J Geriatr Cardiol 2011;8(3):147–58.

# Dilated Cardiomyopathy and $Na_V1.5$

Elena Zaklyazminskaya, MD, PhD[a,*], Sergei Dzemeshkevich, MD, PhD[b]

**KEYWORDS**

- Non-ischemic DCM • *SCN5A* • $Na_V1.5$ • Progressive conduction defect • Cardiac remodeling
- Cardiac resynchronization therapy • CRT • Heart transplantation

**KEY POINTS**

- Mutations in *SCN5A* gene encoding $Na_V1.5$, can cause dilated cardiac myopathy (DCM 1E, MIM: *601154) associated with progressive conduction defect and various supraventricular and ventricular arrhythmias.
- Mutations causing DCM do not share common biophysical properties. The molecular dysfunctions of the $Na_V1.5$ channel may require additional genetic or environmental factors.
- Manifestation of DCM 1E has common features: A wide range of supraventricular and ventricular arrhythmias, and conduction defects. Heart dilatation is age dependent and usually slow progressive.
- DCM 1E patients have benefitted from optimal antiarrhythmic therapy in arrhythmic events risk reduction and also in improvement of heart failure symptoms.

## INTRODUCTION

### *Dilated Cardiomyopathy: Definition, Epidemiology, Genetic Heterogeneity, Natural History, and Treatment Options*

Dilated cardiomyopathy (DCM) is a myocardial disease characterized by ventricular chamber enlargement and decreased myocardial contractility. It is the most common cause of severe congestive heart failure.[1] DCM is also associated with a high rate of sudden death owing to ventricular arrhythmias, and a high mortality rate of 15% to 50% at 5 years after diagnosis.[2] The prevalence of DCM is approximately 36.5 per 100,000 individuals, although this may be an underestimation.[3] Approximately 20% to 30% of DCM cases are familial in origin.[4] The disease is genetically heterogeneous. Currently, mutations in more than 40 genes have been associated with DCM.[5] The implicated genes include, for example, those that encode structural and sarcomeric myocardial proteins, nuclear membrane proteins, and ion channels.[5] Mutations in the largest human gene, *TTN*, have been identified in 25% to 30% of patients on the heart transplant waiting list.[5] Other genes mutations are present in fewer than 5% of patients from DCM cohorts.[6] Obtaining a genetic diagnosis of this disease remains extremely challenging, and data on the genotype–phenotype correlations are very limited. In 2004, the role of *SCN5A* mutations as the cause of DCM accompanied by arrhythmias and conduction disorders was first demonstrated.[7] This form of DCM was defined as DCM 1E variant (MIM: *601154), and was shown to have an autosomal-dominant mode of inheritance.[8] The frequency of *SCN5A*-mediated cases in patients with DCM is only about 2% to 3%[9]; however, the frequency increases to 5% to 10% when

Authors have nothing to disclose.

[a] Medical Genetics Laboratory, Petrovsky Russian Research Centre of Surgery, Abrocosovsky pereulok, Moscow 119991, Russia; [b] Heart Surgery Department, Petrovsky Russian Research Centre of Surgery, Abrocosovsky pereulok, Moscow 119991, Russia
* Corresponding author.
*E-mail address:* zhelene@mail.ru

Card Electrophysiol Clin 6 (2014) 733–740
http://dx.doi.org/10.1016/j.ccep.2014.07.005
1877-9182/14/$ – see front matter 

considering only those patients with progressive cardiac conduction defect and supraventricular and/or ventricular arrhythmias.[10] According to Heart Rhythm Association/European Society of Heart Rhythm recommendations, comprehensive or targeted genetic testing (*SCN5A* and *LMNA* genes) is recommended for patients with either DCM or significant cardiac conduction disease (atrioventricular block of any degree), as well as those with a familial history of premature unexpected sudden death. It is also recommended to screen family members of the proband with the identified disease-causing mutation.[10]

Genetic forms of DCM are typically progressive.[1] Conservative treatment is aimed at slowing the progression to heart failure, preventing thromboembolic complications, introducing antiarrhythmic therapy, and recommending lifestyle modifications. Surgical treatment involves pacemaker and/or cardioverter–defibrillator implantation, cardiac resynchronization therapy (CRT or CRT-D implantation), annuloplasty and/or valve replacement, myocardial reverse remodeling, and left ventricular assist device implantation.[11–13] For advanced stages of DCM, orthotopic cardiac transplantation remains the most effective treatment.

### *Role of $Na_v1.5$ in the Heart in Health and Disease*

The *SCN5A* gene encodes the alpha subunit of the $Na_v1.5$ sodium channel, which is responsible for the inward sodium current ($I_{Na}$). Current $I_{Na}$ is the main component of rapid depolarization in cardiomyocytes.[8] The incoming sodium depolarizing current triggers the action potential, which starts the multistep signal transduction to sarcomeric proteins and the initiation of cardiomyocyte contraction. Because of the intercellular communication between cardiomyocytes and the cardiac conduction system, this periodic depolarization underlies synchronous and rhythmic contraction of the heart chambers.[8]

At present, more than 20 proteins are known to interact with the $Na_v1.5$ alpha subunit, resulting in the regulation of expression and activity of the sodium channel via different molecular mechanisms (**Fig. 1**).[14] The interacting proteins can influence sodium channel function through trafficking, targeting, and stabilization of $Na_v1.5$ subunits to specific cellular compartments, as well as through posttranslational protein processing, and via the modulation of the biophysical properties of the sodium channel upon binding.[15,16]

Genetic alterations in the *SCN5A* gene may affect the structure, function, or level of expression of the $Na_v1.5$ sodium channel. These diverse and often functionally opposite alterations of cardiomyocyte electrical excitability result in various cardiac arrhythmias, such as congenital long QT syndrome, Brugada syndrome, sick sinus syndrome, progressive cardiac conduction defect, idiopathic ventricular fibrillation, sudden infant death syndrome, and mixed arrhythmogenic syndromes, all of which are often associated with a structurally normal heart.[8,17] Currently, several hundred *SCN5A* genetic mutations leading to clinically significant cardiac arrhythmias have been identified.[17] In the most complete online catalog of cardiac ion channel genetic mutations, "The Gene Connection to the Heart," there are 477 mutations associated with the 4 most common cardiac sodium channelopathies.[18]

The $Na_v1.5$ alpha subunit is expressed not only in cardiomyocytes and the limbic system of the brain (excitable cells), but also in various subpopulations of nonexcitable cells, such as astrocytes, microglia, T lymphocytes, endothelial cells, fibroblasts, macrophages, and cancer cells.[15,16] There is some evidence demonstrating that sodium channels can participate in multiple effector functions and may play noncanonical roles in nonexcitable cells.[15] Many of the molecular mechanisms involved in the function of $Na_v1.5$ have yet to be elucidated.

## GENETIC VARIANTS IN THE *SCN5A* GENE ASSOCIATED WITH DILATED CARDIOMYOPATHY: CAUSAL OR CASUAL LINK?

It was recently demonstrated that the phenotypic expression of *SCN5A* genetic mutations could be expanded from electrical disorders with an apparently normal heart to cardiomyopathies. Genetic variations in the *SCN5A* gene that resulted in electrical and structural cardiac remodeling were first described in 2003 by Groenewegen and colleagues[19] in a large family with atrial standstill, a rare form of atrial cardiomyopathy. In 2004 and 2005, the role of *SCN5A* genetic mutations in arrhythmogenic right ventricular cardiomyopathy and DCM accompanied with arrhythmias and conduction disorders was also described.[20,21]

Currently, more than 10 mutations in the *SCN5A* gene (**Table 1**) have been described, which led to the development of DCM in conjunction with a wide range of cardiac arrhythmias and conduction disorders.[7,24,25,29] There is no known hot spot for DCM mutations. Mutations affect almost all protein domains, except for the *N*-terminal region of the protein. The mutations are located in the transmembrane domains, and in the extracellular and intracellular regions. Some variants lead to

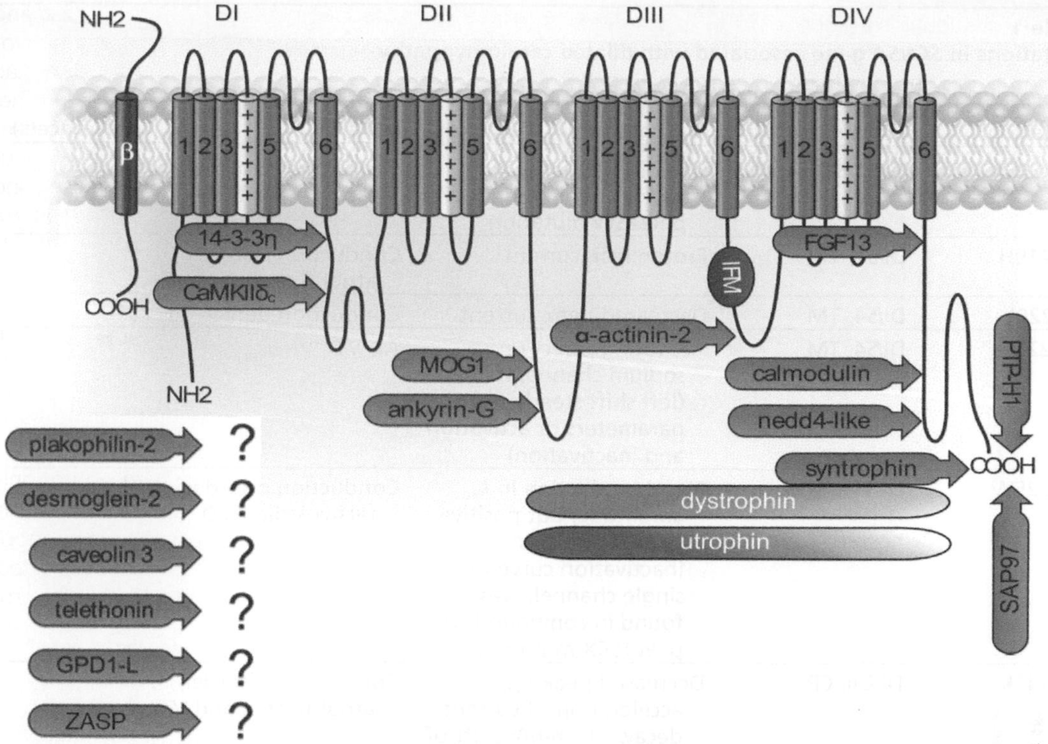


**Fig. 1.** Topology of $Na_V1.5$ and its interaction with various regulatory proteins. The pore-forming alpha subunit of $Na_V1.5$ consists of 4 homologous domains (DI–DIV), connected by intracellular and extracellular loops. Each of these domains contains segments that contribute to the lining of the channel pore (segments S5 and S6) as well as a voltage sensor segment (S4). Several regulatory proteins for $Na_V1.5$ were identified and their sites of interaction have been mapped on the alpha subunit of the $Na_V1.5$ channel. For a few proteins that have been shown (through co-immunoprecipitation) to associate with $Na_V1.5$, the sites of interaction on the $Na_V1.5$ channel are still unknown. (*From* Shy D, Gillet L, Abriel H. Cardiac sodium channel $Na_V1.5$ distribution in myocytes via interacting proteins: the multiple pool model. Biochim Biophys Acta 2013;1833:886–94.)

aberrant splicing. The spectrum of pathophysiologic appearances of the mutations is broad and covers almost all possible effects on sodium channel disturbances, including haploinsufficiency (see **Table 1**). Six of 13 mutations are localized in the highly conserved voltage-sensor mechanism (S3–S4), but they do not seem to share common biophysical properties (see **Table 1**).

Genetic variants have been linked to both an increase in the sodium current through the altered channel as well as to a decrease in sodium conductivity. Several hypotheses linking the multidirectional sodium conductivity alterations and the development of cardiomyopathy are the shifting of tight $Na^+/Ca^{2+}$ homeostasis, changes in contractile changes in myocytes, and the disruption of electromechanical excitation–contraction coupling.[22] These hypotheses, however, cannot explain why the vast majority of the known *SCN5A* mutations, which significantly disturb sodium conductance, do not result in the disruption of calcium homeostasis and DCM. In addition, the development of age-dependent cardiomyopathy in the majority of *SCN5A* mutation carriers has not been demonstrated in clinical practice.

The same dilemma exists regarding the role of *SCN5A* mutations that result in haploinsufficiency in DCM. On the one hand, in series of very convincing experiments Hesse and colleagues[34] demonstrated that the decrease in $Na_v1.5$ expression and the significant reduction in the sodium current results in DCM in dosage-dependent manner in transgenic mice. On the other hand, there are 376 Brugada syndrome mutations listed in the Gene Connection to the Heart Database,[18] and 106 of them (28%) are nonsense, splicing, or frameshift mutations potentially causing haploinsufficiency. Only c.2550–2551insTG and c.3318dupC mutations were shown to be associated with DCM.[9,29] One of the possible explanations could be related to the efficiency of RNA quality control machinery for particular truncating mutations, which result in various levels of $Na_v1.5$ protein expression. The dosage-dependent character of the clinical expression of

**Table 1**
**Mutations in *SCN5A* gene associated with dilated cardiomyopathy**

| Mutation | Protein Domain | Biophysical Properties of Mutant Protein | Features Accompanied DCM | Reference(s) |
|---|---|---|---|---|
| p.W156X | DI/S1-S2, EC | Haploinsufficiency, was found in compound with p.R225W mutation | Conduction disorder, tachycardia, SCD | 21 |
| p.R219H | DI/S4, TM | Proton leak current | Conduction disorder, atrial flutter, and VT | 22 |
| p.T220I | DI/S4, TM | Decreased peak current | Conduction defect, AF | 9,23 |
| p.R222Q | DI/S4, TM | Activating effect on sodium channel function (left shift steady-state parameters of activation and inactivation) | AF, VT | 24–26 |
| p.R225W | DI/S4, TM | 10-fold reduction in $I_{Na}$ amplitude, but positive shift of steady-state inactivation curve of single channel; was found in compound with p. W156X mutation | Conduction disorder, tachycardia, SCD | 21 |
| p.E446K | DI/DII, CP | Decreased peak $I_{Na}$, acceleration of current decay, −6.16-mV shift of steady-state inactivation, slower recovery from inactivation | Conduction disorder, atrial flutter, and VT | 6,25,27 |
| c.2550-2551insTG | Truncating mutation | Haploinsufficiency | Atrial fibrillation, impaired automaticity, and conduction delay | 9 |
| p.R814W | DII/S4, TM | Slower rise times and a hyperpolarized conductance-voltage relationship resulting in an increased "window current", enhanced slow inactivation and greater use-dependent reduction in peak current at fast pulsing frequencies | Atrial and VT | 9,28 |
| c.3318dupC | Truncating mutation | Haploinsufficiency | No data | 29 |
| p.A1180V | DII/DIII, CP | Persistent late $I_{Na}$ current, A1180V could alter calcium homeostasis | Cardiac conduction block | 30 |
| p.D1275N | DIII/S3, CP | No significant changes in biophysical properties (in vitro cellular models), but in vivo mice models are affected | Atrial and VT | 7,9,25,31 |
| p.V1279I | DIII/S3, CP | No data | AF, nonsustained VT | 9,25 |
| p. N1325S | DIII/S4, CP | Late and sustained $I_{Na}$ current | LQT3, SCD, bradycardia, AF | 32 |

(*continued on next page*)

**Table 1**
***(continued)***

| Mutation | Protein Domain | Biophysical Properties of Mutant Protein | Features Accompanied DCM | Reference(s) |
|---|---|---|---|---|
| p.delKPQ1507-1509 | DIII/S6-DIV/S1, CP | Increased rate of inactivation; increased rate of recovery from inactivation; persistent late $I_{Na}$ current | LQT3, conduction disorder | 33 |
| p.F1520L | DIII/S6-DIV/S1, CP | Shift in the activation curve toward more positive voltage | Atrial flatter, atrioventricular block, sinus node dysfunction | 7,25 |
| p.D1595H | DIV/S3, TM | Impaired fast inactivation characterized by slower entry into the inactivated state and a hyperpolarized steady-state inactivation curve | Sinus bradycardia | 9,28 |

*Abbreviations:* CP, cytoplasmic; EC, extracellular; LQT3, Long QT Syndrome type 3; SCD, sudden cardiac death; SSS, Sick Sinus Syndrome; TM, transmembrane; VT, ventricular tachycardia.

arrhythmias and cardiac dilatation[34] may suggest that there is a minimal threshold of remnant $Na_v1.5$ expression required to develop DCM. This hypothesis, however, requires experimental testing.

It is also possible that the prevalence of variants of cardiac remodeling in *SCN5A*-mutations carriers is higher than previously thought. This underestimation may be owing to the fact that there was previously more focus on the ECG arrhythmic phenomena in describing the phenotype of patients with channelopathies, and it could also be related to the reduction in the number of older mutation carriers owing to the increased incidence of sudden cardiac death in the young, which naturally decreases the number of age-dependent complications observed.

The molecular dysfunctions of the $Na_v1.5$ channel that lead to the development of DCM may be more specific or may require the involvement of additional genetic or environmental factors. A unique pathologic mechanism for one of the mutations leading to the development of cardiomyopathy, p.R219H, has been demonstrated. The stable inward proton leakage current passes through the mutated $Na_v1.5$-R219H channel, resulting in the pH reduction and acidification of the cardiomyocyte.[22] Long-term intracellular acidulation might trigger the mechanisms of metabolic and ionic balance disruptions, similar to intracellular disturbances in chronic ischemia. DCM is associated with 16 published genetic variants, illustrating that only 2% to 5% of the currently known mutations in the *SCN5A* gene are characterized by structural changes in the myocardium. Interestingly, the incidence of "double-hit" mutations carriers is comparable between patients with primary cardiomyopathy and those with arrhythmias, which account for approximately 5%.[35–37] The prevalence of cardiomyopathies in the general population is relatively high, with that of hypertrophic cardiomyopathy being 1:500 and DCM 1:2500.[1] It is possible to observe a combined manifestation of 2 diseases: Cardiac arrhythmia resulting from an *SCN5A* mutation and DCM of primary or secondary origin, suggesting a more complex genetic background. Recently published results of extended testing of a DCM proband carrying the *SCN5A*-p.A1180V mutation is an example of the possible complex genetic backgrounds of DCM in *SCN5A*-positive patients.[30] The patient had rare genetic variants in several DCM-related genes: p.G1117S, p.P1119R, p.Y498H in *LAMA4* gene, p.W768S in *RBM20* gene, and p.P398S in *VCL* gene.[30] The search for mutations in all known genes is a low diagnostic yield because DCM is genetically heterogeneous. The introduction of new-generation sequencing technologies might enable more in-depth investigations, resulting in more accurate genotype–phenotype correlations.

## CLINICAL MANIFESTATIONS OF DILATED CARDIOMYOPATHY 1E AND TREATMENT OPTIONS

To date, a few dozen patients with genetically verified forms of DCM 1E have been described. Their clinical manifestations have many common features. The disease often manifests with a wide range of rhythm disorders: Supraventricular tachycardia (more than 85% of patients), atrial fibrillation (40%–60%), progressive cardiac conduction defect (60%), and premature ventricular contractions and ventricular tachycardia (>80%).[9,10,25,27] QT interval prolongation has been observed in a few cases.[33]

Cardiac chamber dilatation is age dependent and usually develops during the third or fourth decade of life. The left ventricular contractile capacity and ejection fraction in *SCN5A*-related DCM patients often remains stable.[9,25,27,38] In 1 family, however, there were 2 patients with the p.F1520L SCN5A mutation who developed rapidly progressing heart failure that required heart transplantation.[25] This form of cardiomyopathy commonly results in progressive atrial dilatation, without obvious predisposing hemodynamic factors, which can develop into atrial standstill.[9,19,25,27]

Genetic forms of DCM are often characterized by a progressive disease course and have a poor prognosis.[39] Cardiotropic and antiarrhythmic therapy are of limited efficacy.[39] About 30% to 40% of patients die within 1 year of being diagnosed, and 60% to 70% die within 5 years.[12,39] The optimization of treatment strategies is the priority for the prolongation of life and transplant-free time for these patients.

Unlike the natural course of primary DCM, an improvement in cardiac output and a reduction in cardiac chamber size was observed in some DCM 1E patients who received antiarrhythmic treatment.[10,26,27]

Mutation p.E446K in the *SCN5A* gene has been described to be associated with DCM with cardiac arrhythmias and conduction defects in 2 unrelated families.[25,27] A 24-year-old patient with DCM had significantly increased left ventricular ejection fraction, 24% to 40%, with effective antiarrhythmic treatment (3-year follow-up).[25] A 46-year-old proband with significant ventricular dyssynchrony had significantly stabilized heart pumping function (ejection fraction of 52%–55%) after CRT implantation over a 6-year follow-up.[20] Another case of myocardial contractile function recovery was described in a patient with DCM, multiple polymorphic premature ventricular contractions and a p.R222Q mutation in *SCN5A* gene.[26] This mutation leads to late inward sodium current (increased total sodium current), and a resultant depolarization of the membrane potential.[26] Standard heart failure therapy for carriers of this mutation was virtually ineffective, but when data on the functional properties of the mutation were obtained, the patients started receiving effective treatment with sodium channel blockers.[26] The treatment resulted in a drastic reduction in premature ventricular contractions number and recovery of left ventricular contractile function within 6 months after the onset of therapy.[26] The relatively slow progression of DCM,[25,27,34] the efficacy of CRT, as well as the reports of myocardial pump function recovery under optimal anti-arrhythmic therapy[26] may be arguments in favor of an arrhythmogenic origin of cardiac remodeling in patients with DCM 1E. Heart chamber dilation may not be a direct consequence of mutant $Na_v1.5$ biophysical properties. It might be owing to an interplay between ventricular and atrial chronic arrhythmia/dyssynchrony caused by mutations in *SCN5A* gene, as well as to a predisposition to cardiac chamber remodeling caused by additional genetic variants in DCM-associated genes (including those which encode $Na_v1.5$ interactors).

## SUMMARY

There is a clear link between $Na_v1.5$ alterations and DCM. *SCN5A* genetic mutations can cause arrhythmias and chamber dilation, but additional genetic factors may also be involved in cardiac remodeling. The important genetic heterogeneity of DCM complicates the clinical picture and understanding of the multiple genetic factors involved. The new-generation sequencing technologies should provide new insight into the genotype–phenotype correlations.

Despite the detailed biophysical characterizations of the mutant variants of $Na_v1.5$ protein, the stages of the molecular pathogenesis leading from the disruption of sodium conductance to the alterations of the conduction system and myocardial remodeling are not fully understood. There might be an "extra"-functional role of $Na_v1.5$ in the cells beside ion conductance, that is, the signaling or stabilization of the dystrophin–sarcoglycan complex and/or Z-discs. Most of the genes encoding protein members of the dystrophin–sarcoglycan complex and Z-discs are causative for DCM by themselves.[1,5]

The altered $Na_v1.5$ channel can increase electrical heterogeneity in the myocardium, and various arrhythmias can facilitate arrhythmogenic cardiac remodeling. Some DCM 1E patients have benefitted from optimal antiarrhythmic therapy, not only from risk reduction of life-threatening arrhythmic events but also through stabilization and improvement of heart failure symptoms. Optimal antiarrhythmic drug control in DCM 1E patients may also lead to the improvement of myocardial contractility. A few publications suggest that mutation-specific therapy directed against $Na_v1.5$ abnormalities can be very effective.[26]

CRT, CRT-P, or CRT-D device implantation is a relatively new approach for the treatment of heart failure. Of patients with heart failure, 20% to 30% do not respond to CRT.[40] It is, therefore, very important to determine the markers that can predict the efficacy of this invasive and costly procedure. Further research is needed to address the question of whether or not DCM 1E patients will respond to CRT.

A detailed understanding of all the phases (molecular, cellular, organ) of myocardial remodeling in DCM 1E is required to select the most effective strategies for personalized therapy based on existing treatments. There is also a need to develop new approaches for the management of rhythm disorders and heart failure.

## REFERENCES


1. Sanbe A. Dilated cardiomyopathy: a disease of the myocardium. Biol Pharm Bull 2013;36(1):18–22.
2. Mestroni L, Maisch B, McKenna WJ, et al. Guidelines for the study of familial dilated cardiomyopathies. Eur Heart J 1999;20:93–102.
3. Olson TM, Thibodeau SN, Lundquist PA, et al. Exclusion of a primary defect at the HLA locus in familial idiopathic dilated cardiomyopathy. J Med Genet 1995;32:876–80.
4. Kimura A. Contribution of genetic factors to the pathogenesis of dilated cardiopathy–the cause of dilated cardiomyopathy: acquired or genetic? (Genetic-side). Circ J 2011;75:1766–73.
5. Hershberger RE, Hedges DJ, Morales A. Dilated cardiomyopathy: the complexity of a diverse genetic architecture. Nat Rev Cardiol 2013;10(9):531–47.
6. Fatkin D, Otway R, Richmond Z. Genetics of dilated cardiomyopathy. Heart Fail Clin 2010;6:129–40.
7. McNair WP, Ku L, Taylor MR, et al, Familial Cardiomyopathy Registry Research Group. SCN5A mutation associated with dilated cardiomyopathy, conduction disorder, and arrhythmia. Circulation 2004;110:2163–7.
8. OMIM (On-line Mendelian Inheritance in Men). Available at: www.ncbi.nlm.nih.gov/omim.
9. Olson TM, Michels VV, Ballew JD, et al. Sodium channel mutations and susceptibility of heart failure and atrial fibrillation. JAMA 2005;293:447–54.
10. Ackerman MJ, Priori SG, Willems S, et al. HRS/EHRA expert consensus statement on the state of genetic testing for the channelopathies and cardiomyopathies. Europace 2011;13:1077–109.
11. Dzemeshkevich S, Korolev S, Frolova J, et al. Isolated replacement of the mitral leaflets and "Mercedes"-plastics of the giant left atrium: surgery for patients with left ventricle dysfunction and left atrium enlargement. J Cardiovasc Surg (Torino) 2001;42(4):505–8.
12. Wohlschlaeger J, Schmitz KJ, Schmid C, et al. Reverse remodeling following insertion of left ventricular assist devices (LVAD): a review of the morphological and molecular changes. Cardiovasc Res 2005;68(3):376–86.
13. Healey JS, Hohnloser SH, Exner DV, et al. Cardiac resynchronization therapy in patients with permanent atrial fibrillation: results from the Resynchronization for Ambulatory Heart Failure Trial (RAFT). Circ Heart Fail 2012;5(5):566–70.
14. Shy D, Gillet L, Abriel H. Cardiac sodium channel NaV1.5 distribution in myocytes via interacting proteins: the multiple pool model. Biochim Biophys Acta 2013;1833:886–94.
15. Black JA, Waxman SG. Noncanonical roles of voltage-gated sodium channels. Neuron 2013;80(2):280–9.
16. Meadows LS, Isom LL. Sodium channels as macromolecular complexes: implications for inherited arrhythmia syndromes. Cardiovasc Res 2005;67(3):448–58.
17. Remme CA. Cardiac sodium channelopathy associated with SCN5A mutations: electrophysiological, molecular and genetic aspects. J Physiol 2013;591(Pt 17):4099–116.
18. The gene connection to the heart. Available at: http://www.fsm.it/cardmoc/.
19. Groenewegen WA, Firouzi M, Bezzina CR, et al. A cardiac sodium channel mutation cosegregates with a rare connexin40 genotype in familial atrial standstill. Circ Res 2003;92(1):14–22.
20. Pérez Riera AR, Antzelevitch C, Schapacknik E, et al. Is there an overlap between Brugada syndrome and arrhythmogenic right ventricular cardiomyopathy/dysplasia? J Electrocardiol 2005;38(3):260–3.
21. Bezzina CR, Rook MB, Groenewegen WA, et al. Compound heterozygosity for mutations (W156X and R225W) in SCN5A associated with severe cardiac conduction disturbances and degenerative changes in the conduction system. Circ Res 2003;92(2):159–68.
22. Gosselin-Badaroudine P, Keller DI, Huang H, et al. A proton leak current through the cardiac sodium channel is linked to mixed arrhythmia and the dilated cardiomyopathy phenotype. PLoS One 2012;7(5):e38331.
23. Olesen MS, Yuan L, Liang B. High prevalence of Long QT syndrome-associated SCN5A variants in patients with early-onset lone atrial fibrillation. Circ Cardiovasc Genet 2012;5(4):450–9.
24. Rampersaud E, Siegfried JD, Norton N, et al. Rare variant mutations identified in pediatric patients with dilated cardiomyopathy. Prog Pediatr Cardiol 2011;31(1):39–47.
25. McNair W, Sinagra G, Taylor M, et al, Familial Cardiomyopathy Registry Research Group. SCN5A

mutations associate with arrhythmic dilated cardiomyopathy and commonly localize to the voltage-sensing mechanism. J Am Coll Cardiol 2011;57:2160–8.
26. Mann SA, Castro ML, Ohanian M, et al. R222Q SCN5A mutation is associated with reversible ventricular ectopy and dilated cardiomyopathy. J Am Coll Cardiol 2012;60(16):1566–73.
27. Zaklyazminskaya EV, Chapurnykh AV, Voronina TS, et al. Dilated cardiomyopathy caused by p.E446K mutation in *SCN5A* gene. Kardiologiia (Russian) 2014;3:102–6.
28. Nguyen TP, Wang DW, Rhodes TH, et al. Divergent biophysical defects caused by mutant sodium channels in dilated cardiomyopathy with arrhythmia. Circ Res 2008;102(3):364–71.
29. van Spaendonck-Zwarts KY, van Rijsingen IA, van den Berg MP, et al. Genetic analysis in 418 index patients with idiopathic dilated cardiomyopathy: overview of 10 years' experience. Eur J Heart Fail 2013;15(6):628–36.
30. Shen C, Xu L, Yang Z, et al. A1180V of cardiac sodium channel gene (SCN5A): is it a risk factor for dilated cardiomyopathy or just a common variant in Han Chinese? Dis Markers 2013;35(5):531–5.
31. Watanabe H, Yang T, Stroud DM, et al. Striking in vivo phenotype of a disease-associated human *SCN5A* mutation producing minimal changes in vitro. Circulation 2011;124:1001–11.
32. Young SN, Ni Y, Zhang T, et al. Characterization of the cardiac sodium channel SCN5A mutation, N1325S, in single murine ventricular myocytes. Biochem Biophys Res Commun 2007;352:372–83.
33. Shi R, Zhang Y, Yang C, et al. The cardiac sodium channel mutation delQKP 1507-1509 is associated with the expanding phenotypic spectrum of LQT3, conduction disorder, dilated cardiomyopathy, and high incidence of youth sudden death. Europace 2008;10(11):1329–35.
34. Hesse M, Kondo CS, Clark RB, et al. Dilated cardiomyopathy is associated with reduced expression of the cardiac sodium channel Scn5a. Cardiovasc Res 2007;75(3):498–509.
35. Girolami F, Ho CY, Semsarian C, et al. Clinical features and outcome of hypertrophic cardiomyopathy associated with triple sarcomere protein gene mutations. J Am Coll Cardiol 2010;55:1444–53.
36. Maron BJ, Maron MS, Semsarian C. Double or compound sarcomere mutations in hypertrophic cardiomyopathy: a potential link to sudden death in the absence of conventional risk factors. Heart Rhythm 2012;9:57–66.
37. Abriel H, Zaklyazminskaya EV. Cardiac channelopathies: genetic and molecular mechanisms. Gene 2013;517(1):1–11.
38. Ge J, Sun A, Paajanen V, et al. Molecular and clinical characterization of a novel SCN5A mutation associated with atrioventricular block and dilated cardiomyopathy. Circ Arrhythm Electrophysiol 2008;1(2):83–92.
39. Larson LW, Gerbert DA, Herman LM, et al, American College of Cardiology; American Heart Association. ACC/AHA 2005 guideline update: chronic heart failure in the adult. JAAPA 2006;19(4):53–6.
40. Castellant P, Fatemi M, Bertault-Valls V, et al. Cardiac resynchronization therapy: "nonresponders" and "hyperresponders". Heart Rhythm 2008;5(2):193–7.

# Atrial Fibrillation and *SCN5A* Variants

Eleonora Savio-Galimberti, MD, PhD*, Dawood Darbar, MD

**KEYWORDS**

• Atrial fibrillation • *SCN5A* mutations • Electrophysiology • *SCN5A* • Gain of function • Loss of function • Action potential • "Two-hit" hypothesis

**KEY POINTS**

- The incidence and prevalence of atrial fibrillation (AF) continues to increase and may in part be explained by the aging of the population.
- Recent data suggest that both genetic and acquired risk factors increase susceptibility to AF and their simultaneous occurrence has given rise to the "two-hit" hypothesis for the development of AF.
- *SCN5A* variants have also been linked with an increasing number of cardiac arrhythmia syndromes including long QT syndrome, Brugada syndrome, sick-sinus syndrome, conduction disease, AF, atrial standstill, overlap syndromes with mixed arrhythmia phenotypes, and drug-induced arrhythmias.
- Common and rare genetic variants in *SCN5A*, which encode the α-subunit of human cardiac sodium channel, have been associated with AF with both gain- and loss-of-function variants modulating susceptibility to AF.
- *SCN5A* genetic variants have not only provided important insights into AF mechanisms but also uncovered novel therapeutic targets for the treatment of this common and morbid condition.

## DEFINITION AND EPIDEMIOLOGY OF ATRIAL FIBRILLATION

Atrial fibrillation (AF) is the most frequent sustained cardiac arrhythmia encountered in the clinical practice. It is described as a rapid irregular and chaotic electrical activation of atria that results in highly variable ventricular rates.[1] The AF electrocardiogram is characterized by the absence of P waves and irregularities in the R-R intervals.

AF is clinically and genetically a highly heterogeneous disease. Both acquired[2] and genetic[3] risk factors for AF have been identified. About 10% of patients older than 80 years develop AF. Up to 30% of AF cases occur in individuals with no prior history of cardiac or systemic conditions, a group that has previously been defined as "lone" or early-onset AF. Cristophersen and colleagues[4] have estimated this number to be as high as 60% of total AF cases. Although the number of patients with true "lone" AF is probably very few,[5] not all the patients with early-onset AF can be categorized as having a monogenic/Mendelian form of AF[6] because only approximately 35% have a positive family history.[5] Genome-wide association studies (GWAS) have identified common genetic variants at 9 different chromosomal loci that are significantly associated with AF.[7–10] However, most of the heritability of AF still remains unexplained.[11] The recognition that both acquired and genetic AF risk factors are associated with increased risk for AF has fundamentally altered

This work was supported by the National Institutes of Health (U19 HL65962, HL092217, awarded to D. Darbar), and MMPC MicroMouse grant (MMPC/NIH, awarded to E. Savio-Galimberti). CTSA award (UL1TR000445).
Disclosures: None.
Division of Cardiovascular Medicine, Vanderbilt University, 2215B Garland Avenue, Medical Research Building IV, Nashville, TN 37232, USA
* Corresponding author.
*E-mail address:* eleonora.savio.galimberti@vanderbilt.edu

Card Electrophysiol Clin 6 (2014) 741–748
http://dx.doi.org/10.1016/j.ccep.2014.07.006
1877-9182/14/$ – see front matter 

the authors' perception of this arrhythmia. Due to its clinical and genetic heterogeneity, AF should be considered a syndrome rather than a homogeneous disease entity, where the arrhythmia represents the culmination of diverse causes and pathways.

In 1994, using the Framingham cohort, Benjamin and colleagues[2] identified independent risk factors for AF. The strongest predictor of development of AF was age. AF prevalence increased from 0.5% in the age group of 50 to 60 years to 8.8% in patients older than 80 years.[12] This study also demonstrated that common risk factors for cardiovascular disease, such as diabetes, hypertension, and cardiac valve disease, are associated with increased risk for AF and modification of these risk factors may reduce incidence of AF.[2] Importantly however, only some patients with these risk factors develop AF. One possible explanation for this apparent paradox is that both acquired and genetic risk factors are required to develop AF—the so-called two-hit hypothesis.[13]

## GENETICS OF ATRIAL FIBRILLATION

Despite AF being the most common arrhythmia in clinical practice requiring pharmacologic treatment, response to antiarrhythmic drugs (AADs) is highly unpredictable with approximately 50% of patients experiencing a symptomatic recurrence of AF within 6 to 12 months of starting therapy. The limited success of AADs is related to poor understanding of the molecular pathophysiology of AF, interindividual differences in underlying mechanisms, and inability to target mechanism-based therapies. There is increasing support for the idea that variability in drug and ablation therapy may in part reflect heterogeneity of the underlying AF mechanisms.[13]

Over the last decade, the authors and other investigators have applied diverse genetic approaches to define the genetic architecture of AF and better define the underlying genetic mechanisms. Although a comprehensive review of the genetic basis of AF is beyond the scope of this article, many excellent reviews have recently been published.[13,14] Linkage and positional cloning approaches have identified family-specific rare mutations that encode not only cardiac ion channels including *SCN5A* but also signaling molecules such as atrial natriuretic peptide and nucleoporins (NUP155). Furthermore, a candidate gene approach has uncovered both common and rare genetic variants linked with AF. A more contemporary approach that has been used is the identification of common genetic variants (or single nucleotide polymorphioms [SNPs]) by GWAS. These studies have uncovered novel genes and loci that are important for the initiation and maintenance of AF.[13]

## NORMAL ATRIAL ELECTROPHYSIOLOGY AND ROLE OF *SCN5A*/$Na_V1.5$

As cardiac myocytes are excitable cells, they are capable of generating rapid changes in the cell membrane polarity due to changes in their ionic conductance. These cells are characteristically activated by an electrical "all-or-none" response, the action potential (AP). These changes in the electrical potential across the plasma membrane of the cardiomyocytes are a consequence of an orchestrated sequence of openings and closings of cardiac ion channels. The electronegative resting membrane potential in atrial cells (of approximately −80 mV) is critical for the normal propagation of the atrial AP across cells. Cardiomyocytes heavily depend mainly on the electrogenic Na/K-ATPase but also inward rectifying potassium currents (mainly, $I_{K1}$) to maintain the electronegativity of the resting membrane potential. The potassium currents facilitate termination of the AP by repolarizing the depolarized membrane back to resting levels.[15]

A typical atrial AP can be divided into 5 phases: phase 0 (upstroke), phase 1 ("early repolarization" phase), phase 2 (or "plateau"), phase 3 (or repolarization phase), and phase 4 (resting potential) (**Fig. 1**). The sodium ($I_{Na}$) and the L-type calcium ($I_{Ca\text{-}L}$) currents are the 2 main inward currents that participate in the upstroke (phase 0) of atrial AP.[16] One consequence of the dual participation of these 2 ionic currents during phase 0 is that the $[dV/dt]_{max}$ of atrial AP is less steep than that of ventricular myocytes.[15] Although these 2 depolarizing inward currents participate in the generation of phase 0 of the atrial AP, the main determinant of the plateau for both atrial and the ventricular cells is $I_{Ca\text{-}L}$.[15] In addition to its contribution to phases 0 and 2 of the AP, $I_{Ca\text{-}L}$ triggers the release of additional $Ca^{2+}$ from the sarcoplasmic reticulum, which is central for activation of atrial contraction. Moreover, a transient outward aminopyridine-sensitive potassium current ($I_{to1}$) contributes to the low membrane potential during the plateau phase. Phase 1 of AP ("early repolarization") is due to activation of $I_{to2}$, a transient outward $Ca^{2+}$-dependent chloride current that is 4-aminopyridine sensitive.[17] Once $I_{to1}$ is inactivated, the ultrarapid delayed rectifier potassium current ($I_{Kur}$) remains active. $I_{Kur}$ is selectively expressed in the atria and is generated by the $K_V1.5$ channel. During the repolarization phase (phase 3 of AP), several other transient inward potassium

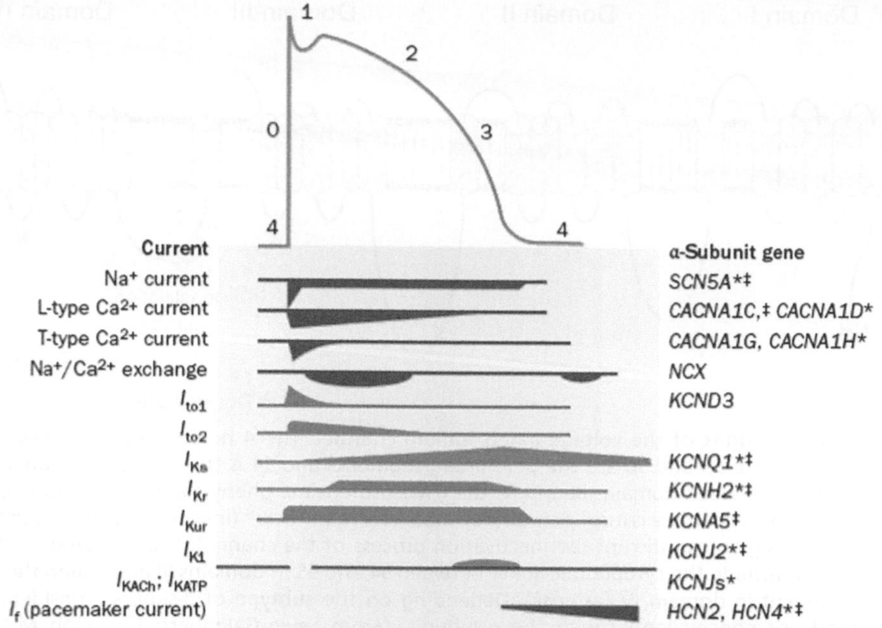


**Fig. 1.** The relationship between ionic currents and the duration of the atrial action potential (AP). The AP is initiated by a rapid influx of Na+ ions (phase 0), followed by early (phases 1 and 2) and late (phase 3) stages of repolarization, before returning to the resting membrane potential (phase 4). * Function-modifying subunit. ‡ Mutations in this gene were associated with atrial fibrillation. (*From* Darbar D, Roden DM. Genetic mechanisms of atrial fibrillation: impact on response to treatment. Nat Rev Cardiol 2013;10(6):317–29.)

currents ($I_{Ks}$, $I_{Kr}$, $I_{KACh}$, $I_{KATP}$, $I_{K1}$) ensure return of the membrane potential back to resting levels.[13,15]

The main sodium channel involved in the upstroke of the atrial AP is the canonical $Na_V1.5$ cardiac channel, which is part of a group of ion channels called voltage-gated sodium channels (VGSCs) (a detailed review of all the VGSCs has recently been published in a book edited by Peter C Ruben: *Handbook of Experimental Pharmacology*, vol. 221. 2014).[18] Similar to other channels, VGSCs activate, deactivate, and inactivate in response to changes in the membrane potential. VGSCs conform to a universal ion channel structure consisting of an α-subunit that is organized into 4 homologous domains (DI-DIV). Each domain comprises of 6 transmembrane segments (S1–S6). These 24 α-helical transmembrane segments arranged in 4 domains surround a central aqueous pore that allows sodium ions to flow from the extracellular space into the cytosol of the myocyte, causing depolarization of the myocyte. Each of the 4 domains of the sodium channel contains a voltage-sensing domain formed by the first 4 transmembrane segments S1 to S4 and a pore domain consisting of segments S5 and S6 and the extracellular linker between these 2 segments (the p-loop) (**Fig. 2**).[19]

Although the α-subunit of the cardiac sodium channel is normally associated with one or more β regulatory subunits, the α-subunit itself conducts sodium.[19–21] The β-subunits are integral proteins of the cardiac myocytes sarcolemma. There are 4 different types of β-subunits, β1 to β4. Each β-subunit is composed of an N-terminal domain, one transmembrane domain, and one intracellular C-terminal domain. In addition to being cell adhesion molecules, the cardiac sodium channel β-subunits also modulate cell surface expression of the α-subunits, enhancing sodium current density and cell excitability.[20,21] The α-subunit of the $Na_V1.5$ channel is encoded by the *SCN5A* gene. The β-subunits are encoded by *SCN1B* through *SCN4B*. Mutations in both the α- and β-subunits have been linked with increased susceptibility to atrial and ventricular arrhythmias.[20]

Although the main cardiac sodium channel isoform expressed in cardiomyocytes is $Na_V1.5$ (which is tetrodotoxin [TTX]-resistant), there are several other sodium (TTX-sensitive) channel isoforms expressed in the myocardium. These isoforms account for a smaller fraction of the total sodium channel transcripts and include isoforms $Na_V1.1$ to $Na_V1.4$ and $Na_V1.6$. The TTX-sensitive component of the sodium channel contributes to approximately 8% of the total $I_{Na}$.[15,22] TTX-resistant $Na_V1.8$ messenger RNA has also been detected and quantified in the atria of mice.[23] Facer and colleagues[24] were able to identify the

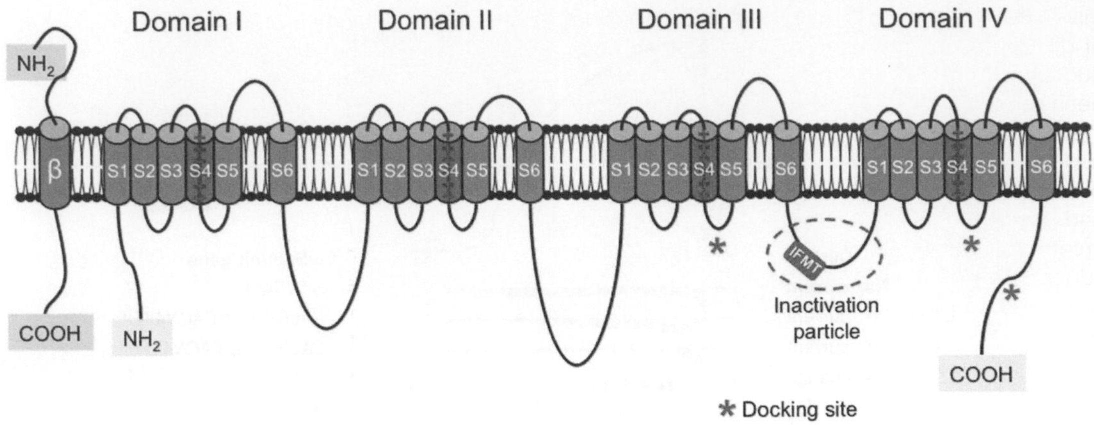


**Fig. 2.** The α- and β-subunits of the voltage-gated sodium channel. The 4 homologous domains (I–IV) of the α-subunit are represented; S5 and S6 are the pore-lining segments and S4 is the core of the voltage-sensor. In the cytoplasmic linker between domains III and IV, the IFMT (isoleucine, phenylalanine, methionine, and threonine) region is indicated, which is a critical part of the "inactivation particle" (inactivation gate), and substitution of aminoacids in this region can disrupt the inactivation process of the channel. The "docking site" consists of multiple regions that include the cytoplasmic linker between S4 and S5 in domains III and IV and the cytoplasmic end of the S6 segment in domain IV (*asterisk*). Depending on the subtype of β-subunit considered, they can interact (covalently or noncovalently) with the α-subunit. (*From* Savio-Galimberti E, Gollob MH, Darbar D. Voltage-gated sodium channels: biophysics, pharmacology, and related channelopathies. Front Pharmacol 2012;3:124. http://dx.doi.org/10.3389/fphar.2012.00124. eCollection 2012.)

$Na_V1.8$ channel in human atrial samples collected during surgery for valve disease using immunohistochemistry.

## ROLE OF CARDIAC POTASSIUM AND SODIUM CHANNEL MUTATIONS IN INCREASED SUSCEPTIBILITY TO ATRIAL FIBRILLATION

The clinical and genetic heterogeneity of AF may in part be related to the poor understanding of the underlying pathophysiology of AF. Although most cases of AF are acquired and related to structural remodeling of the atria, in approximately 30% of patients AF occurs without structural heart disease. It is in this group of patients with early-onset AF that common and rare *SCN5A* variants may not only play an important role in the pathophysiology of AF but also identify underlying mechanisms.[25] However, it should be appreciated that the familial monogenic AF is an uncommon disease.

The first mutations linked with AF were identified in genes encoding cardiac potassium channels. A mutation in *KCNQ1* (S140G), encoding the α-subunit of the slowly repolarizing potassium channel current $I_{Ks}$, was identified in a large Chinese family with 16 members who developed early-onset AF. When the *KCNQ1* S140G mutation was expressed in a heterologous expression system, a marked increase in $I_{Ks}$ was discovered. It is postulated that this gain-of-function mutation may lead to shortening of the atrial AP duration (APD) and the effective refractory period (ERP) of the atria.[26] Several gain-of-function mutations in *KCNQ1* have subsequently been reported.[14] Identification of *KCNQ1* as an AF-causative gene led to screening of other cardiac potassium channels as potential candidate genes for familial AF. Mutations in *KCNE1*,[27] *KCNE2*,[28] *KCNE3*,[29] *KCNE5*,[30] *KCND3*,[31] *KCNJ2*,[32,33] and *KCNA5*[34] have now all been associated with increased susceptibility to AF. Most potassium channel variants associated with AF exhibit a gain-of-function cellular phenotype and predispose to AF by shortening of the atrial APD and ERP.[13,14] However, loss-of-function mutations in *KCNA5*, encoding the $K_V1.5$ channel, have also been reported.[35–37] These loss-of-function mutations are postulated to prolong atrial APD and trigger early afterdepolarizations and thereby provide an electrophysiologic substrate for AF. Although mutations in cardiac potassium channels modulate atrial APD and likely generate an electrophysiologic substrate for AF, large-scale resequencing has not identified genes encoding cardiac potassium channels as a common cause for AF.[38,39]

## ROLE OF *SCN5A* MUTATIONS IN MIXED INHERITED ARRHYTHMIA SYNDROMES

Both common and rare genetic variants in the cardiac sodium channel have also been associated with the development of AF. *SCN5A* was considered a strong candidate gene for AF after the publication of 2 studies that showed that mutations in this gene were linked with a syndrome comprising of dilated cardiomyopathy, AF, and cardiac conduction disease.[40,41] AF-causing variants have been reported in both the α-subunit (encoded by the *SCN5A* gene) and associated β-subunits (encoded by the genes *SCN1B–SCN4B*). Similar to potassium channel genetic variants, both gain- and loss-of-function mutations are capable of creating a proarrhythmogenic substrate, further supporting the idea that mutations in cardiac sodium channel genes are also candidate genes for AF.

*SCN5A* mutations are associated not only with AF but also with ventricular inherited syndromes such long-QT syndrome (LQTS), sudden infant death syndrome, and Brugada syndrome, as well as progressive cardiac conduction disease, and more complex overlapping inherited arrhythmia syndromes. There is a high incidence (20%–40%) of AF in Brugada patients presenting with *SCN5A* mutations.[42,43] As would be expected with loss of function of the cardiac sodium channel, these patients often also have evidence of progressive conduction disease with prolonged atrioventricular and atrial-His conduction. There is also a high incidence (~2%) of AF in patients with the LQTS.[44] Benito and colleagues[45] identified a moderate-sized kindred where an *SCN5A* gain of function mutation was associated with a mixed phenotype of prolonged QT intervals and AF. Although the precise electrophysiologic mechanisms by which an *SCN5A* mutation gives rise to a mixed phenotype such as LQTS and AF, Brugada syndrome, and progressive conduction disease have not been completely determined, one explanation may relate to differential expression or chamber-specific interactions between the $Na_V1.5$ protein and its partners; these may be β-subunits, other sodium channels such as *SCN10A*, which encodes $Na_V1.8$ or proteins that have not yet been identified.

## *SCN5A* MUTATIONS AND ATRIAL FIBRILLATION

The first comprehensive resequencing of the entire coding region of *SCN5A* in patients with AF was performed in 2008. Here, the authors screened 375 subjects with early-onset AF (n = 118) or AF associated with traditional risk factors (n = 257) and identified 8 novel *SCN5A* mutations, not found in a control population, in 10 familial AF probands.[39] These variants were in highly conserved residues and cosegregated with AF in 6 familial AF kindreds. Furthermore, when these variants were expressed in a heterologous expression system, they modulated the biophysics of the $Na_V1.5$ channel.[46] Although 4 of the 8 novel variants were identified in probands with early-onset AF (age 36 ± 14 years), AF in the other 4 probands was associated with underlying structural heart disease (cardiomyopathy, hypertension, or ischemic heart disease). The authors also identified 12 rare *SCN5A* variants that have previously been reported and 3 common SNPs.[39]

Since then, other studies have confirmed the association between *SCN5A* variants and increased susceptibility to AF. In 2008, Ellinor and colleagues[38] reported the results of a study where they showed that an *SCN5A* mutation contributes to the development of early-onset AF. However, this study was limited by the small size; out of a total cohort of 189 patients with early-onset AF, only 57 AF probands with family history underwent further evaluation. A single *SCN5A* mutation (N1986K), absent in 600 control chromosomes, was identified in a small familial AF kindred. The expression of this mutant in Xenopus oocytes demonstrated a hyperpolarizing shift in the steady state inactivation of the N1986K mutant channel, which would be expected to result in an effective loss of function of the sodium channel and prolongation of the atrial APD.

Although shortening of the atrial APD is the most common postulated mechanism for the initiation of AF, an alternative mechanism may relate to prolongation of the atrial APD.[35] This mechanism is supported by several studies where *SCN5A* gain-of-function mutations have been linked with increased susceptibility to AF. In 2009, Li and colleagues[47] reported an *SCN5A* gain-of-function mutation in AF patients that can enhance cellular excitability and lowered the AP threshold.[13] Most recently, Ziyadeh-Isleem and colleagues[48] reported an *SCN5A* C-terminal truncating mutation (R1860Gfs*12) identified in a family presenting with a complex clinical phenotype of sick-sinus syndrome and AF or atrial flutter. The mutation was a 1 bp (A) deletion at position 5578 in exon 28. This deletion induced a frameshift mutation, R1860Gfs*12, which changed the arginine in position 1860 to glycine followed by 10 frameshift amino acids before a premature stop codon. The heterologous expression of the mutant channels alone or in combination with the wild-type channel demonstrated an approximately 70% reduction in the sodium current density. As this mutation involved the C-terminus, inactivation of the channel was markedly impaired giving rise to persistent late sodium current; this was described as both a combined loss- and gain-of-function mutation, because the mutation not only decreased the peak current but also exhibited a persistent late current. The increased persistent late $I_{Na}$ can disrupt repolarization of atrial myocytes and prolong APD, thereby providing another potential mechanism by which the mutation may increase susceptibility to AF.

## CHALLENGES ASSOCIATED WITH LINKING *SCN5A* VARIANTS WITH INCREASED SUSCEPTIBILITY TO ATRIAL FIBRILLATION

The authors and other investigators have identified *SCN5A* mutations that have been linked with mixed phenotypes and postulated potential mechanisms to explain the diverse arrhythmia syndromes.[13,49] However, these studies clearly highlight some of the challenges encountered when trying to determine the pathogenicity of an *SCN5A* mutation and uncovering the underlying mechanisms.

Multiple approaches have been used to distinguish between benign rare polymorphisms and pathogenic mutations: screening a large ethnically matched control population in a large kindred evaluating if the variant cosegregates with AF; determining whether the variant is evolutionary conserved using in silico prediction models; and functionally characterizing the variant in vitro.[50] Although heterologous expression systems and in vitro studies can contribute to the characterization of the variants, these systems tend to be oversimplified models that fail to recapitulate the electrical milieu in which the variants function and do not necessarily provide clarification of how both loss- and gain-of-function *SCN5A* mutations may cause a diverse array of clinical arrhythmia phenotypes.

Although other expression modeling systems, such as cardiac myocytes and induced pluripotent stem cell (iPSc)-derived myocytes, have also been proposed as suitable models to dissect the underlying mechanisms associated with *SCN5A* mutations, these approaches also have several limitations. One of the techniques used to transfer a gene into mammalian cells (like cardiomyocytes) is using adenoviral or retroviral/lentiviral vectors. As retroviral vectors only accommodate approximately 8kb of DNA, this poses problems when attempting to insert the complete coding region of a gene like *SCN5A*, whose size is approximately 10,161 kb, and its promoter elements.[51,52] An alternate approach is the transfection of sodium channels in neonatal cardiomyocytes instead of adult myocytes. Neonatal cells are less committed and more "plastic" in terms of gene expression. However, the disadvantage of transfecting neonatal cells is that they exhibit an immature electrophysiologic phenotype that does not completely recapitulate the adult atrial AP. The use of iPSc-derived cardiomyocytes (iPSc-CM) is even more technically challenging, with the major obstacle related to the lack of clear atrial structure and electrophysiologic phenotype of these early cardiomyocytes. Although criticized, the use of iPSc-CM is a new approach that is actively developing and has been adopted by many scientific groups as the more approachable disease model that can provide an improved inside in diseases based on genotype specificity.[53,54]

Genetically modified mice have also been proposed as a complimentary approach to in vitro electrophysiology to explore and improve our understanding of the pathophysiologic consequences of *SCN5A* mutations. Although many *SCN5A* mouse models generated express either an LQT type 3 or Brugada syndrome phenotypes, some do also exhibit mixed phenotypes.[55] Furthermore, many mouse models of SCN5A mutations also demonstrate inducible AF.[56] The lack of mouse models of *SCN5A* genetic variants exhibiting purely an AF phenotype highlights some of the challenges and complexities of dissecting the underlying pathophysiology of AF related to cardiac sodium channel mutations.

## REFERENCES


1. Brugada R, Kaab S. Genetics of AF. Chapter 6. In: Natale A, Jalife J, editors. Atrial fibrillation: from bench to bedside. Totowa (NJ): Humana Press; 2008. p. 69–76.
2. Benjamin EJ, Levy D, Vaziri SM, et al. Independent risk factors in a population-based cohort. The Framingham heart study. JAMA 1994;271(11): 840–4.
3. Sinner MF, Ellinor PT, Meitinger T, et al. Genome-wide association studies of atrial fibrillation: past, present, and future. Cardiovasc Res 2011;89(4): 701–9.
4. Cristophersen IE, Ravn LS, Budtz-Joergensen E, et al. Familial aggregation of atrial fibrillation: a study in Danish twins. Circ Arrhythm Electrophysiol 2009;4:378–83.
5. Wyse DG, Van Gelder IC, Ellinor PT, et al. Lone atrial fibrillation: does it exist? J Am Coll Cardiol 2014;63(17):1715–23.
6. Kirchhof P, Breithardt G, Aliot E, et al. Personalized management of atrial fibrillation: proceedings from the fourth atrial fibrillation competence NETwork/European Heart Rhythm Association consensus conference. Europace 2013;11:1540–56.
7. Gudbjartsson DF, Arnar DO, Helgadottir A, et al. Variants conferring risk of atrial fibrillation on chromosome 4q25. Nature 2007;448:353–7.
8. Ellinor PT, Lunetta KL, Albert CM, et al. Meta-analysis identifies six new susceptibility loci for atrial fibrillation. Nat Genet 2012;44(6):670–5.

9. Ellinor PT, Lunetta KL, Glazer NL, et al. Common variants in *KCNN3* are associated with lone atrial fibrillation. Nat Genet 2010;42(3):240–4.
10. Benjamin EJ, Rice KM, Arking DE, et al. Variants in *ZFHX3* are associated with atrial fibrillation in individuals of European ancestry. Nat Genet 2009; 41(8):879–81.
11. Parvez B, Darbar D. The "missing" link in atrial fibrillation heritability. J Electrocardiol 2011;44(6):641–4. http://dx.doi.org/10.1016/j.electrocard.2011.07.027.
12. Wolf PA, Abbott RD, Kannel WB. Atrial fibrillation as an independent risk factor for stroke: the Framingham Study. Stroke 1991;22(8):983–8.
13. Darbar D, Roden DM. Genetic mechanisms of atrial fibrillation: impact on response to treatment. Nat Rev Cardiol 2013;10(6):317–29.
14. Tucker NR, Ellinor PT. Emerging directions in the genetics of atrial fibrillation. Circ Res 2014;114(9): 1469–82.
15. Hatem SN, Coulombe A, Balse E. Specificities of atrial electrophysiology: clues to a better understanding of cardiac function and the mechanisms of arrhythmias. J Mol Cell Cardiol 2010;48(1):90–5.
16. Li GR, Nattel S. Properties of human atrial ICa at physiological temperatures and relevance to action potential. Am J Physiol 1997;272(1 Pt 2):H227–35.
17. Escande D, Coulombe A, Faivre JF, et al. Two types of transient outward currents in adult human atrial cells. Am J Physiol 1987;252(1 Pt 2):H142–8.
18. Ruben PC. Handbook of Experimental Pharmacology, vol. 221. Springer-Verlag Berlin Heidelberg; 2014.
19. Payandeh J, Scheuer T, Zheng N, et al. The crystal structure of a voltage-gated sodium channel. Nature 2011;475(7356):353–8.
20. Savio-Galimberti E, Gollob MH, Darbar D. Voltage-gated sodium channels: biophysics, pharmacology, and related channelopathies. Front Pharmacol 2012; 3:124. http://dx.doi.org/10.3389/fphar.2012.00124. eCollection 2012.
21. Patino GA, Isom LL. Electrophysiology and beyond: multiple roles of Na+ channel beta subunits in development and disease. Neurosci Lett 2010;486(2):53–9.
22. Haufe V, Chamberland C, Dumaine R. The promiscuous nature of the cardiac sodium channel. J Mol Cell Cardiol 2007;42(3):469–77.
23. Yang T, Atack T, Stroud DM, et al. Blocking Scn10a channels in heart reduces late sodium current and is antiarrhythmic. Circ Res 2012;111(3):322–32.
24. Facer P, Punjabi PP, Abrari A, et al. Localisation of *SCN10A* gene product Na(v)1.8 and novel pain-related ion channels in human heart. Int Heart J 2011;52(3):146–52.
25. Darbar D, Hardy A, Haines JL, et al. Prolonged signal-averaged P-wave duration as an intermediate phenotype for familial atrial fibrillation. J Am Coll Cardiol 2008;51(11):1083–9.
26. Chen YH, Xu SJ, Bendahhou S, et al. *KCNQ1* gain-of-function mutation in familial atrial fibrillation. Science 2003;299(5604):251–4.
27. Oleson MS, Bentzen BH, Nielsen JB, et al. Mutations in the potassium channel subunit *KCNE1* are associated with early-onset familial atrial fibrillation. BMC Med Genet 2012;13:24.
28. Yang Y, Xia M, Jin Q, et al. Identification of a *KCNE2* gain-of-function mutation in patients with familial atrial fibrillation. Am J Hum Genet 2004; 75(5):899–905.
29. Lundby A, Ravn LS, Svendsen JH, et al. *KCNE3* mutation V17M identified in a patient with lone atrial fibrillation. Cell Physiol Biochem 2008;21(1–3): 47–54.
30. Ravn LS, Aizawa Y, Pollevick GD, et al. Gain of function in IKs secondary to a mutation in *KCNE5* associated with atrial fibrillation. Heart Rhythm 2008;5(3):427–35.
31. Olesen MS, Refsgaard L, Hoist AG, et al. A novel *KCND3* gain-of-function mutation associated with early-onset of persistent lone atrial fibrillation. Cardiovasc Res 2013;98(3):488–95.
32. Deo M, Ruan Y, Padit SV, et al. *KCNJ2* mutation in short QT syndrome 3 results in atrial fibrillation and ventricular proarrhythmia. Proc Natl Acad Sci U S A 2013;110(11):4291–6.
33. Xia M, Jin Q, Bendahhou S, et al. A Kir2.1 gain-of-function mutation underlies familial atrial fibrillation. Biochem Biophys Res Commun 2005;332(4): 1012–9.
34. Christophensen IE, Olesen MS, Liang B, et al. Genetic variation in *KCNA5*: impact on the atrial-specific potassium current IKur in patients with lone atrial fibrillation. Eur Heart J 2013;34(20): 1517–25.
35. Olson TM, Alekseev AE, Liu XK, et al. Kv1.5 channelopathy due to *KCNA5* loss-of-function mutation causes human atrial fibrillation. Hum Mol Genet 2006;15(14):2185–91.
36. Yang Y, Li J, Lin X, et al. Novel *KCNA5* loss-of-function mutations responsible for atrial fibrillation. J Hum Genet 2009;54(5):277–83.
37. Yang T, Yang P, Roden DM, et al. Novel *KCNA5* mutation implicates tyrosine kinase signaling in human atrial fibrillation. Heart Rhythm 2010;7(9): 1246–52.
38. Ellinor PT, Nam EG, Shea MA, et al. Cardiac sodium channel mutation in atrial fibrillation. Heart Rhythm 2008;5(1):99–105.
39. Darbar D, Kannankeril PJ, Donahue BS, et al. Cardiac sodium channel (*SCN5A*) variants associated with atrial fibrillation. Circulation 2008;117(15): 1927–35.
40. McNair WP, Ku L, Taylor MR, et al. Familial Cardiomyopathy Registry Research Group. SCN5A mutation associated with dilated cardiomyopathy,

conduction disorder, and arrhythmia. Circulation 2004;110(15):2163–7.
41. Olson TM, Michels VV, Ballew JD, et al. Sodium channel mutations and susceptibility to heart failure and atrial fibrillation. JAMA 2005;293(4): 447–54.
42. Morita H, Kusano-Fukushima K, Nagase S, et al. Atrial fibrillation and atrial vulnerability in patients with Brugada syndrome. J Am Coll Cardiol 2002; 40(8):1437–44.
43. Antzelevitch C, Brugada P, Borggrefe M, et al. Brugada syndrome: report of the second consensus conference: endorsed by the Heart Rhythm Society and the European Heart Rhythm Association. Circulation 2005;111(5):659–70.
44. Johnson JN, Tester DJ, Perry J, et al. Prevalence of early-onset atrial fibrillation in congenital long QT syndrome. Heart Rhythm 2008;5(5):704–9.
45. Benito B, Brugada R, Perich RM, et al. A mutation in the sodium channel is responsible for the association of long QT syndrome and familial atrial fibrillation. Heart Rhythm 2008;5(10):1434–40.
46. Wang DW, Gillani N, Roden DM, et al. Sodium channel variants associated with atrial fibrillation exhibit abnormal fast and slow inactivation. Biophys J 2010;98:S1–10.
47. Li Q, Huang H, Liu G, et al. Gain-of-function mutation in Nav1.5 in atrial fibrillation enhances cellular excitability and lowers the threshold for action potential firing. Biochem Biophys Res Commun 2009;380(1):132–7.
48. Ziyadeh-Isleem A, Clatot J, Duchatelet S, et al. A truncated *SCN5A* mutation combined with genetic variability causes sick sinus syndrome and early atrial fibrillation. Heart Rhythm 2014; 11(6):1015–23. http://dx.doi.org/10.1016/j.hrthm.2014.02.021.
49. Remme CA, Wilde AA, Bezzina CR. Cardiac sodium channel overlap syndromes: different faces of *SCN5A* Mutations. Trends Cardiovasc Med 2008;18:78–87.
50. Darbar D. IS it time to develop a "pathogenicity" score to distinguish long QT syndrome causing mutations from "background" genetic noise? Heart Rhythm 2009;6(9):1304–5.
51. Dale JW, Von Schantz M, Plant N. Modifying organisms. Transgenics. Chapter 11. In: From genes to genomes. 3rd edition. United Kingdom: Wiley & Sons, Ltd; 2012.
52. Louch WE, Sheehan KA, Wolska BM. Methods in cardiomyocyte isolation, culture, and gene transfer. J Mol Cell Cardiol 2011;51:288–98.
53. Josowitz R, Carvajal-Vergara X, Lemischka IR, et al. Induced pluripotent stem cell-derived cardiomyocytes as models for genetic cardiovascular disorders. Curr Opin Cardiol 2011;26:223–9.
54. Knollmann BC. Induced pluripotent stem cell-derived cardiomyocytes. Boutique science or valuable arrhythmia model? Circ Res 2013;112:969–76.
55. Carpentier F, Bourge A, Merot J. Mouse models of *SCN5A*-related cardiac arrhythmias. Prog Biophys Mol Biol 2008;98(2–3):230–7.
56. Watanabe H, Yang T, Stroud DM, et al. Striking in vivo phenotype of a disease-associated human *SCN5A* mutation producing minimal changes in vitro. Circulation 2011;124(9):1001–11.

# The Role of the Cardiac Sodium Channel in Perinatal Early Infant Mortality

Lia Crotti, MD, PhD[a,b,c,d,*], Alice Ghidoni, PhD[b,c], Roberto Insolia, PhD[c], Peter J. Schwartz, MD[a,b]

**KEYWORDS**

• Sodium channel • SIDS • Stillbirth • IUFD • Long QT syndrome • Perinatal mortality • Genetics

**KEY POINTS**

- The cardiac sodium channel plays an important role in arrhythmias of genetic origin and is implicated in perinatal mortality.
- Channelopathies have been implicated in 15% of sudden infant death syndrome (SIDS) cases, and genetic variants with a functional effect on *SCN5A* or in sodium channel ancillary proteins are present in most of them.
- Genetic variants with a functional effect on long QT syndrome [LQTS] genes are present in 8.8% of intrauterine unexplained fetal death [IUFD] cases and *SCN5A* plays a major role.
- Patients with severe LQTS type 3 (LQT3) manifesting in the perinatal early infant period are associated with very marked QT prolongations, which make them easily identifiable by electrocardiogram screening in the first month of life, thus enhancing the chances of effective preventive therapies.
- There are differences between *SCN5A* mutations producing severe early-onset LQT3 and SIDS/IUFD in terms of topology and frequency in the general population. This observation translates in pathophysiologic considerations.

## INTRODUCTION

Mortality in the perinatal and infant period is an important public health issue and indeed, their rate of occurrence represents a commonly used indicator of the health status of any given population.[1] A wide range of causes are associated with such a tragic event (ie, a variety of diseases including infections and congenital defects, poor nutritional status, etc.), and their relative importance varies significantly in different countries according to the socioeconomic conditions.[2] The identification of the causes is essential to allow the implementation of focused preventive approaches.[2] However, still a significant number of these deaths (25%–40% of stillbirths and approximately 10% of neonatal demises) are unexplained after a thorough postmortem examination[3,4]; it is among these that sodium channel dysfunctions play a role.

Ion channel diseases, the so-called *channelopathies*, are a group of genetically transmitted heart diseases, characterized by a morphologic normal heart and a predisposition to life-threatening arrhythmias, which could cause sudden cardiac

Disclosure: None of the authors have conflicts of interest to disclose.

[a] Center for Cardiac Arrhythmias of Genetic Origin, IRCCS Istituto Auxologico Italiano, Casa di Cura San Carlo, Via Pier Lombardo 22, Milan 20135, Italy; [b] Laboratory of Cardiovascular Genetics, IRCCS Istituto Auxologico Italiano, via Zucchi 18, Cusano Milanino (MI), Milan 20095, Italy; [c] Department of Molecular Medicine, University of Pavia, IRCCS Fondazione Policlinico San Matteo, Viale Golgi 19, Pavia 27100, Italy; [d] Helmholtz Zentrum München, Institute of Human Genetics, Ingolstaedter Landstrasse 1, Neuherberg 85764, Germany
* Corresponding author. Center for Cardiac Arrhythmias of Genetic Origin, IRCCS Istituto Auxologico Italiano, Casa di Cura San Carlo, Via Pier Lombardo 22, Milan 20135, Italy.
*E-mail address:* liacrotti@yahoo.it

Card Electrophysiol Clin 6 (2014) 749–759
http://dx.doi.org/10.1016/j.ccep.2014.07.009
1877-9182/14/$ – see front matter 

death (SCD) even very early in life.[5] Whenever SCD is the first clinical manifestation of the disease, these cases would be labeled according to the age of occurrence, as sudden unexplained deaths (SUD),[5,6] sudden infant death syndrome (SIDS),[7,8] or intrauterine unexplained fetal deaths (IUFD).[3] Channelopathies have been recognized as the cause of the SCD in approximately 35% of SUD, 15% of SIDS, and 9% of IUFD[3,6–8] and mutations in *SCN5A* have been identified in all subgroups.

## THE CARDIAC SODIUM CHANNEL

The cardiac sodium channel, a member of the voltage-dependent family of ion channels, is a transmembrane protein involved in the generation and transmission of action potential. It is a large molecular complex containing an $\alpha$-subunit, 4 ancillary $\beta$-subunits, and several regulatory proteins.[9] The $\alpha$-subunit of the channel (designated $Na_v1.5$) forming the ion conducting pore is encoded by the *SCN5A* gene (UCSC uc021wvo.1; OMIM #603830) located on the short arm of chromosome 3 (3p21–24).[10] $Na_v1.5$ consists of 4 homologous domains, from DI to DIV, with 3 interdomain linkers. These linkers, as well as the N- and C-terminus of the protein, are located inside the cytoplasm of the cell.

The $Na^+$ channel isoform $Na_v1.5$ is the predominant $\alpha$-subunit in the human heart[11]; however, other 4 splice variants are recognized, known respectively as $Na_v1.5a$ (exon 18 deletion), $Na_v1.5c$ (glutamine 1077 insertion), $Na_v1.5d$ (deletion in exon 17), and $Na_v1.5e$ (alternative neonatal exon 6a).[12] Specifically, exon 6, encoding part of the S3/S4 region in DI, is known to be alternatively spliced through developmental stages, being different in neonatal and adult heart.[13] The neonatal ($Na_v1.5e$) and the adult isoforms ($Na_v1.5$) behave differently in patch-clamp experiments[14] and this should be considered when studying sodium channel mutations implicated in perinatal mortality.

Sodium channel mutations causing an increase in persistent inward $Na^+$ current during myocardial repolarization are referred to as gain-of-function mutations and are responsible for the type 3 variant of long QT syndrome (LQT3).[15] In this subgroup of LQTS patients, most cardiac events occur while patients are at rest or asleep (**Fig. 1**),[16] consistent with what observed in SIDS cases. Loss-of-function mutations in the sodium channel gene can result in different channelopathies, the main one being Brugada syndrome (BrS).[5] Currently there are more than 300 known *SCN5A* mutations associated with the Brugada phenotype, whereas among the minor genes implicated in the disease,[17] around half are proteins modulating the sodium channel function. Because the clinical manifestations of BrS usually occur in adulthood, loss-of-function mutations in the sodium channel gene are usually less implicated in perinatal mortality compared with gain-of-function mutations.

## ROLE OF *SCN5A* IN NEONATAL SUDDEN UNEXPECTED DEATHS

SIDS remains the leading cause of mortality in the first year of life and its actual prevalence is around 0.5 to 0.6 per 1000 live births.[7] During the Second

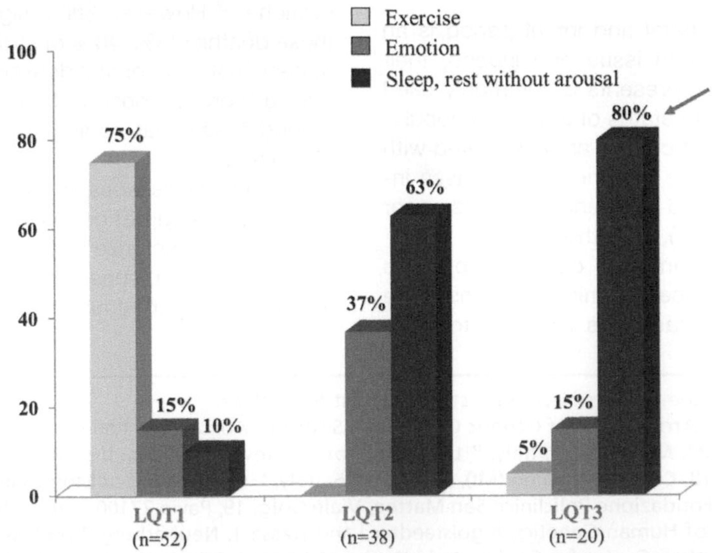


**Fig. 1.** Triggers for lethal and nonlethal cardiac events in the 3 main LQTS genotypes. The arrow indicates that patients carrying a mutation in *SCN5A* (LQT3) have most of the cardiac events at rest or during sleep. (*Adapted from* Schwartz PJ, Priori SG, Spazzolini C, et al. Genotype-phenotype correlation in the long-QT syndrome: gene-specific triggers for life-threatening arrhythmias. Circulation 2001;103:89–95.)

International Conference on Causes of Sudden Death in Infants, held in Seattle in 1970,[18] Beckwith provided its first classic definition: *SIDS is the sudden death of any infant or young child which is unexpected by history, and in which a thorough postmortem examination fails to demonstrate an adequate cause of death*. This definition remains valid, despite several revisions by the National Institute of Child Health and Human Development (NICHD), with the specification that the victim had to be younger than the age of 1 year, the death had to occur during sleep, and had to include not only a complete postmortem examination but also an evaluation of clinical history and a review of the death scene.[19]

Many different theories have been developed during the years to explain these deaths *sine materia* and many different risk factors have been identified, some maternal (ie, multiple pregnancies, young age, smoking, drug intake, alcohol use), some infant-specific (ie, prone sleeping, prematurity, low birth weight), and some environmental (ie, bed-sharing with parents or siblings, winter months, low socioeconomic status, lack of breastfeeding).[7] Progressively it has been accepted that SIDS is a multifactorial disease, that is, many different causes can provoke the SCD of an infant and multiple factors, by themselves insufficient, may act synergistically to induce sudden death. The latter concept represents the so-called *triple risk model*[20] that hypothesizes that SIDS may occur only if a vulnerable infant is exposed to one or more exogenous stressors, during a critical developmental period.[20] Not in contrast with the *triple risk model* is the *cardiac hypothesis*, formally advanced in 1976.[21] According to this hypothesis, some cases of SIDS may be due to a lethal cardiac arrhythmia, that is, ventricular fibrillation, through a mechanism similar to the one acting in the congenital LQTS. In this context, a mutation in a cardiac ion channel gene may render an infant vulnerable, and whenever a trigger is present, during a critical developmental period, SIDS may occur.[7]

The proof of concept that LQTS can cause SIDS came in 2000,[22] when a 44-day-old infant was found by the parents cyanotic, apneic, and pulseless. If this infant had not been found by the parents in time to be rushed to a nearby hospital and resuscitated from documented ventricular fibrillation, it would have been a typical SIDS case. The infant had a corrected QT interval of 648 ms, and a *de novo* mutation (S941N) in *SCN5A* was identified (**Fig. 2**).[22] In the following years, the relevance of LQTS was evaluated in different cohorts of SIDS cases[23–26] and the presence of functional mutations in the LQTS genes was identified in 10% to 15% of cases. The $Na^+$ channel in particular plays a major role in SIDS. Indeed, more than half of the mutations identified in population-based cohort studies are related to the $Na^+$ channel.[23–27] Specifically, in addition to mutations in the $\alpha$-subunit of the $Na^+$ channel (encoded by the *SCN5A* gene), mutations in the $\beta$-subunit–encoding genes (*SCN1Bb*, *SCN3B*, *SCN4B*) and in $Na_v1.5$ regulatory genes (*CAV3*, *SNTA1*, *GPD1L*) were identified (**Fig. 3**). The relevance of $Na^+$ channel dysfunctions in the genesis of SIDS is also in line with the clinical evidence that both in LQT3 and SIDS the life-threatening events occur at rest or during sleep.[7,16]

As previously mentioned, an impaired cardiac $Na^+$ channel can lead to both LQTS (gain-of-function) and BrS (loss-of-function), depending on the functional effect of the specific mutation. In the literature there are also some examples of SIDS in which the electrophysiologic properties of the SCN5A mutations are associated with a more Brugada-like phenotype.[26]

**Table 1** provides the list of *SCN5A* mutations and mutations in $Na_v1.5$-related genes[23,26,28–35] identified in SIDS cases.

Recently, Andreasen and colleagues[36] questioned the role of *SCN5A* variants identified in SIDS cases, because they observed their presence also in the general population, as reported in the Exome Variant Server (EVS) database.[37] In the authors' view, this could simply mean that variants present in the EVS are not sufficient to cause SCD by themselves, but they could act as favoring factors, according to the triple risk model.[20]

## ROLE OF *SCN5A* IN INTRAUTERINE UNEXPLAINED FETAL DEATH

IUFD, including miscarriages (fetal losses $<$20th week of gestation) and stillbirths (fetal losses $\geq$20th week), is a major public health problem with significant impact especially on the mothers. Stillbirth has an incidence of 6.05 per 1000 live births.[38] In 70% of cases a probable or a possible cause to explain the demise can be identified (40% placental, 21.5% fetal, 12.7% maternal causes), whereas the remaining cases are unexplained.[39,40] Cardiac channelopathies have been shown to contribute to sudden death in children and infants with an inconclusive autopsy.[7,8,24] Therefore, it was logical to think that the same mechanism causing SCD in the first few months of life could cause SCD also just before birth.[41] The first proof of this concept came from a study by Hoorntje and colleagues,[42] which found a homozygous premature truncation of the *KCNH2*

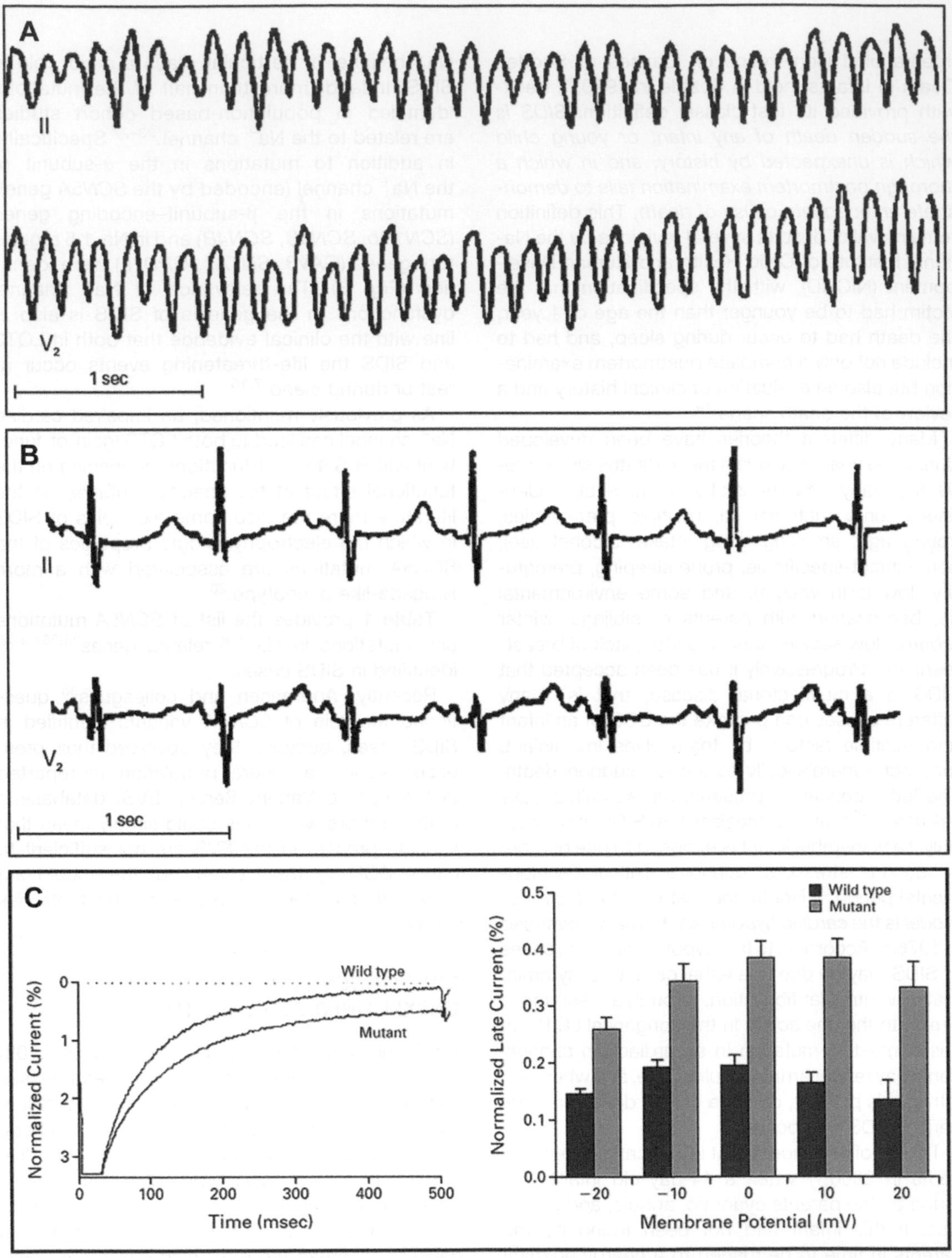


**Fig. 2.** Electrocardiograms (ECGs) at the time of admission to the hospital (*A*) and after the restoration of sinus rhythm by countershock (*B*). At hospital admission, this 44-day-old infant had ventricular fibrillation (*A*). After return to sinus rhythm, the ECG showed a QT interval extremely prolonged (QTc 648 ms) (*B*) and also a clear T wave alternans. He was found to carry SCN5A-S941N, a *de novo* mutation. Whole-cell current traces measured in *Xenopus laevis* oocytes and recorded with a voltage-clamp protocol (*C*). Representative wild-type and mutant (SCN5A-S941N) late Na+ currents, expressed as the percentage of the peak current that was tetrodotoxin-sensitive and recorded at 0 mV, are shown on the left. The relative amplitudes of the wild-type and mutant late sodium currents measured at 300 ms are showed on the right at different membrane potentials ($P<.001$). Values are means (+SD) of 7 experiments. (*Modified from* Schwartz PJ, Priori SG, Dumaine R, et al. A molecular link between the sudden infant death syndrome and the long-QT syndrome. N Engl J Med 2000;343:263–5; with permission.)

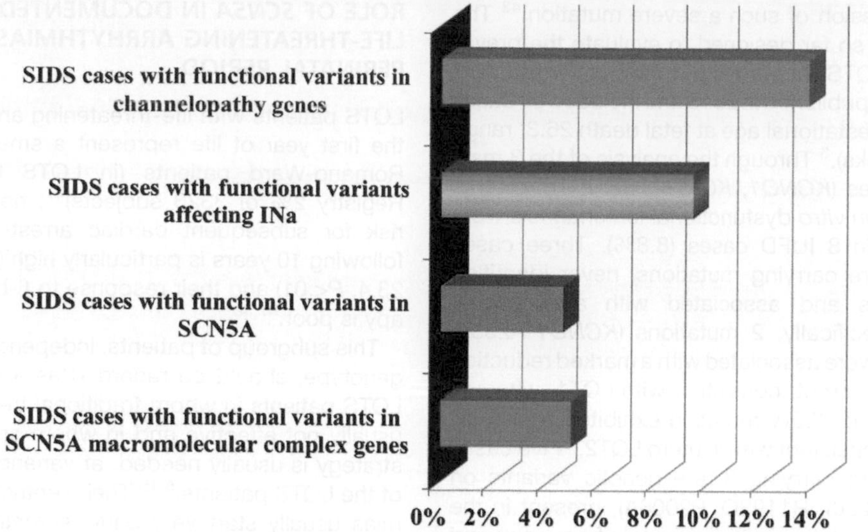


**Fig. 3.** Percentage of SIDS cases with functional genetic variants identified in cardiac channelopathy genes and reported in population-based cohort studies. Comparison among SIDS carriers of mutations in channelopathy-associated genes, SIDS cases with functional variants affecting INa, SIDS cases with functional variants located in *SCN5A* or in ancillary proteins forming the SCN5A macromolecular complex. The percentages are obtained according to **Table 1**.

protein in a stillbirth case and in the sister who was born premature in distress, due to ventricular arrhythmia in the presence of severe QT prolongation. Later on, the *SCN5A*-R1623Q mutation was identified as the cause of 2 stillbirths and of a malignant perinatal LQTS, requiring cardiac transplantation, in the 3 siblings[43]; the mother had a mosaicism and this explains the possibility

**Table 1**
**SIDS-associated genetic variants in the cardiac sodium channel gene and in its ancillary proteins**

| Gene | Protein | Cardiac Functional Role | Genetic Variant | Reported Study [Ref] |
|---|---|---|---|---|
| *SCN5A* | $Na_v1.5$ | α-subunit of $I_{Na}$ channel | **S216L, delAL586–587, R680H, R1193Q (2 cases), T1304M, F1486L, V1951L, F2004L (3 cases), P2006A (2 cases)** | 23 |
| | | | **F532C, G1084S, F1705S** | 26 |
| | | | **A997S, R1826H** | 28 |
| | | | S524Y (2 cases), **R689H, E1107K** | 29 |
| | | | Q692K, R975W, **S1333Y** | 30 |
| *CAV3* | Caveolin-3 | Caveolar coating | **V14L, T78M, L79R** | 31 |
| | | | C72W, **T78M** | 23 |
| *SNTA1* | α1-syntrophin | Scaffolding protein | G54R, P56S, T262P, **S287R, T372M, G460S** | 32 |
| *SCN1Bb* | Navβ1B | β-subunit of $I_{Na}$ channel | **R214Q** | 33 |
| *SCN3B* | Navβ3 | β-subunit of $I_{Na}$ channel | **V36M, V54G** | 34 |
| *SCN4B* | Navβ4 | β-subunit of $I_{Na}$ channel | **S206L** | 34 |
| *GPD1-L* | G3PD1L | Glycerol-3-phosphate dehydrogenase 1-like | **I124V, R273C** | 35 |

Note: Functionally significant variants are in bold; homozygous and double/triple mutation carriers are excluded.

of transmission of such a severe mutation.[43] The only study so far designed to evaluate the prevalence of LQTS mutations in a population of IUFD cases was published in 2013 and included 91 cases (average gestational age at fetal death 26.3; range 14–41 weeks).[3] Through the analysis of the 3 main LQTS genes (*KCNQ1*, *KCNH2*, *SCN5A*), variants leading to *in vitro* dysfunctional ion channels were identified in 8 IUFD cases (8.8%). Three cases (3.3%) were carrying mutations, never identified in controls and associated with a functional effect; specifically, 2 mutations (*KCNQ1*-A283T, -R397W), were associated with a marked reduction of the $I_{Ks}$ current, consistent with LQT1, whereas the HERG1b-R25W mutation exhibited a loss-of-function consistent with in utero LQT2.[3] Five cases (5.5%) were carrying 3 rare genetic variants on *SCN5A* (T220I, R1193Q, P2006A), present in the general population with a very low frequency and demonstrated to be functionally relevant.[3] As observed in SIDS, most of the genetic variants with a functional effect identified are located on *SCN5A* (**Fig. 4**); and even if these variants are also present in the general population,[36,37] they are significantly more prevalent in IUFD cases ($P = .0001$), again suggesting their role as predisposing factors.

## ROLE OF *SCN5A* IN DOCUMENTED LIFE-THREATENING ARRHYTHMIAS IN THE PERINATAL PERIOD

LQTS patients with life-threatening arrhythmias in the first year of life represent a small subset of Romano-Ward patients (in LQTS International Registry 2% of 3323 subjects)[47]; however, their risk for subsequent cardiac arrest/SCD in the following 10 years is particularly high (hazard ratio 23.4, $P<.01$) and their response to β-blocker therapy is poor.[47,48]

This subgroup of patients, independently on the genotype, should be regarded as a subgroup of LQTS patients in whom traditional treatments are usually not effective and in whom an aggressive strategy is usually needed, at variance with most of the LQTS patients.[5,15] Their ventricular arrhythmias usually start very early, sometimes also in the fetal period. Cuneo and colleagues[49] studied 43 subjects exhibiting fetal arrhythmias potentially linked to LQTS (torsades de pointes, second-degree atrioventricular [AV] block, and sinus bradycardia) and evaluated the correlation with the LQTS genotype. Disease-causing variants in known LQTS genes were found in 95% (38/40) of tested cases, 35 of them carrying a mutation in one of the major LQTS genes (23 *KCNQ1*, 6 *KCNH2*, and

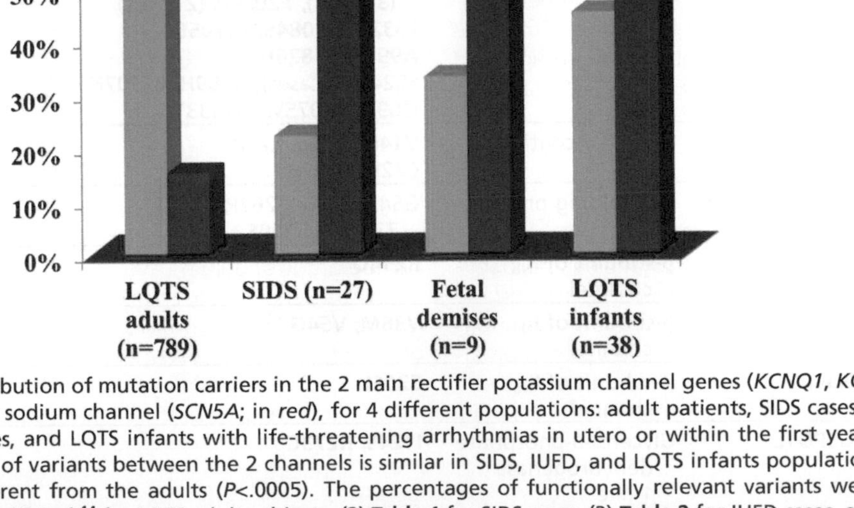

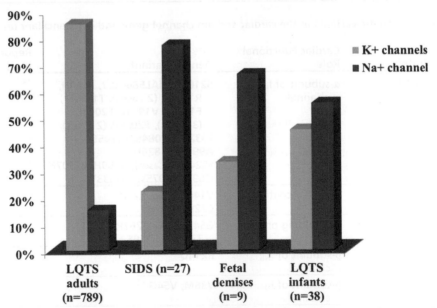


**Fig. 4.** Distribution of mutation carriers in the 2 main rectifier potassium channel genes (*KCNQ1*, *KCNH2*; in *light blue*) and in sodium channel (*SCN5A*; in *red*), for 4 different populations: adult patients, SIDS cases, intrauterine fetal demises, and LQTS infants with life-threatening arrhythmias in utero or within the first year of life. The distribution of variants between the 2 channels is similar in SIDS, IUFD, and LQTS infants populations, all significantly different from the adults ($P<.0005$). The percentages of functionally relevant variants were calculated according to (1) Ref.[44] for LQTS adult subjects, (2) **Table 1** for SIDS cases, (3) **Table 2** for IUFD cases, and (4) **Table 2** and Refs.[45,46] for LQTS infants.

6 *SCN5A*). Excluding the fetuses with only second-degree AV block and sinus bradycardia, and focusing on the infants with life-threatening arrhythmias, who in the study were 7, it is interesting to observe that 5/7 (71%) were carrying a *SCN5A* mutation.[49] Another interesting observation from this study was the overrepresentation of the *SCN5A*-R1623Q mutation, present in 4 of the 5 LQT3 cases with life-threatening arrhythmias[49] and already identified in association with very severe and early-onset phenotypes.[43,50] In the literature, other very severe cases associated with *de novo* mutation in *SCN5A* have been reported,[51–55] all presenting very prolonged QT and sign of electrical instability, such as 2:1 AV block and T-wave alternans.

Horigome and colleagues[56] using a questionnaire collected 58 cases of LQTS from 33 institutions in Japan in which the diagnosis has been done in fetal, neonatal, or infant life (up to 1 year). Among these, 41 underwent genetic testing and 19 had life-threatening arrhythmias. In this cohort, at variance with what mainly present in literature, a greater prevalence of *KCNH2* mutations was observed, whereas *SCN5A* mutations were identified in 26% of the cases.

In the authors' own internal database, among 11 severe early-onset LQTS cases, 5 have a mutation on *SCN5A*[48] (unpublished) (45%), 3 on calmodulin genes[57] (27%), and the remaining 3 are distributed equally among *KCNH2*, *KCNQ1*, and unknown genotype. Calmodulin mutations associated with these severe forms of LQTS cause impaired calcium affinity[57]; however, how this produces severe cases of LQTS and arrhythmias is still under investigation, given the multiple ion channels, including the sodium channel[58] targeted by calmodulin. **Table 2** summarizes all the *SCN5A* mutations identified so far in association with malignant early-onset LQT3.

In summary, these data show the prominent role of *SCN5A* in inducing life-threatening conditions in the perinatal period (see **Fig. 4**). Given the observation that in adult life *SCN5A* mutations are present only in a minority of genotype-positive LQTS patients, it is reasonable to postulate a negative selection for *SCN5A* carriers in the perinatal and early infant period.

## DIFFERENCES AMONG THE *SCN5A* MUTATIONS IDENTIFIED IN SUDDEN INFANT DEATH SYNDROME, INTRAUTERINE UNEXPLAINED FETAL DEATH, AND LONG QT SYNDROME TYPE 3 PATIENTS WITH LIFE-THREATENING ARRHYTHMIAS IN THE PERINATAL PERIOD

In SIDS, IUFD, and neonatal LQT3, most of the genetic variants identified with a functional effect are located on *SCN5A*, and probably these variants are responsible for an adverse selection, as the picture is completely reversed in adult life (see **Fig. 4**). However, the genetic variants identified in SIDS, IUFD, and neonatal LQT3 have a different topological distribution. Indeed, as shown in **Fig. 5**, mutations located in the transmembrane and linker regions (the regions where variants present in controls are less frequently observed)[59] are

**Table 2**
**Genetic variants in the cardiac sodium channel gene found respectively in LQT3 infants with early malignant arrhythmias in utero or within the first year of life and in intrauterine fetal demises**

| Gene | Protein | Cardiac Functional Role | Genetic Variant | Reported Study [Ref] |
|---|---|---|---|---|
| **LQT3 infants** | | | | |
| *SCN5A* | $Na_v1.5$ | α-subunit of $I_{Na}$ channel | **G1631D (2 cases)** | 51 |
| | | | **R1623Q (7 cases)** | The authors' group unpublished[43,49,50] |
| | | | **L409P, F1473C** | 49 |
| | | | **P1332L** | 53 |
| | | | **S941N, A1330D** | 52 |
| | | | **V1763M (2 cases)** | 48 |
| | | | **A1330P** | 48,55 |
| | | | **L1772V, N1774D, V176M, N406K** | 54,56 |
| **IUFD** | | | | |
| *SCN5A* | $Na_v1.5$ | α-subunit of $I_{Na}$ channel | **R1623Q** | 43 |
| | | | **T220I**, S524Y, D772N, R1116Q, **R1193Q (2 cases)**, **P2006A (2 cases)** | 3 |

Note: Functionally significant variants are in bold; homozygous and double/triple mutation carriers are excluded.

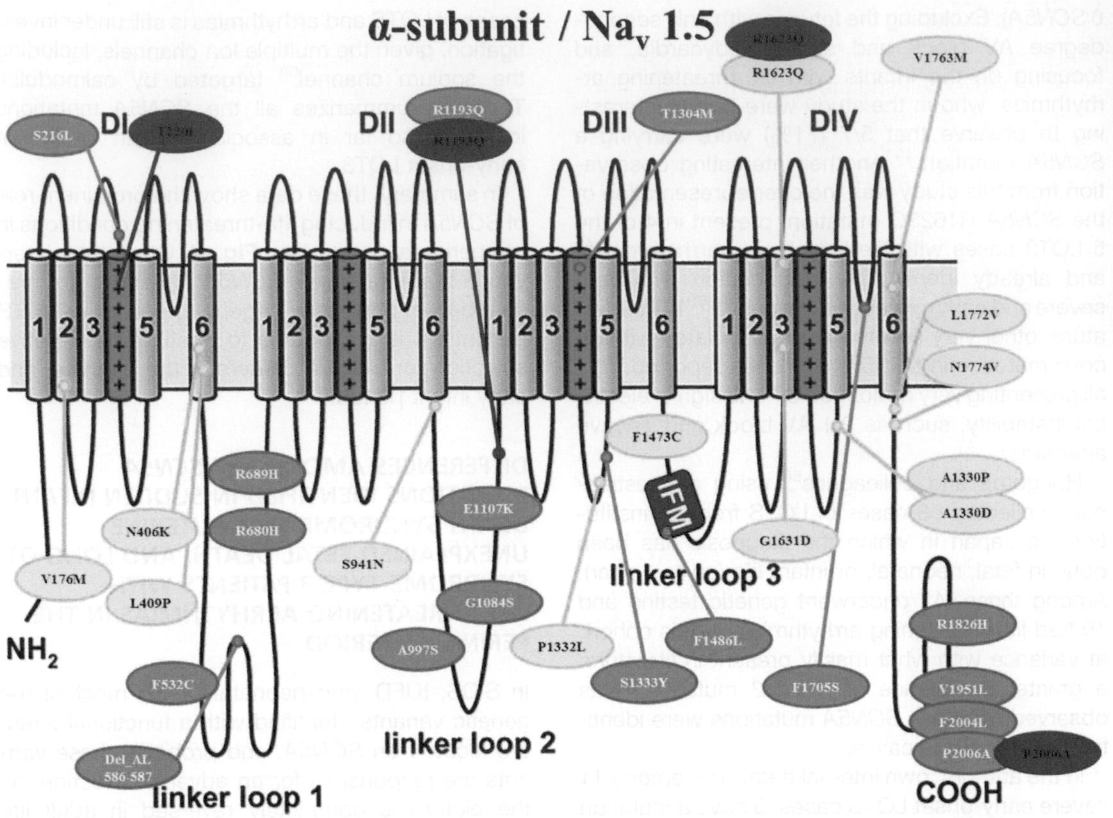


**Fig. 5.** Distribution and location of functional variants reported in SIDS (*light blue circles*), IUFD (*red circles*), and LQT3 infants with life-threatening arrhythmias in utero or within the first year of life (*yellow circles*) in structural/functional domains of Na$_v$1.5. (*Adapted from* Abriel H. Cardiac sodium channel Nav1.5 and interacting proteins: physiology and pathophysiology. J Mol Cell Cardiol 2010;48:2–11.)

significantly more present in neonatal LQT3 patients than in SIDS/IUFD patients (86% vs 22%, $P$ = .002), whereas the variants located in the N-terminal and in the interdomain linkers (the regions where variants present in controls are more frequently observed)[59] are 9.5% in neonatal LQT3 versus 44.4% in SIDS/IUFD, $P$ = .01. Furthermore, although none of the mutations identified in the cases with severe neonatal LQT3 are present in the EVS database, 47% of functional variants associated with SIDS/IUFD are also observed in the general population. These considerations support the concept that severe neonatal LQT3 cases are caused by mutations able *per se* to cause such a severe phenotype and are therefore not compatible with survival to adulthood. Indeed, the mutations identified in this subgroup of patients are mainly *de novo*. By contrast, the genetic variants identified in SIDS and IUFD cases have a wider range of clinical severity and some of them, identified also in the general population, are probably not able per se to cause SCD, although they can act as favoring factors. In further support of this view, the authors have observed that the *SCN5A* rare variants with a functional effect identified in SIDS and IUFD, also present in the EVS database, are significantly more prevalent in the SIDS/IUFD cohorts than in the general population (2.8% vs 1.5%, $P$ = .01). This observation is strengthened by the removal of *SCN5A*-V1951L and *SCN5A*-F2004L, the most prevalent variants in EVS that were initially considered as potentially detrimental variants in the SIDS cohort,[23] but not in the more recent IUFD cohort.[3] Indeed, while the prevalence of these 2 variants is similar in the SIDS cohort and in EVS, thus not supporting their role in increasing the risk of SCD, all the others are much more prevalent in SIDS and IUFD, compared with the general population (12/634, 1.9% vs 45/6261, 0.7%; $P$ = .0019).

## CLINICAL IMPLICATIONS

The concepts discussed earlier contribute to a better understanding of the mechanisms underlying several sudden deaths occurring shortly before or after birth. Importantly, they also carry practical clinical implications.

It is evident that the cardiac sodium channel mutations associated with the highest risk and with the more malignant clinical course are those accompanied by very marked QT interval prolongations. As such, they could be easily identified even before the onset of the first episode of life-threatening arrhythmias, provided an ECG is performed in the first weeks after birth. The European Society of Cardiology has published[60] guidelines for the interpretation of neonatal ECG and has clearly supported an ECG screening program to be performed in the first 2 to 3 weeks of life with the main objective to identify early on infants affected by LQTS, thus allowing to anticipate initiation of protective therapeutic strategies. A prospective ECG study in more than 40,000 2- to 3-week-old infants has demonstrated that neonatal ECG screening can identify the affected infants with subsequent genetic confirmation.[61] The cost-benefit ratio in Europe is very favorable,[62] and it is difficult to justify the still ongoing resistance to what would be a simple and very effective screening program which, by the early use of appropriate therapeutic strategies, could lead to a significant reduction of avoidable tragedies.[63]

## ACKNOWLEDGMENTS

We are grateful to Pinuccia De Tomasi for expert editorial support, Elisa Mastantuono for helping with Medline searches, and Carla Spazzolini for statistical support.

## REFERENCES


1. Zeitlin J, Wildman K, Bréart G, et al. Indicators for monitoring and evaluating perinatal health in Europe. Eur J Public Health 2003;13(Suppl 3):29–37.
2. Walker N, Yenokyan G, Friberg IK, et al. Patterns in coverage of maternal, newborn, and child health interventions: projections of neonatal and under-5 mortality to 2035. Lancet 2013;382:1029–38.
3. Crotti L, Tester DJ, White WM, et al. Long QT syndrome-associated mutations in intrauterine fetal death. JAMA 2013;309:1473–82.
4. Mathews TJ, MacDorman MF. Infant mortality statistics from the 2005 period linked birth/infant death data set. Natl Vital Stat Rep 2008;57:1–32.
5. Priori SG, Wilde AA, Horie M, et al. HRS/EHRA/APHRS expert consensus statement on the diagnosis and management of patients with inherited primary arrhythmia syndromes: document endorsed by HRS, EHRA, and APHRS in May 2013 and by ACCF, AHA, PACES, and AEPC in June 2013. Heart Rhythm 2013;10:1932–63.
6. Schwartz PJ, Crotti L. Can a message from the dead save lives? J Am Coll Cardiol 2007;49:247–9.
7. Insolia R, Ghidoni A, Dossena C, et al. Sudden infant death syndrome and cardiac channelopathies: from mechanism to prevention of avoidable tragedies. Cardiogenetics 2011;1(s1):e6.
8. Schwartz PJ, Crotti L. Cardiac arrhythmias of genetic origin are important contributors to sudden infant death syndrome. Heart Rhythm 2007;4:740–2.
9. Abriel H. Cardiac sodium channel Nav1.5 and interacting proteins: physiology and pathophysiology. J Mol Cell Cardiol 2010;48:2–11.
10. Wang Q, Li Z, Shen J, et al. Genomic organization of the human SCN5A gene encoding the cardiac sodium channel. Genomics 1996;34:9–16.
11. Gellens ME, George AL Jr, Chen LQ, et al. Primary structure and functional expression of the human cardiac tetrodotoxin-insensitive voltage-dependent sodium channel. Proc Natl Acad Sci U S A 1992; 89:554–8.
12. Makielski JC, Ye B, Valdivia CR, et al. A ubiquitous splice variant and a common polymorphism affect heterologous expression of recombinant human SCN5A heart sodium channels. Circ Res 2003;93:821–8.
13. Chioni AM, Fraser SP, Pani F, et al. A novel polyclonal antibody specific for the Na(v)1.5 voltage-gated Na(+) channel 'neonatal' splice form. J Neurosci Methods 2005;147:88–98.
14. Onkal R, Mattis JH, Fraser SP, et al. Alternative splicing of Nav1.5: an electrophysiological comparison of 'neonatal' and 'adult' isoforms and critical involvement of a lysine residue. J Cell Physiol 2008;216:716–26.
15. Schwartz PJ, Crotti L, Insolia R. Long-QT syndrome: from genetics to management. Circ Arrhythm Electrophysiol 2012;5:868–77.
16. Schwartz PJ, Priori SG, Spazzolini C, et al. Genotype-phenotype correlation in the long-QT syndrome: gene-specific triggers for life-threatening arrhythmias. Circulation 2001;103:89–95.
17. Crotti L, Marcou CA, Tester DJ, et al. Spectrum and prevalence of mutations involving BrS1- through BrS12-susceptibility genes in a cohort of unrelated patients referred for Brugada syndrome genetic testing: implications for genetic testing. J Am Coll Cardiol 2012;60:1410–8.
18. Beckwith JB. Discussion of terminology and definition of the sudden infant death syndrome. In: Bergman AB, Beckwith JB, Ray CG, editors. Sudden infant death syndrome: proceedings of the Second International Conference on the Causes of Sudden Death in Infants. Seattle (WA): University of Washington Press; 1970. p. 14–22.
19. Krous HF, Beckwith JB, Byard RW, et al. Sudden infant death syndrome and unclassified sudden infant deaths: a definitional and diagnostic approach. Pediatrics 2004;114:234–8.

20. Filiano JJ, Kinney HC. A perspective on neuropathologic findings in victims of the sudden infant death syndrome: the triple-risk model. Biol Neonate 1994; 65:194–7.
21. Schwartz PJ. Cardiac sympathetic innervation and the sudden infant death syndrome. A possible pathogenic link. Am J Med 1976;60:167–72.
22. Schwartz PJ, Priori SG, Dumaine R, et al. A molecular link between the sudden infant death syndrome and the long-QT syndrome. N Engl J Med 2000;343:262–7.
23. Arnestad M, Crotti L, Rognum TO, et al. Prevalence of long-QT syndrome gene variants in sudden infant death syndrome. Circulation 2007;115:361–7.
24. Wilders R. Cardiac ion channelopathies and the sudden infant death syndrome. ISRN Cardiol 2012;2012:846171.
25. Klaver EC, Versluijs GM, Wilders R. Cardiac ion channel mutations in the sudden infant death syndrome. Int J Cardiol 2011;152:162–70.
26. Otagiri T, Kijima K, Osawa M, et al. Cardiac ion channel gene mutations in sudden infant death syndrome. Pediatr Res 2008;64:482–7.
27. Wang DW, Desai RR, Crotti L, et al. Cardiac sodium channel dysfunction in sudden infant death syndrome. Circulation 2007;115:368–76.
28. Ackerman MJ, Siu BL, Sturner WQ, et al. Postmortem molecular analysis of SCN5A defects in sudden infant death syndrome. JAMA 2001;286:2264–9.
29. Plant LD, Bowers PN, Liu Q, et al. A common cardiac sodium channel variant associated with sudden infant death in African Americans, SCN5A S1103Y. J Clin Invest 2006;116:430–5.
30. Millat G, Kugener B, Chevalier P, et al. Contribution of long-QT syndrome genetic variants in sudden infant death syndrome. Pediatr Cardiol 2009;30:502–9.
31. Cronk LB, Ye B, Kaku T, et al. Novel mechanism for sudden infant death syndrome: persistent late sodium current secondary to mutations in caveolin-3. Heart Rhythm 2007;4:161–6.
32. Cheng J, van Norstrand DW, Medeiros-Domingo A, et al. α1-syntrophin mutations identified in sudden infant death syndrome cause an increase in late cardiac sodium current. Circ Arrhythm Electrophysiol 2009;2:667–76.
33. Hu D, Barajas-Martínez H, Medeiros-Domingo A. A novel rare variant in SCN1Bb linked to Brugada syndrome and SIDS by combined modulation of Na(v)1.5 and K(v)4.3 channel currents. Heart Rhythm 2012;9:760–9.
34. Tan BH, Pundi KN, Van Norstrand DW, et al. Sudden infant death syndrome-associated mutations in the sodium channel β subunits. Heart Rhythm 2010;7:771–8.
35. Van Norstrand DW, Valdivia CR, Tester DJ, et al. Molecular and functional characterization of novel glycerol-3-phosphate dehydrogenase 1 like gene (GPD1-L) mutations in sudden infant death syndrome. Circulation 2007;116:2253–9.
36. Andreasen C, Refsgaard L, Nielsen JB, et al. Mutations in genes encoding cardiac ion channels previously associated with sudden infant death syndrome (SIDS) are present with high frequency in new exome data. Can J Cardiol 2013;29:1104–9.
37. National Heart, Lung, and Blood Institute Exome Sequencing Project (ESP). Exome variant server: Seattle WA. Available at: http://evs.gs.washington.edu/EVS. Accessed February, 2014.
38. Macdorman MF, Kirmeyer SE, Wilson EC. Fetal and perinatal mortality, United States, 2006. Natl Vital Stat Rep 2012;60:1–22.
39. VanderWielen B, Zaleski C, Cold C, et al. Wisconsin stillbirth services program: a multifocal approach to stillbirth analysis. Am J Med Genet A 2011;155A(5): 1073–80.
40. Stillbirth Collaborative Research Network Writing Group. Causes of death among stillbirths. JAMA 2011;306:2459–68.
41. Schwartz PJ. Stillbirth, sudden infant deaths, and long-QT syndrome: puzzle or mosaic, the pieces of the Jigsaw are being fitted together. Circulation 2004;109:2930–2.
42. Hoorntje T, Alders M, van Tintelen P, et al. Homozygous premature truncation of the HERG protein: the human HERG knockout. Circulation 1999;100: 1264–7.
43. Miller TE, Estrella E, Myerburg RJ, et al. Recurrent third-trimester fetal loss and maternal mosaicism for long-QT syndrome. Circulation 2004;109:3029–34.
44. Kapplinger JD, Tester DJ, Salisbury BA, et al. Spectrum and prevalence of mutations from the first 2,500 consecutive unrelated patients referred for the FAMILION long QT syndrome genetic test. Heart Rhythm 2009;6:1297–303.
45. Lupoglazoff JM, Denjoy I, Villain E, et al. Long QT syndrome in neonates: conduction disorders associated with HERG mutations and sinus bradycardia with KCNQ1 mutations. J Am Coll Cardiol 2004;43: 826–30.
46. Lin MT, Wu MH, Chang CC, et al. In utero onset of long QT syndrome with atrioventricular block and spontaneous or lidocaine-induced ventricular tachycardia: compound effects of hERG pore region mutation and SCN5A N-terminus variant. Heart Rhythm 2008;5:1567–74.
47. Spazzolini C, Mullally J, Schwartz PJ, et al. Clinical implications for patients with long QT syndrome who experience a cardiac event during infancy. J Am Coll Cardiol 2009;54:832–7.
48. Schwartz PJ, Spazzolini C, Crotti L. All LQT3 patients need an ICD. True or false? Heart Rhythm 2009;1: 113–20.
49. Cuneo BF, Etheridge SP, Horigome H, et al. Arrhythmia phenotype during fetal life suggests

long-QT syndrome genotype: risk stratification of perinatal long-QT syndrome. Circ Arrhythm Electrophysiol 2013;6:946–51.
50. Ten Harkel AD, Witsenburg M, de Jong PL, et al. Efficacy of an implantable cardioverter- defibrillator in a neonate with LQT3 associated arrhythmias. Europace 2005;7:77–84.
51. Wang DW, Crotti L, Shimizu W, et al. Malignant perinatal variant of long-QT syndrome caused by a profoundly dysfunctional cardiac sodium channel. Circ Arrhythm Electrophysiol 2008;1:370–8.
52. Schulze-Bahr E, Fenge H, Etzrodt D, et al. Long QT syndrome and life threatening arrhythmia in a newborn: molecular diagnosis and treatment response. Heart 2004;90:13–6.
53. Bankston JR, Yue M, Chung W, et al. A novel and lethal de novo LQT-3 mutation in a newborn with distinct molecular pharmacology and therapeutic response. PLoS One 2007;2:e1258.
54. Wedekind H, Smits JP, Schulze-Bahr E, et al. De novo mutation in SCN5A gene associated with early onset of sudden infant death. Circulation 2001;104:1158–64.
55. Chang CC, Acharfi S, Wu MH, et al. A novel SCN5A mutation manifests as a malignant form of long QT syndrome with perinatal onset of tachycardia/bradycardia. Cardiovasc Res 2004;64:268–78.
56. Horigome H, Nagashima M, Sumitomo N, et al. Clinical characteristics and genetic background of congenital Long-QT syndrome diagnosed in fetal, neonatal, and infantile life. A nationwide questionnaire survey in Japan. Circ Arrhythm Electrophysiol 2010;3:10–7.
57. Crotti L, Johnson CN, Graf E, et al. Calmodulin mutations associated with recurrent cardiac arrest in infants [abstract]. Circulation 2013;127:1009–17.
58. Murphy LL, Campbell CM, Crotti L, et al. Calmodulin mutation associated with neonatal long-QT syndrome evokes increased persistent sodium current from a fetal Nav1.5 splice variant. Circulation 2013;128:A14999.
59. Kapa S, Tester DJ, Salisbury BA, et al. Genetic testing for long-QT syndrome. Distinguishing pathogenic mutations from benign variants. Circulation 2009;120:1752–60.
60. Schwartz PJ, Garson A Jr, Paul T, et al. Guidelines for the interpretation of the neonatal electrocardiogram. Eur Heart J 2002;23:1329–44.
61. Schwartz PJ, Stramba-Badiale M, Crotti L, et al. Prevalence of the congenital long-QT syndrome. Circulation 2009;120:1761–7.
62. Quaglini S, Rognoni C, Spazzolini C, et al. Cost-effectiveness of neonatal ECG screening for the Long QT-Syndrome. Eur Heart J 2006;27:1824–32.
63. Schwartz PJ. Newborn ECG screening to prevent sudden cardiac death. Heart Rhythm 2006;3:1353–5.

# Cardiac Sodium Channel Overlap Syndrome

Carol Ann Remme, MD, PhD

**KEYWORDS**

• Sodium channel • *SCN5A* • Mutation • Sudden cardiac death • Arrhythmia • Brugada syndrome • Long QT syndrome type 3 (LQT3) • Sodium channel overlap syndrome

**KEY POINTS**

- Cardiac sodium channels play a central role in excitability of myocardial cells and proper conduction of the electrical impulse within the heart.
- Mutations in the *SCN5A* gene encoding the cardiac sodium channel are associated with a wide range of arrhythmia syndromes that potentially lead to fatal arrhythmias in relatively young individuals.
- A single *SCN5A* mutation can result in multiple clinical phenotypes and rhythm disturbances within the same family, a phenomenon now referred to as "cardiac sodium channel overlap syndrome."
- Various clinical, environmental, and genetic modifiers modulate variable disease expressivity and severity in sodium channel overlap syndrome.

## INTRODUCTION

Influx of sodium ions through cardiac voltage-gated sodium channels is responsible for the initial fast upstroke of the cardiac action potential, and consequently plays a central role in excitability of myocardial cells and proper conduction of the electrical impulse within the heart (**Fig. 1**). During common pathologic conditions, such as myocardial ischemia and heart failure, decreased sodium current function may cause conduction disturbances and potentially life-threatening arrhythmias.[1,2] In addition, sodium channel dysfunction secondary to mutations in the *SCN5A* gene, encoding the major sodium channel in heart, underlie a number of inherited arrhythmia syndromes associated with fatal arrhythmias in otherwise healthy young individuals. Over the past 20 years, an increasing number of *SCN5A* mutations have been described in patients with long QT syndrome type 3 (LQT3), Brugada syndrome (BrS), (progressive) conduction disease, sick sinus syndrome, atrial standstill, atrial fibrillation, and dilated cardiomyopathy.[3,4] Moreover, a single *SCN5A* mutation can result in multiple clinical phenotypes and rhythm disturbances within the same family (including features of LQT3, BrS, and/or conduction disease), a phenomenon now referred to as "cardiac sodium channel overlap syndrome."[5] The complexity of these overlap syndromes is further underlined by the large variability in type and severity of clinical symptoms within affected families. Multiple biophysical defects of single *SCN5A* mutations are considered instrumental to the observed overlapping clinical manifestations.[5,6] Furthermore, genetic modifiers and environmental factors are suspected to determine variable disease expressivity and severity. Here, an overview is provided of the current knowledge

This work was supported by the Netherlands Heart Institute (grant 061.02), and the Division for Earth and Life Sciences (ALW; project 836.09.003) with financial aid from the Netherlands Organization for Scientific Research (NWO).

Department of Experimental Cardiology, Academic Medical Center, University of Amsterdam, Meibergdreef 15, Room K2-110, PO Box 22660, Amsterdam 1100 DD, The Netherlands
*E-mail address:* c.a.remme@amc.uva.nl

Card Electrophysiol Clin 6 (2014) 761–776
http://dx.doi.org/10.1016/j.ccep.2014.08.005
1877-9182/14/$ – see front matter 

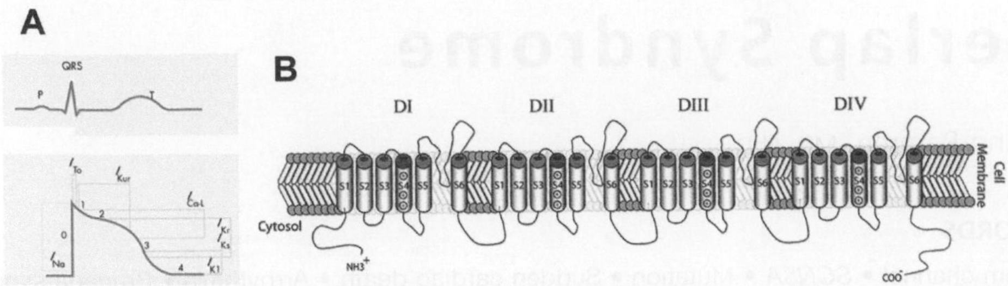


**Fig. 1.** (*A*) Ion currents underlying the cardiac action potential. (*B*) Structure of the cardiac sodium channel. (*From* [*A*] Remme CA, Bezzina CR. Sodium channel (dys)function and cardiac arrhythmias. Cardiovasc Ther 2010;28:288; with permission.)

on inherited sodium channelopathies and *SCN5A* mutations associated with sodium channel overlap syndromes.

## CARDIAC SODIUM CHANNEL STRUCTURE, FUNCTION, DISTRIBUTION, AND REGULATION

The voltage-dependent cardiac sodium channel consists of a transmembrane pore-forming α-subunit protein associated with a small ancillary modulatory β-subunit. The α-subunit protein $Na_V1.5$ (encoded by the *SCN5A* gene) is made up of a cytoplasmic N terminus, 4 internally homologous domains (DI-DIV; each consisting of 6 transmembrane segments S1–S6) interconnected by cytoplasmic linkers, and a cytoplasmic C terminal domain (see **Fig. 1**). The positively charged fourth transmembrane segment (S4) acts as the voltage sensor responsible for increased channel permeability (channel activation) during membrane depolarization.[7] The ion-conducting pore of the channel is formed by the S5 and S6 segments of all 4 domains, and their interconnecting P-loops contain the channels' selectivity filter for sodium ions.[8] Channel inactivation is a more complicated process involving multiple parts of $Na_V1.5$, including the intracellular DIII–DIV linker, the intracellular S4–S5 linkers of both DIII and DIV, the C terminal domain, and the S5–S6 P-loops.[8,9] Secondary to mutations in *SCN5A*, sodium channel activation and/or inactivation properties may be altered, depending on the location of the mutation. Consequently, sodium channel availability and peak sodium current may be decreased, setting the stage for conduction slowing. Alternatively, the channel may not be properly inactivated, resulting in a persistent (sustained), noninactivating sodium current during the action potential plateau phase, thereby prolonging repolarization (**Fig. 2**).[10]

Cardiac sodium channels are not homogeneously distributed throughout the myocardium. Within the cardiac conduction system, low to absent $Na_V1.5$ protein expression is observed in the

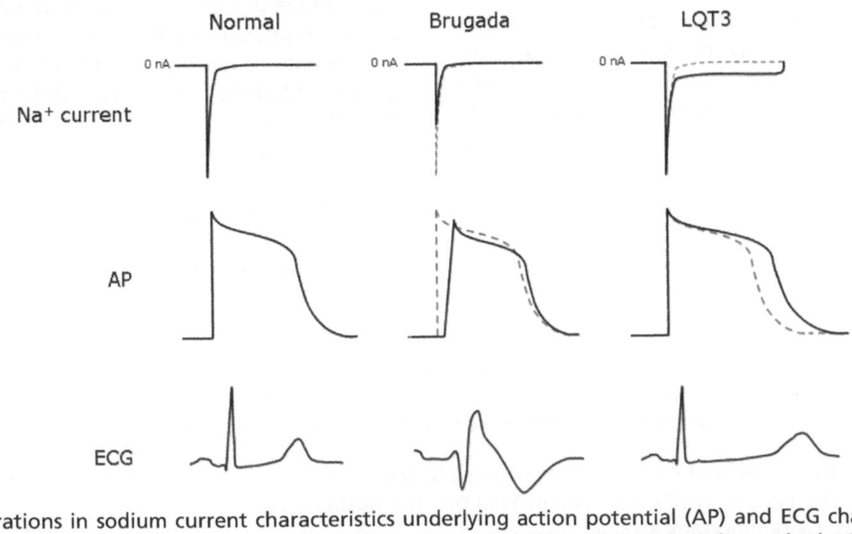


**Fig. 2.** Alterations in sodium current characteristics underlying action potential (AP) and ECG characteristics in LQT3 and BrS. (*From* Remme CA, Bezzina CR. Sodium channel (dys)function and cardiac arrhythmias. Cardiovasc Ther 2010;28:290; with permission.)

sinoatrial and atrioventricular nodes, whereas $Na_V1.5$ is abundant in the His bundle, bundle branches, and Purkinje fibers.[11] Furthermore, a transmural gradient is present in ventricular tissue, with lower $Na_V1.5$ expression and decreased functional sodium channel availability observed in the subepicardium as compared with the subendocardium.[11,12] Differences in sodium channel (in)activation properties also have been described between atrial and ventricular myocytes.[13]

Cardiac sodium channel properties are regulated by physiologic and metabolic factors, including intracellular calcium levels, extracellular protons and pH, reactive oxygen species, temperature, and stretch (see Ref.[14]). Furthermore, $Na_V1.5$ expression and function also may be modulated by posttranslational modifications, including phosphorylation, glycosylation, and ubiquitination.[15] Finally, sodium channel expression, trafficking, and function are importantly regulated by a large number of interacting proteins.[16]

## CLINICAL DISORDERS ASSOCIATED WITH *SCN5A* MUTATIONS

Over the past 15 to 20 years, an increasing number of *SCN5A* mutations have been identified in patients presenting with a diverse range of clinical symptoms and syndromes (**Box 1**, **Fig. 3**). Although caused by mutations in the same ion channel, these clinical syndromes each display distinct phenotypical and biophysical characteristics.

### *Long QT Syndrome Type 3*

Long QT syndrome (LQTS) is characterized by a prolongation of the QT interval on the electrocardiogram (ECG) accompanied by an increased risk for sudden death due to ventricular tachyarrhythmias, in particular torsades de pointes. Patients with LQT3 (associated with *SCN5A* mutations) are often relatively bradycardic and display arrhythmias predominantly during rest or sleep (at slow heart rates).[4,17] Compared with other LQT subtypes, patients with LQT3 are particularly at risk for sudden death, and cardiac arrest (rather than syncope) is often the first clinical event.[17] Biophysical alterations observed secondary to *SCN5A* mutations associated with LQT3 include disruption of sodium current fast inactivation (allowing for channels to re-open, resulting in a persistent inward current during the action potential plateau phase), slowed inactivation (resulting in channel openings of longer duration), faster recovery from inactivation (causing increased sodium channel availability), and increased peak sodium current density.[18,19] As a consequence, delayed repolarization and action potential prolongation may set the stage for early after-depolarizations, torsades de pointes arrhythmias, and sudden death.

**Box 1**
**Clinical entities associated with *SCN5A* mutations**

- Long QT syndrome type 3 (LQT3)
- Brugada syndrome
- (Progressive) cardiac conduction disease
- Sick sinus syndrome
- Atrial standstill
- Atrial fibrillation
- Dilated cardiomyopathy
- Overlap syndrome

### *Brugada Syndrome*

BrS is associated with the occurrence of ventricular arrhythmias and sudden cardiac death (mostly during rest and sleep) in relatively young (age <40 years) and apparently healthy individuals. The ECG hallmark of BrS comprises ST-segment elevation in the right-precordial leads V1 to V3. This typical ECG pattern may be variably present, and can be unmasked or increased after administration of Class 1A or 1C anti-arrhythmic sodium channel blocking drugs (ajmaline, flecainide) or during exercise (see Ref.[20]). Cardiac conduction disease is often also observed in patients with BrS, evidenced by prolonged PQ and QRS duration on the ECG in the presence of a normal QT interval.[4] *SCN5A* mutations associated with BrS are typically "loss-of-function" mutations, leading to reduced sodium channel availability, either through decreased trafficking and membrane surface channel expression, or through altered channel gating properties, including disruption of activation, accelerated inactivation, and impaired recovery from inactivation.[3,6,21]

### *Progressive Cardiac Conduction Defect and Sick Sinus Syndrome*

Mutations in *SCN5A* have been associated with conduction disorders affecting the cardiac conduction system, including progressive cardiac conduction defect (PCCD; also called Lenègre or Lev disease) and inherited sick sinus syndrome.[22] PCCD is characterized by progressive conduction slowing through the His-Purkinje system associated with right and/or left bundle branch block and QRS widening, complete AV block, syncope,

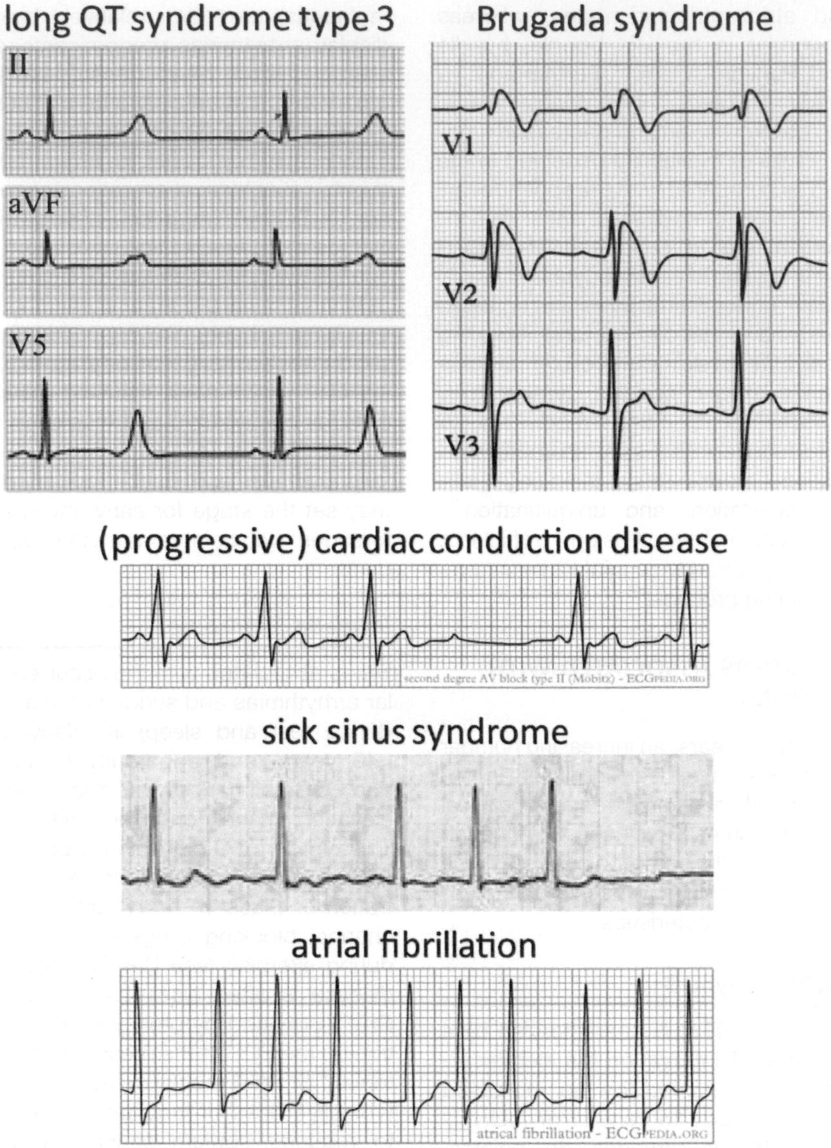


**Fig. 3.** ECG examples of clinical signs and syndromes associated with mutations in the SCN5A gene encoding the cardiac sodium channel. (*From* ECGpedia, with permission; sick sinus syndrome example courtesy of Dr. R.W. Koster, MD, PhD, AMC, The Netherlands).

and sudden death. *SCN5A* mutations underlying both PCCD and inherited sick sinus syndrome typically lead to reduced sodium channel availability (loss-of-function) similar to BrS,[22–24] and considerable overlap exists between these clinical entities (see also later in this article).[25]

### *Atrial Fibrillation*

Atrial fibrillation is commonly observed in mostly elderly patients with underlying structural cardiac abnormalities, but it may also occur as a hereditary disease in young patients with structurally normal hearts. Both loss-of-function and gain-of-function mutations in *SCN5A* have been described in the familial form of atrial fibrillation.[26–29]

### *Dilated Cardiomyopathy*

In rare cases, familial forms of dilated cardiomyopathy (DCM) are reported in patients with *SCN5A* mutations.[30,31] Because this type of DCM often presents in combination with atrial arrhythmias and/or fibrillation,[32] it is unclear whether the observed structural defects are a direct effect of sodium current alterations, or merely secondary to long-standing cardiac abnormalities. Interestingly, biophysical properties consistent with both loss and gain of sodium channel function have been observed in *SCN5A* mutations associated with DCM.[31,33–35]

## CARDIAC SODIUM CHANNEL OVERLAP SYNDROME: CLINICAL AND GENETIC PERSPECTIVE

The previously mentioned clinical disorders comprise separate clinical entities, each caused by different mutations in *SCN5A*. In some instances, however, a single *SCN5A* mutation can result in multiple disease phenotypes, even within one affected family. In 1999, our group identified the first such mutation, *SCN5A*-1795insD, in a large Dutch family presenting with extensive variability in type and severity of symptoms, including ECG features of sinus node dysfunction, bradycardia, conduction disease, BrS (ST-segment elevation), and LQT3 (QT-interval prolongation), in addition to nocturnal sudden death.[36,37]

Since our description of this unique family, other mutations with similar clinical overlap of LQT3, BrS, and conduction disease have been reported, now collectively referred to as "sodium channel overlap syndrome." These include a deletion of a lysine in the intracellular DIII–DIV linker (delK1500; located close to the LQT3-associated mutation delKPQ1505-1507),[38] a missense mutation (D1114N) in the intracellular DII–DIII linker,[39,40] a deletion of a phenylalanine at position 1617 (delF1617) in the extracellular S3–S4 linker in domain IV,[41] and missense mutations E1784K and L1786Q in the C-terminal domain (**Fig. 4**).[42,43] In addition, combined clinical features of LQT3 and conduction disease have been described for the delKPQ deletion and the missense mutations V411M, P1332L, V1763M, M1766L, V1777M, and P2005A.[44–51]

Other commonly observed combinations of clinical symptoms for single *SCN5A* mutations include the simultaneous presence of Brugada syndrome and various forms of cardiac conduction disease, including sick sinus syndrome, atrial standstill, and (atrio-)ventricular conduction slowing or block (among others, E161K, T187I, P336L, D356N, R376H, G1406R, R1623X) (see **Fig. 4**).[24,25,52–55] Furthermore, familial forms of DCM combined with conduction disease, atrial arrhythmias, and/or fibrillation have been reported in patients with the *SCN5A* mutations T220I, R222Q, R814W, S851fs, A1180V, D1275N, V1279I, and D1595H.[31–34,56] More recently, a possible genetic overlap between BrS and arrhythmogenic right ventricular cardiomyopathy (ARVC) has been suggested. Clinical features of both syndromes were observed in patients who did not carry mutations in ARVC-related desmosomal proteins, but were found to have a mutation in *SCN5A* (ie, I137M, R367H, E746K, R1023H, R1644C, I1968S).[57–59] ARVC and BrS are both diseases considered to affect predominantly the right ventricle, and an increasing overlap between these entities has been suggested.[60] Taken together, these clinical and genetic findings indicate that single *SCN5A* mutations may be associated with a wide

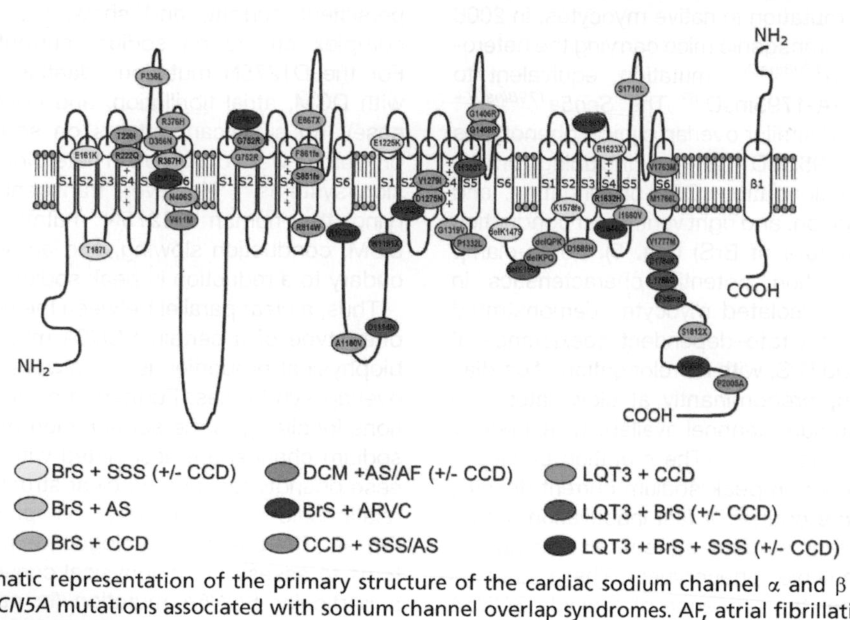


**Fig. 4.** Schematic representation of the primary structure of the cardiac sodium channel α and β subunit with location of *SCN5A* mutations associated with sodium channel overlap syndromes. AF, atrial fibrillation; AS, atrial standstill; SSS, sick sinus syndrome. (*From* Remme CA, Wilde AA, Bezzina CR. Cardiac sodium channel overlap syndromes: different faces of SCN5A mutations. Trends Cardiovasc Med 2008;18:79; with permission.)

spectrum of complex disease phenotypes, as summarized in **Fig. 4**.

## CARDIAC SODIUM CHANNEL OVERLAP SYNDROME: BIOPHYSICAL PERSPECTIVE

It may not be immediately clear how a single *SCN5A* mutation causes the observed overlap in clinical disease phenotypes, as specific mutations typically affect particular biophysical properties of the sodium channel (see **Fig. 2**).[6] In LQT3, mutations classically disrupt fast inactivation of the sodium current, allowing for sodium channels to re-open, resulting in a persistent inward current during the action potential plateau phase, with subsequent delayed repolarization and QT-prolongation (gain-of-function mutations).[18] In contrast, loss-of-function *SCN5A* mutations underlying BrS and conduction disease reduce the total amount of available sodium current, either due to impaired intracellular trafficking and decreased membrane surface channel expression, or through altered channel gating properties, including disruption of activation, accelerated inactivation, and impaired recovery from inactivation (see Ref.[3]). Thus, the simultaneous presence of LQT3 (ie, gain of function) and BrS or conduction disease (ie, loss of function) due to one single *SCN5A* mutation was considered improbable before our description of the 1795insD family.

Patch-clamp studies of the 1795insD mutation in 2 separate expression systems revealed opposing and inconclusive effects on sodium current density and kinetics.[36,61] To assess the biophysical properties of this mutation in native myocytes, in 2006 we generated transgenic mice carrying the heterozygous $Scn5a^{1798insD/+}$ mutation, equivalent to human *SCN5A*-1795insD.[62] The $Scn5a^{1798insD/+}$ mice displayed similar overlap clinical phenotypes as human 1795insD carriers, including bradycardia, PR-prolongation, QRS-prolongation, and QTc-prolongation, and right ventricular conduction slowing (a feature of BrS) (**Fig. 5**). Patch-clamp analysis of action potential characteristics in $Scn5a^{1798insD/+}$ isolated myocytes demonstrated a potential heart rate–dependent coexistence of both LQT3 and BrS, with a prolongation of cardiac repolarization, predominantly at slow rates and decreased sodium channel availability, especially at high frequencies.[61,63] The mutation caused a drastic reduction in peak sodium current density, a delayed time course of fast inactivation, and a small persistent sodium current, explaining the observed multiple phenotypes. These findings confirmed that the presence of a single *SCN5A* mutation is indeed sufficient to cause an overlap syndrome of cardiac sodium channel disease.

Other mutant *SCN5A* channels also display multiple biophysical defects that can potentially lead to various clinical disease manifestations. Both E1784K and delK1500 (mutations associated with LQT3, BrS, and conduction disease) enhance channel inactivation and reduce peak current density, but also significantly increase persistent current magnitude.[38,42] The delF1617 mutation (observed in LQT3 and BrS) displays reduced peak sodium current density and impaired recovery from inactivation (loss of function) versus delayed inactivation (gain of function).[23] In addition, delF1617 causes a membrane potential–dependent magnitude of persistent current, further contributing to biophysical and clinical heterogeneity.[41] *SCN5A* mutations associated with both BrS and conduction disease (and/or sick sinus syndrome) invariably lead to decreased peak sodium current density when studied in heterologous expression systems.[24,25,53–55] For mutations presenting with both LQT3 and conduction disease, the biophysical defects underlying the overlapping clinical phenotypes are not as clearly defined. For instance, *SCN5A* mutations V1777M and V1763M both increase persistent current magnitude, but do not affect peak sodium current density or any other biophysical property consistent with loss of sodium channel function.[49,50] For *SCN5A* mutations associated with DCM, A1180V resulted in enhanced inactivation and slower recovery, leading to a rate-dependent sodium current reduction, in addition to a moderate increase in persistent sodium current.[33] In contrast, DCM-associated mutations R814W and D1595H did not enhance persistent current, and showed divergent and complex effects on sodium current kinetics.[34] For the D1275N mutation (identified in patients with DCM, atrial fibrillation, and conduction disease), no significant effects on sodium current properties were observed in heterologous expression systems.[64] However, transgenic mice carrying the human D1275N mutation displayed DCM, conduction slowing, and arrhythmias secondary to a reduction in peak sodium current.[64]

Thus, a clear parallel between the mixed clinical phenotype of a certain *SCN5A* mutation and its biophysical properties is not always observed in overlap syndromes. Furthermore, different mutations localizing to the same region of the cardiac sodium channel are associated with various disease phenotypes, and no clear structure-function relationship can therefore be predicted (see **Fig. 4**). The use of heterologous expression systems to assess the biophysical consequences of a particular *SCN5A* mutation (in particular one associated with a mixed clinical phenotype) should be viewed with caution, as evidenced by

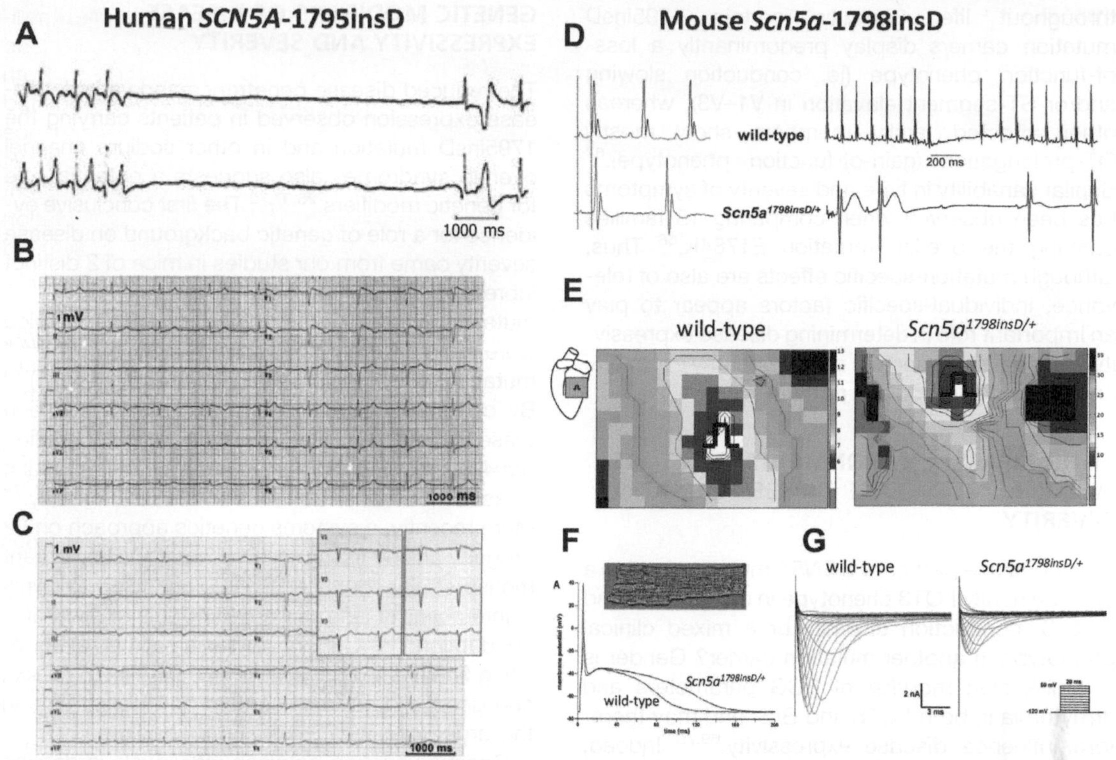


**Fig. 5.** Mixed clinical phenotype with characteristics of both LQT3, BrS, and conduction disease in patients with the *SCN5A*-1795insD$^{+/-}$ mutation, as well as transgenic mice carrying the *Scn5a*$^{1798insD/+}$ mutation. (*A*) Prolonged sinus arrest observed in a symptomatic carrier of the *SCN5A*-1795insD$^{+/-}$ mutation. (*B, C*) ECG examples of a patient carrying the *SCN5A*-1795insD$^{+/-}$ mutation, displaying increased PQ and QRS duration in addition to marked ST-segment elevation in precordial leads V1–V3 (*B*), pronounced QTc prolongation during sinus bradycardia (*C*), and increase in ST-segment elevation after administration of 250 mg procainamide (inset in *C*). (*D*) Examples of traces from telemetry recordings showing an episode of extreme bradycardia and AV block in *Scn5a*$^{1798insD/+}$ mice. (*E*) Epicardial mapping experiments in Langendorff-perfused mouse hearts indicate conduction slowing in the right ventricle of *Scn5a*$^{1798insD/+}$ mice compared with wild-type mice. (*F, G*) Isolated cardiomyocytes from *Scn5a*$^{1798insD/+}$ mice display action potential prolongation (*F*) and reduced peak sodium current (*G*). (*From* [*A–C*] Remme CA, Wilde AA, Bezzina CR. Cardiac sodium channel overlap syndromes: different faces of SCN5A mutations. Trends Cardiovasc Med 2008;18:80; and [*D–G*] Remme CA, Verkerk AO, Nuyens D, et al. Overlap syndrome of cardiac sodium channel disease in mice carrying the equivalent mutation of human SCN5A-1795insD. Circulation 2006;114:2586–90; with permission.)

the contrasting findings observed in the limited available transgenic mouse models of sodium channel overlap syndrome.

## MUTATION-SPECIFIC VERSUS INDIVIDUAL-SPECIFIC DISEASE EXPRESSIVITY AND SEVERITY

A large variety of mixed clinical phenotypes are now known to form part of sodium overlap syndromes. However, patients harboring (overlap) mutations in *SCN5A* may display profound variability in the clinical expression of the disease, complicating clinical and genetic diagnosis.[65] Clearly, variability in disease severity may stem from different severities of the biophysical defect associated with the various mutations, with truncating loss-of-function mutations in *SCN5A* causing more severe conduction disease than missense mutations.[66] Similarly, the range of biophysical alterations induced by a particular *SCN5A* mutation defines the potential of that mutation to cause complex clinical phenotypes. However, variability in disease expressivity and severity is also observed among family members carrying the same primary genetic defect. In the *SCN5A*-1795insD family for instance, some family members display pronounced ECG abnormalities, whereas others appear unaffected in spite of carrying the same familial mutation.[36] Moreover, among the electrocardiographically affected family members, some individuals present with arrhythmia whereas others remain symptom-free throughout life. Similarly, certain 1795insD mutation carriers display predominantly a loss-of-function phenotype (ie, conduction slowing and/or ST-segment elevation in V1–V3), whereas other affected family members show mostly QT-prolongation (gain-of-function phenotype).[67] Similar variability in type and severity of symptoms has been observed when comparing 15 families carrying the overlap mutation E1784K.[68] Thus, although mutation-specific effects are also of relevance, individual-specific factors appear to play an important role in determining disease expressivity and severity in sodium channelopathy in general and overlap syndrome in particular.

## CLINICAL AND ENVIRONMENTAL FACTORS INFLUENCING DISEASE EXPRESSIVITY AND SEVERITY

Why does one particular *SCN5A* mutation lead to a predominantly LQT3 phenotype in one patient, and to BrS, conduction disease, or a mixed clinical phenotype in another mutation carrier? Gender is a well-known modifier of ECG parameters and arrhythmia in both LQTS and BrS, and may therefore influence disease expressivity.[69,70] Indeed, Kyndt and colleagues[25] showed that the G1406R mutation caused gender-dependent differences in disease expressivity; affected female carriers displayed predominantly conduction defects whereas male mutation carriers presented mostly with clinical features of BrS. Age may constitute another clinical determinant of both disease severity and expressivity. Carriers of the 1795insD mutation show age-dependent penetrance of ECG characteristics, with QT-prolongation and signs of conduction disease present from birth, whereas ECG features of BrS usually develop at later stages.[71] In patients with progressive cardiac conduction disease, age-related fibrosis is thought to play a major role in exacerbating cardiac conduction with advancing age.[72] Importantly, transgenic mice haploinsufficient for the cardiac sodium channel *Scn5a* display similar age-dependent structural abnormalities.[73] Some *SCN5A* mutations have been shown to induce symptoms of BrS specifically during episodes of fever, with channel-gating properties affected by increasing temperature.[74,75] Furthermore, membrane expression of certain trafficking-deficient loss of function *SCN5A* mutations may be improved by drugs, such as the sodium channel blocker mexiletine and the $I_{Kr}$ blocker cisapride.[76,77] However, the QT-prolonging drug cisapride has been shown to not only (partly) rescue cell surface expression of a mutated channel, but at the same time also increased the persistent current.[77]

## GENETIC MODIFIERS OF DISEASE EXPRESSIVITY AND SEVERITY

The reduced disease penetrance and variable disease expression observed in patients carrying the 1795insD mutation and in other sodium channel overlap syndromes also suggests a potential role for genetic modifiers.[25,37,72] The first conclusive evidence for a role of genetic background on disease severity came from our studies in mice of 2 distinct inbred strains carrying the same *Scn5a*$^{1798insD/+}$ mutation, where we observed that 129P2 mice were more severely affected by the *Scn5a*$^{1798insD/+}$ mutation as compared with FVB/N mice (**Fig. 6**).[78] By comparing cardiac gene expression between these 2 strains of mice we subsequently identified *Scn4b*, encoding the sodium channel beta subunit 4, as a modifier of conduction disease severity.[78] More recently, a systems genetics approach on F2 progeny arising from the 129P2 and FVB/N mutant mouse strains identified *Tnni3k* encoding troponin 1–interacting kinase as a novel modulator of cardiac conduction.[79,80] Current studies are aimed at correlating findings from these mouse studies to clinical and genetic data from carriers and noncarriers in the large *SCN5A*-1795insD family pedigree.

Genetic variation between individuals is derived from the presence of single nucleotide polymorphisms (SNPs, "snips"), which are frequently observed and by definition occur in at least 1% of the population. H558R is the most common amino-acid changing polymorphism in *SCN5A*, and has a reported prevalence (minor allelic frequency) of 9% to 36% in the general population, with a specific distribution among different ethnic populations.[81] A number of studies have demonstrated that an interaction between this polymorphism and *SCN5A* mutations may exert relevant effects on the functional consequences of mutant sodium channels. In fact, the presence of the H558R polymorphism was able to mitigate the biophysical defect associated with the *SCN5A*-T512I mutation,[82] rescue the plasma membrane–targeting defect associated with the *SCN5A*-M1766L mutation,[83] and increase the current density of *SCN5A*-R282H mutant channels.[84] However, H558R does not affect all *SCN5A* mutations and its electrophysiological effects are mutation-specific.[85] H558R also has been suggested to affect gating characteristics of mutant channels and modulate sodium channel disease expressivity.[86,87] Clinically, the H558R variant also affects ECG parameters and symptoms in patients with BrS.[88] A combination of certain polymorphisms (haplotype) within the regulatory (promoter) region of *SCN5A* also has been shown to modulate cardiac conduction. This haplotype (HapB), commonly observed in Asians but

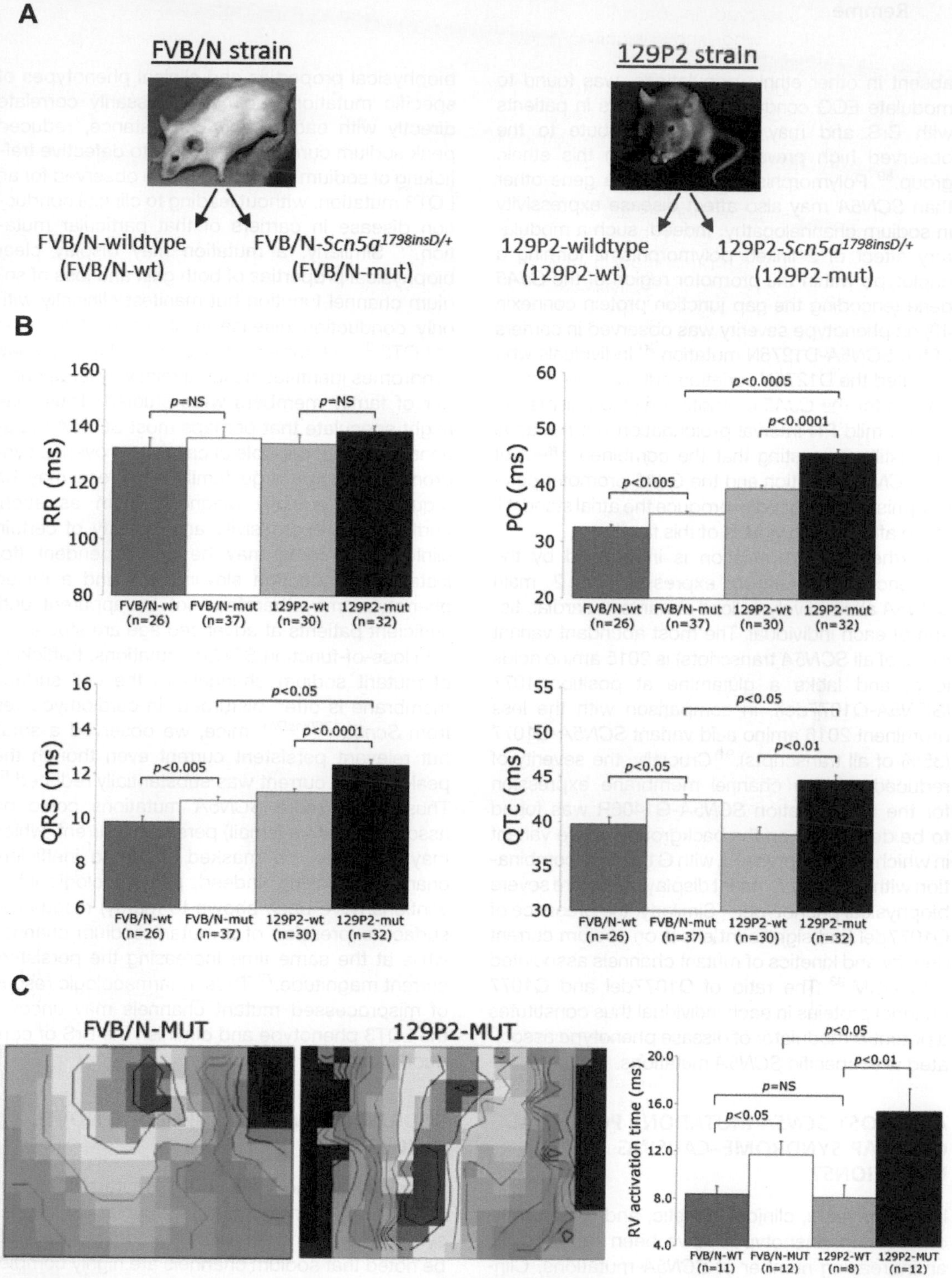


**Fig. 6.** (*A*) Wild-type (wt) and *Scn5a*$^{1798insD/+}$ (mut) mice of both the FVB/N and 129P2 inbred mouse strains were generated. (*B*) The 129P2 mice were more severely affected by the mutation. Mean values of RR, PQ, QRS, and QTc duration at baseline for wild-type (FVB/N-wt, 129P2-wt) and *Scn5a*$^{1798insD/+}$ (FVB/N-mut, 129P2-mut) mice of both strains. (*C*) The 129P2 mutant mice of the 129P2 strain showed more severe right ventricular conduction slowing on epicardial mapping in Langendorff-perfused hearts. The left panel shows typical examples of ventricular activation maps during stimulation from the center of the electrode, the right panel shows mean values for total right ventricular (RV) activation time during pacing from the center of the electrode grid at a basic cycle length of 120 ms. (*From* Remme CA, Scicluna BP, Verkerk AO, et al. Genetically determined differences in sodium current characteristics modulate conduction disease severity in mice with cardiac sodium channelopathy. Circ Res 2009;104:1285–6; with permission.)

absent in other ethnic populations, was found to modulate ECG conduction parameters in patients with BrS and may therefore contribute to the observed high prevalence of BrS in this ethnic group.[89] Polymorphisms residing in a gene other than *SCN5A* may also affect disease expressivity in sodium channelopathy. Indeed, such a modulatory effect of 2 linked polymorphisms forming a haplotype within the promotor region of the *GJA5* gene (encoding the gap junction protein connexin 40) on phenotype severity was observed in carriers of the *SCN5A*-D1275N mutation.[90] Individuals who inherited the D1275N variation but were not homozygous for the *GJA5* promoter polymorphisms exhibited mild PR interval prolongation but not atrial standstill, suggesting that the combined effect of the *SCN5A* mutation and the *GJA5* promoter polymorphisms conspired to produce the atrial standstill in the affected individuals of this family.

Further genetic variation is introduced by the presence and relative expression of 2 main *SCN5A* alternatively spliced variants in cardiac tissue of each individual. The most abundant variant (65% of all *SCN5A* transcripts) is 2015 amino acids long, and lacks a glutamine at position 1077 (*SCN5A*-Q1077del), in comparison with the less prominent 2016 amino acid variant *SCN5A*-Q1077 (35% of all transcripts).[91] Crucially, the severity of reduced sodium channel membrane expression for the BrS mutation *SCN5A*-G1406R was found to be dependent on the background splice variant in which it was expressed, with G1406R in combination with the Q1077 variant displaying a more severe biophysical phenotype.[92] Similarly, the presence of Q1077del had significant effect on sodium current density and kinetics of mutant channels associated with DCM.[93] The ratio of Q1077del and Q1077 channel proteins in each individual thus constitutes a potential modulator of disease phenotype associated with specific *SCN5A* mutations.

## ARE MOST *SCN5A* MUTATIONS POTENTIAL OVERLAP SYNDROME–CAUSING MUTATIONS?

In recent years, clinical, genetic, and/or biophysical overlap phenotypes have been reported for an increasing number of *SCN5A* mutations. Clinical overlap between gain and loss of sodium channel function was further evidenced by the observation by Priori and colleagues[94] that the sodium channel blocker flecainide induced ST-segment elevation in the right precordial leads not only in BrS but also in patients with LQT3 syndrome. The question thus arises whether in fact most (if not all) *SCN5A* mutations are theoretically capable of causing overlap syndromes. Clearly, biophysical properties and clinical phenotypes of specific mutations do not necessarily correlate directly with each other. For instance, reduced peak sodium current density due to defective trafficking of sodium channels may be observed for an LQT3 mutation, without leading to clinical conduction disease in carriers of that particular mutation.[77] Similarly, a mutation may display clear biophysical properties of both gain and loss of sodium channel function but manifest clinically with only conduction disease in absence of features of LQT3.[95] In families with *SCN5A*-related overlap syndromes identified so far, a relatively large number of family members were studied. Thus, one might speculate that perhaps most *SCN5A* mutations are in fact capable of causing an overlap syndrome, although large family pedigrees may be required to actually diagnose them as such. Furthermore, expressivity and severity of certain clinical symptoms may be age-dependent (for instance, conduction slowing)[71,72] and a mixed phenotype may therefore not be apparent until sufficient patients at advanced age are studied.

In loss-of-function *SCN5A* mutations, trafficking of mutant sodium channels to the cell surface membrane is often disturbed. In cardiomyocytes from $Scn5a^{1798insD/+}$ mice, we observed a small but relevant persistent current even though the peak sodium current was substantially reduced.[62] Thus, many more *SCN5A* mutations could be associated with a (small) persistent current, which may, however, be masked owing to inefficient channel trafficking. Indeed, pharmacologic interventions have been shown to (partly) rescue cell surface expression of a mutant sodium channel, while at the same time increasing the persistent current magnitude.[77] Thus, pharmacologic rescue of misprocessed mutant channels may uncover the LQT3 phenotype and diminish the BrS or conduction disorder phenotype.

## SODIUM CHANNEL COMPLEXITY: NOVEL INSIGHTS

When translating results on (mutated) sodium channel function from heterologous expression systems to the myocardial environment, it should be noted that sodium channels are highly complex proteins. As mentioned previously, cardiac sodium channels show inhomogeneous expression within the cardiac conduction system and across the ventricular wall.[11] In addition, differences in sodium channel properties and pharmacologic responsiveness have been described between atrial and ventricular myocytes.[96] Hence, the effects of *SCN5A* mutations may vary throughout regions of the heart, depending on the (effects on) biophysical properties of the cell types involved. More recently, 2 distinct functional pools of sodium channels within the cardiomyocyte have been described, one at the intercalated discs region in close approximation with gap junctional proteins (connexins), the other at the lateral membrane (**Fig. 7**).[97] Sodium channels located at the lateral membrane are associated with the syntrophin-dystrophin complex, whereas those located in the intercalated disc region (which is devoid of syntrophin) interact with synapse-associated protein 97 (SAP97), a member of the membrane-associated guanylate kinase family.[97,98] Functionally, differences in peak sodium current amplitude and kinetics between channels located at the intercalated discs and at the cardiomyocyte lateral membrane have been observed (see **Fig. 7**).[99] Thus, various sodium channels likely have distinct functional roles depending on their composition, subcellular location, and local interaction with proteins and pathways within the myocyte. The consequences of these complexities of sodium channel distribution,

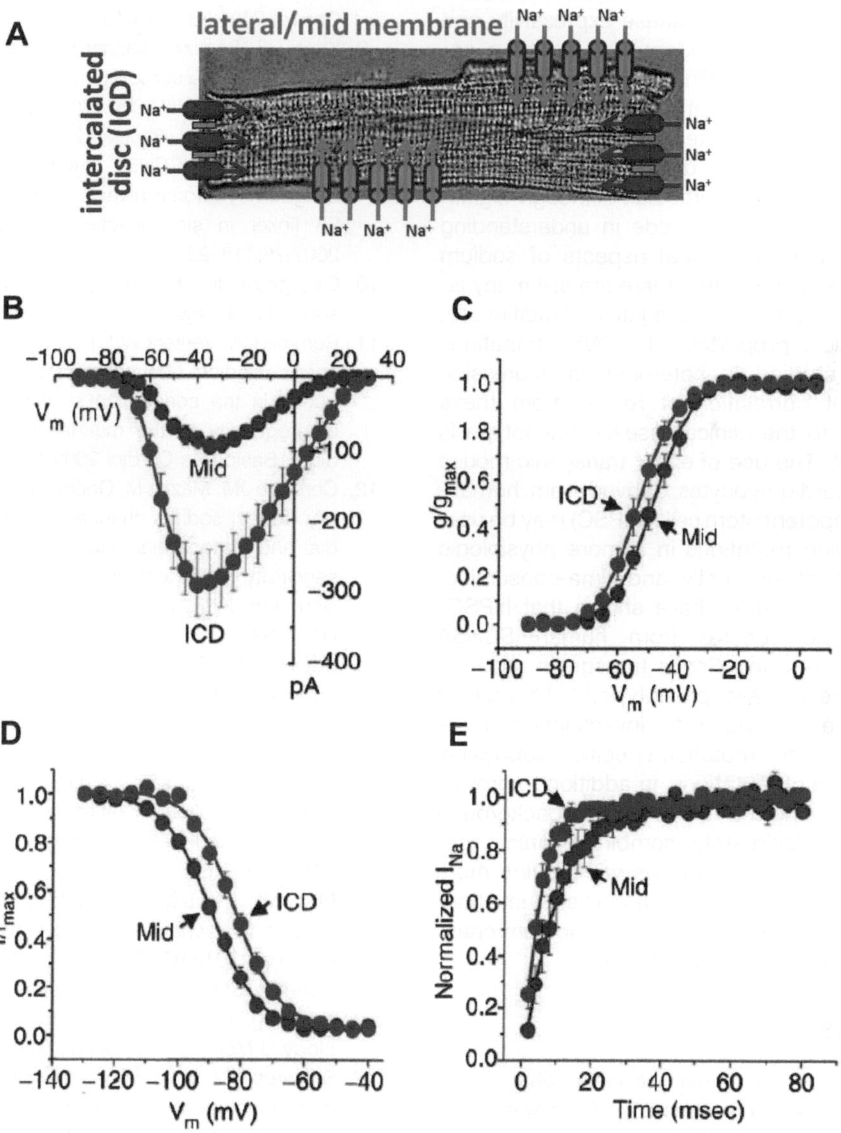


**Fig. 7.** (*A*) Schematic representation of the 2 major subcellular pools of sodium channels, located at the lateral/mid-membrane and at the intercalated disc (ICD) region of the myocyte. (*B–E*) Macropatch measurements in rat ventricular myocytes reveal significant differences in peak sodium current magnitude (*B*), steady-state activation (*C*), steady-state inactivation (*D*), and reactivation (*E*) between the ICD region and the lateral side (Mid) of the cell. (*From* [*Panels B–E*] Lin X, Liu N, Lu J, et al. Subcellular heterogeneity of sodium current properties in adult cardiac ventricular myocytes. Heart Rhythm 2011;8:1927; with permission.)

composition, and function for disease severity and expressivity of *SCN5A* mutations associated with sodium channelopathy and overlap syndrome are as yet unclear, but form a challenging topic for future investigations.

## SUMMARY

Cardiac sodium channel overlap syndrome is increasingly recognized among carriers of *SCN5A* mutations. Multiple biophysical defects of single *SCN5A* mutations are often found to underlie the overlapping clinical manifestations. However, other determinants of variable disease expressivity and severity also have been identified, including genetic background and clinical and environmental factors. Further identification of these modifiers represents an essential step in research related to cardiac sodium channel disease in general, and overlap syndromes in particular. Although significant progress has been made in understanding the genetic and biophysical aspects of sodium channel overlap syndrome, there are still many issues requiring further investigation. Traditionally, the biophysical properties of *SCN5A* mutations have been studied in heterologous expression systems, but correlation of results from these experiments to the clinical disease phenotype is often difficult. The use of either transgenic mouse models or cardiomyocytes derived from human-induced pluripotent stem cells (hiPSC) may be useful for studying mutations in a more physiologic environment, albeit costly and time-consuming. Indeed, we and others have shown that hiPSC-derived cardiomyocytes from human *SCN5A* mutation carriers and *Scn5a* transgenic mice recapitulate the disease phenotype,[100–102] making them suitable candidates for investigation of patient-specific and mutation-specific biophysical consequences of mutations, in addition to providing a tool studying the role of genetic background and modifiers. Ultimately, combined clinical, genetic, and translational studies will provide more insight into the complexity of cardiac sodium channel function and regulation, cardiac sodium channelopathy, and overlap syndromes.

## REFERENCES

1. Cascio WE. Myocardial ischemia: what factors determine arrhythmogenesis? J Cardiovasc Electrophysiol 2001;12:726–9.
2. Tomaselli GF, Zipes DP. What causes sudden death in heart failure? Circ Res 2004;95:754–63.
3. Tan HL, Bezzina CR, Smits JP, et al. Genetic control of sodium channel function. Cardiovasc Res 2003;57:961–73.
4. Wilde AA, Brugada R. Phenotypical manifestations of mutations in the genes encoding subunits of the cardiac sodium channel. Circ Res 2011;108(7):884–97.
5. Remme CA, Wilde AA, Bezzina CR. Cardiac sodium channel overlap syndromes: different faces of SCN5A mutations. Trends Cardiovasc Med 2008;18:78–87.
6. Viswanathan PC, Balser JR. Inherited sodium channelopathies: a continuum of channel dysfunction. Trends Cardiovasc Med 2004;14:28–35.
7. Balser JR. The cardiac sodium channel: gating function and molecular pharmacology. J Mol Cell Cardiol 2001;33:599–613.
8. Kass RS. Sodium channel inactivation in heart: a novel role of the carboxyterminal domain. J Cardiovasc Electrophysiol 2006;17(Suppl 1):S21–5.
9. Casini S, Tan HL, Bhuiyan ZA, et al. Characterization of a novel SCN5A mutation associated with Brugada syndrome reveals involvement of DIIIS4-S5 linker in slow inactivation. Cardiovasc Res 2007;76:418–29.
10. George AL Jr. Inherited disorders of voltage-gated sodium channels. J Clin Invest 2005;115:1990–9.
11. Remme CA, Verkerk AO, Hoogaars WM, et al. The cardiac sodium channel displays differential distribution in the conduction system and transmural heterogeneity in the murine ventricular myocardium. Basic Res Cardiol 2009;104:511–22.
12. Cordeiro JM, Mazza M, Goodrow R, et al. Functionally distinct sodium channels in ventricular epicardial and endocardial cells contribute to a greater sensitivity of the epicardium to electrical depression. Am J Physiol Heart Circ Physiol 2008;295:H154–62.
13. Li GR, Lau CP, Shrier A. Heterogeneity of sodium current in atrial vs epicardial ventricular myocytes of adult guinea pig hearts. J Mol Cell Cardiol 2002;34:1185–94.
14. Remme CA. Cardiac sodium channelopathy associated with SCN5A mutations: electrophysiological, molecular and genetic aspects. J Physiol 2013;591:4099–116.
15. Rook MB, Evers MM, Vos MA, et al. Biology of cardiac sodium channel Nav1.5 expression. Cardiovasc Res 2012;93:12–23.
16. Abriel H. Cardiac sodium channel Na(v)1.5 and interacting proteins: physiology and pathophysiology. J Mol Cell Cardiol 2010;48:2–11.
17. Schwartz PJ. The congenital long QT syndromes from genotype to phenotype: clinical implications. J Intern Med 2006;259:39–47.
18. Bennett PB, Yazawa K, Makita N, et al. Molecular mechanism for an inherited cardiac arrhythmia. Nature 1995;376:683–5.
19. Clancy CE, Tateyama M, Liu H, et al. Non-equilibrium gating in cardiac $Na^+$ channels: an original

mechanism of arrhythmia. Circulation 2003;107: 2233–7.
20. Meregalli PG, Wilde AA, Tan HL. Pathophysiological mechanisms of Brugada syndrome: depolarization disorder, repolarization disorder, or more? Cardiovasc Res 2005;67:367–78.
21. Kapplinger JD, Tester DJ, Alders M, et al. An international compendium of mutations in the SCN5A-encoded cardiac sodium channel in patients referred for Brugada syndrome genetic testing. Heart Rhythm 2010;7:33–46.
22. Schott JJ, Alshinawi C, Kyndt F, et al. Cardiac conduction defects associate with mutations in SCN5A. Nat Genet 1999;23:20–1.
23. Benson DW, Wang DW, Dyment M, et al. Congenital sick sinus syndrome caused by recessive mutations in the cardiac sodium channel gene (*SCN5A*). J Clin Invest 2003;112:1019–28.
24. Smits JP, Koopmann TT, Wilders R, et al. A mutation in the human cardiac sodium channel (E161K) contributes to sick sinus syndrome, conduction disease and Brugada syndrome in two families. J Mol Cell Cardiol 2005;38:969–81.
25. Kyndt F, Probst V, Potet F, et al. Novel *SCN5A* mutation leading either to isolated cardiac conduction defect or Brugada syndrome in a large French family. Circulation 2001;104:3081–6.
26. Darbar D, Kannankeril PJ, Donahue BS, et al. Cardiac sodium channel (SCN5A)variants associated with atrial fibrillation. Circulation 2008;117:1927–35.
27. Ellinor PT, Nam EG, Shea MA, et al. Cardiac sodium channel mutation in atrial fibrillation. Heart Rhythm 2008;5:99–105.
28. Makiyama T, Akao M, Shizuta S, et al. A novel SCN5A gain-of-function mutation M1875T associated with familial atrial fibrillation. J Am Coll Cardiol 2008;52:1326–34.
29. Li Q, Huang H, Liu G, et al. Gain-of-function mutation of Nav1.5 in atrial fibrillation enhances cellular excitability and lowers the threshold for action potential firing. Biochem Biophys Res Commun 2009;380:132–7.
30. Bezzina CR, Rook MB, Groenewegen WA, et al. Compound heterozygosity for mutations (W156X and R225W) in SCN5A associated with severe cardiac conduction disturbances and degenerative changes in the conduction system. Circ Res 2003;92:159–68.
31. McNair WP, Ku L, Taylor MR, et al. SCN5A mutation associated with dilated cardiomyopathy, conduction disorder, and arrhythmia. Circulation 2004; 110:2163–7.
32. Olson TM, Michels VV, Ballew JD, et al. Sodium channel mutations and susceptibility to heart failure and atrial fibrillation. JAMA 2005;293:447–54.
33. Ge J, Sun A, Paajanen V, et al. Molecular and clinical characterization of a novel SCN5A mutation associated with atrioventricular block and dilated cardiomyopathy. Circ Arrhythm Electrophysiol 2008;1:83–92.
34. Nguyen TP, Wang DW, Rhodes TH, et al. Divergent biophysical defects caused by mutant sodium channels in dilated cardiomyopathy with arrhythmia. Circ Res 2008;102:364–71.
35. Olesen MS, Yuan L, Liang B, et al. High prevalence of long QT syndrome-associated SCN5A variants in patients with early-onset lone atrial fibrillation. Circ Cardiovasc Genet 2012;5(4):450–9.
36. Bezzina CR, Veldkamp MW, van den Berg MP, et al. A single $Na^+$ channel mutation causing both long-QT and Brugada syndromes. Circ Res 1999;85:1206–13.
37. Van den Berg MP, Wilde AA, Viersma JW, et al. Possible bradycardic mode of death and successful pacemaker treatment in a large family with features of long QT syndrome type 3 and Brugada syndrome. J Cardiovasc Electrophysiol 2001;12:630–6.
38. Grant AO, Carboni MP, Neplioueva V, et al. Long QT syndrome, Brugada syndrome, and conduction system disease are linked to a single sodium channel mutation. J Clin Invest 2002;110:1201–9.
39. Splawski I, Shen J, Timothy KW, et al. Spectrum of mutations in long-QT syndrome genes. KVLQT1, HERG, SCN5A, KCNE1, and KCNE2. Circulation 2000;102:1178–85.
40. Priori SG, Napolitano C, Gasparini M, et al. Clinical and genetic heterogeneity of right bundle branch block and ST-segment elevation syndrome: a prospective evaluation of 52 families. Circulation 2000;102:2509–15.
41. Chen T, Inoue M, Sheets MF. Reduced voltage dependence of inactivation in the SCN5A sodium channel mutation delF1617. Am J Physiol Heart Circ Physiol 2005;288:H2666–76.
42. Makita N, Behr E, Shimizu W, et al. The E1784K mutation in SCN5A is associated with mixed clinical phenotype of type 3 long QT syndrome. J Clin Invest 2008;118(6):2219–29.
43. Kanters JK, Yuan L, Hedley PL, et al. Flecainide provocation reveals concealed Brugada syndrome in a long QT syndrome family with a novel L1786Q mutation in SCN5A. Circ J 2014;78:1136–43.
44. Kehl HG, Haverkamp W, Rellensmann G, et al. Images in cardiovascular medicine. Life-threatening neonatal arrhythmia: successful treatment and confirmation of clinically suspected extreme long QT-syndrome-3. Circulation 2004;109:e205–6.
45. Zareba W, Sattari MN, Rosero S, et al. Altered atrial, atrioventricular, and ventricular conduction in patients with the long QT syndrome caused by the DeltaKPQ SCN5A sodium channel gene mutation. Am J Cardiol 2001;88:1311–4.
46. Shim SH, Ito M, Maher T, et al. Gene sequencing in neonates and infants with the long QT syndrome. Genet Test 2005;9:281–4.

47. Tester DJ, Will ML, Haglund CM, et al. Compendium of cardiac channel mutations in 541 consecutive unrelated patients referred for long QT syndrome genetic testing. Heart Rhythm 2005;2: 507–17.
48. Valdivia CR, Ackerman MJ, Tester DJ, et al. A novel SCN5A arrhythmia mutation, M1766L, with expression defect rescued by mexiletine. Cardiovasc Res 2002;55:279–89.
49. Chang CC, Acharfi S, Wu MH, et al. A novel SCN5A mutation manifests as a malignant form of long QT syndrome with perinatal onset of tachycardia/ bradycardia. Cardiovasc Res 2004;64:268–78.
50. Lupoglazoff JM, Cheav T, Baroudi G, et al. Homozygous SCN5A mutation in long-QT syndrome with functional two-to-one atrioventricular block. Circ Res 2001;89:E16–21.
51. Horne AJ, Eldstrom J, Sanatani S, et al. A novel mechanism for LQT3 with 2:1 block: a pore-lining mutation in Nav1.5 significantly affects voltage-dependence of activation. Heart Rhythm 2011; 8(5):770–7.
52. Schulze-Bahr E, Eckardt L, Breithardt G, et al. Sodium channel gene (SCN5A) mutations in 44 index patients with Brugada syndrome: different incidences in familial and sporadic disease. Hum Mutat 2003;21:651–2.
53. Rossenbacker T, Carroll SJ, Liu H, et al. Novel pore mutation in SCN5A manifests as a spectrum of phenotypes ranging from atrial flutter, conduction disease, and Brugada syndrome to sudden cardiac death. Heart Rhythm 2004;1:610–5.
54. Makiyama T, Akao M, Tsuji K, et al. High risk for bradyarrhythmic complications in patients with Brugada syndrome caused by SCN5A gene mutations. J Am Coll Cardiol 2005;46:2100–6.
55. Cordeiro JM, Barajas-Martinez H, Hong K, et al. Compound heterozygous mutations P336L and I1660V in the human cardiac sodium channel associated with the Brugada syndrome. Circulation 2006;114:2026–33.
56. McNair WP, Sinagra G, Taylor MR, et al, Familial Cardiomyopathy Registry Research Group. SCN5A mutations associate with arrhythmic dilated cardiomyopathy and commonly localize to the voltage-sensing mechanism. J Am Coll Cardiol 2011;57(21):2160–8.
57. Yu J, Hu J, Dai X, et al. SCN5A mutation in Chinese patients with arrhythmogenic right ventricular dysplasia. Herz 2014;39(2):271–5.
58. Peters S. Arrhythmogenic right ventricular dysplasia-cardiomyopathy and provocable coved-type ST-segment elevation in right precordial leads: clues from long-term follow-up. Europace 2008;10(7): 816–20.
59. Frustaci A, Priori SG, Pieroni M, et al. Cardiac histological substrate in patients with clinical phenotype of Brugada syndrome. Circulation 2005;112(24):3680–7.
60. Agullo-Pascual E, Cerrone M, Delmar M. Arrhythmogenic cardiomyopathy and Brugada syndrome: diseases of the connexome. FEBS Lett 2014;588: 1322–30.
61. Veldkamp MW, Viswanathan PC, Bezzina C, et al. Two distinct congenital arrhythmias evoked by a multidysfunctional $Na^+$ channel. Circ Res 2000; 86:e91–7.
62. Remme CA, Verkerk AO, Nuyens D, et al. Overlap syndrome of cardiac sodium channel disease in mice carrying the equivalent mutation of human SCN5A-1795insD. Circulation 2006;114:2584–94.
63. Clancy CE, Rudy Y. $Na^+$ channel mutation that causes both Brugada and long-QT syndrome phenotypes. A simulation study of mechanism. Circulation 2002;105:1208–13.
64. Watanabe H, Yang T, Stroud DM, et al. Striking in vivo phenotype of a disease-associated human SCN5A mutation producing minimal changes in vitro. Circulation 2011;124(9):1001–11.
65. Probst V, Wilde AA, Barc J, et al. SCN5A mutations and the role of genetic background in the pathophysiology of Brugada syndrome. Circ Cardiovasc Genet 2009;2(6):552–7.
66. Meregalli PG, Tan HL, Probst V, et al. Type of SCN5A mutation determines clinical severity and degree of conduction slowing in loss-of-function sodium channelopathies. Heart Rhythm 2009;6(3): 341–8.
67. Postema PG, Van den Berg M, Van Tintelen JP, et al. Founder mutations in the Netherlands: SCN5a 1795insD, the first described arrhythmia overlap syndrome and one of the largest and best characterised families worldwide. Neth Heart J 2009;17(11):422–8.
68. Makita N. Phenotypic overlap of cardiac sodium channelopathies: individual-specific or mutation-specific? Circ J 2009;73(5):810–7.
69. Priori SG, Schwartz PJ, Napolitano C, et al. Risk stratification in the long-QT syndrome. N Engl J Med 2003;348:1866–74.
70. Gehi AK, Duong TD, Metz LD, et al. Risk stratification of individuals with the Brugada electrocardiogram: a meta-analysis. J Cardiovasc Electrophysiol 2006;17: 577–83.
71. Beaufort-Krol GC, van den Berg MP, Wilde AA, et al. Developmental aspects of long QT syndrome type 3 and Brugada syndrome on the basis of a single SCN5A mutation in childhood. J Am Coll Cardiol 2005;46:331–7.
72. Probst V, Kyndt F, Potet F, et al. Haploinsufficiency in combination with aging causes SCN5A-linked hereditary Lenègre disease. J Am Coll Cardiol 2003;41:643–52.
73. Royer A, van Veen TA, Le Bouter S, et al. Mouse model of SCN5A-linked hereditary Lenègre's

disease: age-related conduction slowing and myocardial fibrosis. Circulation 2005;111:1738–46.
74. Mok NS, Priori SG, Napolitano C, et al. A newly characterized SCN5A mutation underlying Brugada syndrome unmasked by hyperthermia. J Cardiovasc Electrophysiol 2003;14:407–11.
75. Keller DI, Rougier JS, Kucera JP, et al. Brugada syndrome and fever: genetic and molecular characterization of patients carrying SCN5A mutations. Cardiovasc Res 2005;67:510–9.
76. Valdivia CR, Tester DJ, Rok BA, et al. A trafficking defective, Brugada syndrome-causing SCN5A mutation rescued by drugs. Cardiovasc Res 2004;62:53–62.
77. Liu K, Yang T, Viswanathan PC, et al. New mechanism contributing to drug-induced arrhythmia: rescue of a misprocessed LQT3 mutant. Circulation 2005;112:3239–46.
78. Remme CA, Scicluna BP, Verkerk AO, et al. Genetically determined differences in sodium current characteristics modulate conduction disease severity in mice with cardiac sodium channelopathy. Circ Res 2009;104:1283–92.
79. Scicluna BP, Tanck MW, Remme CA, et al. Quantitative trait loci for electrocardiographic parameters and arrhythmia in the mouse. J Mol Cell Cardiol 2011;50:380–9.
80. Lodder EM, Scicluna BP, Milano A, et al. Dissection of a quantitative trait locus for PR interval duration identifies Tnni3k as a novel modulator of cardiac conduction. PLoS Genet 2012;8:e1003113.
81. Ackerman MJ, Splawski I, Makielski JC, et al. Spectrum and prevalence of cardiac sodium channel variants among black, white, Asian, and Hispanic individuals: implications for arrhythmogenic susceptibility and Brugada/long QT syndrome genetic testing. Heart Rhythm 2004;15:600–7.
82. Viswanathan PC, Benson DW, Balser JR. A common SCN5A polymorphism modulates the biophysical effects of an SCN5A mutation. J Clin Invest 2003;111:341–6.
83. Ye B, Valdivia CR, Ackerman MJ, et al. A common human SCN5A polymorphism modifies expression of an arrhythmia causing mutation. Physiol Genomics 2003;12:187–93.
84. Poelzing S, Forleo C, Samodell M, et al. SCN5A polymorphism restores trafficking of a Brugada syndrome mutation on a separate gene. Circulation 2006;114:368–76.
85. Gui J, Wang T, Trump D, et al. Mutation-specific effects of polymorphism H558R in SCN5A-related sick sinus syndrome. J Cardiovasc Electrophysiol 2010;21(5):564–73.
86. Marangoni S, Di Resta C, Rocchetti M, et al. A Brugada syndrome mutation (p.S216L) and its modulation by p.H558R polymorphism: standard and dynamic characterization. Cardiovasc Res 2011;91(4):606–16.
87. Shinlapawittayatorn K, Du XX, Liu H, et al. A common SCN5A polymorphism modulates the biophysical defects of SCN5A mutations. Heart Rhythm 2011;8(3):455–62.
88. Lizotte E, Junttila MJ, Dube MP, et al. Genetic modulation of Brugada syndrome by a common polymorphism. J Cardiovasc Electrophysiol 2009;20(10):1137–41.
89. Bezzina CR, Shimizu W, Yang P, et al. A common sodium channel promoter haplotype in Asian subjects underlies variability in cardiac conduction. Circulation 2006;113:338–44.
90. Groenewegen WA, Firouzi M, Bezzina CR, et al. A cardiac sodium channel mutation cosegregates with a rare connexin40 genotype in familial atrial standstill. Circ Res 2003;92:14–22.
91. Makielski JC, Ye B, Valdivia CR, et al. A ubiquitous splice variant and a common polymorphism affect heterologous expression of recombinant human SCN5A heart sodium channels. Circ Res 2003;93:821–8.
92. Tan BH, Valdivia CR, Song C, et al. Partial expression defect for the SCN5A missense mutation G1406R depends on splice variant background Q1077 and rescue by mexiletine. Am J Physiol Heart Circ Physiol 2006;291:H1822–8.
93. Cheng J, Morales A, Siegfried JD, et al. SCN5A rare variants in familial dilated cardiomyopathy decrease peak sodium current depending on the common polymorphism H558R and common splice variant Q1077del. Clin Transl Sci 2010;3(6):287–94.
94. Priori SG, Napolitano C, Schwartz PJ, et al. The elusive link between LQT3 and Brugada syndrome. The role of flecainide challenge. Circulation 2000;102:945–7.
95. Zumhagen S, Veldkamp MW, Stallmeyer B, et al. A heterozygous deletion mutation in the cardiac sodium channel gene SCN5A with loss- and gain-of-function characteristics manifests as isolated conduction disease, without signs of Brugada or long QT syndrome. PLoS One 2013;8(6):e67963.
96. Burashnikov A, Di Diego JM, Zygmunt AC, et al. Atrium-selective sodium channel block as a strategy for suppression of atrial fibrillation: differences in sodium channel inactivation between atria and ventricles and the role of ranolazine. Circulation 2007;116:1449–57.
97. Shy D, Gillet L, Abriel H. Cardiac sodium channel $Na_V1.5$ distribution in myocytes via interacting proteins: the multiple pool model. Biochim Biophys Acta 2013;1833:886–94.
98. Petitprez S, Zmoos AF, Ogrodnik J, et al. SAP97 and dystrophin macromolecular complexes determine two pools of cardiac sodium channels Nav1.5 in cardiomyocytes. Circ Res 2011;108:294–304.

99. Lin X, Liu N, Lu J, et al. Subcellular heterogeneity of sodium current properties in adult cardiac ventricular myocytes. Heart Rhythm 2011;8:1923–30.
100. Davis RP, Casini S, van den Berg CW, et al. Cardiomyocytes derived from pluripotent stem cells recapitulate electrophysiological characteristics of an overlap syndrome of cardiac sodium channel disease. Circulation 2012;125:3079–91.
101. Malan D, Friedrichs S, Fleischmann BK, et al. Cardiomyocytes obtained from induced pluripotent stem cells with long-QT syndrome 3 recapitulate typical disease-specific features in vitro. Circ Res 2011;109:841–7.
102. Terrenoire C, Wang K, Tung KW, et al. Induced pluripotent stem cells used to reveal drug actions in a long QT syndrome family with complex genetics. J Gen Physiol 2013;141:61–72.

# Cardiac Sodium Channel $Na_v1.5$ and Drug-Induced Long QT Syndrome

Hugues Abriel, MD, PhD

**KEYWORDS**

• Sodium channel • $Na_v1.5$ • Long QT syndrome • Drugs • Arrhythmia • hERG

**KEY POINTS**

- Genetic and acquired factors may increase the cardiac late sodium current ($I_{Na}$), thus prolonging the cardiac action potential duration and QT interval of the electrocardiogram.
- An increase in late $I_{Na}$ reduces the cardiac repolarization reserve of patients.
- Patients with increased late $I_{Na}$ are more likely to present with symptomatic drug-induced long QT syndrome.
- Drug-induced long QT syndrome is one of the manifestations of genetic variants found in the gene *SCN5A* encoding the cardiac sodium channel $Na_v1.5$.

## INTRODUCTION

The duration of the action potential (AP) of cardiac cells mainly depends on the balance between the inward (depolarizing) and outward (repolarizing) currents during the plateau phase of the AP, so-called phase 2 (**Fig. 1**). Because total membrane conductance is least during phase 2,[1] small changes in inward or outward currents may have major consequences on AP duration.[2] Consequently, any increase in the inward currents, mediated by either sodium or calcium voltage-gated channels, or decrease of the outward potassium currents prolongs AP duration. The prolongation of the AP duration of ventricular cells is reflected by a prolongation of the QT interval duration on the body surface electrocardiogram (ECG).[3] QT interval prolongation above the normal range is, in itself, not a problem for the patient, but is well known to be a marker of a specific type of polymorphic ventricular arrhythmia known as Torsades de pointes (TdP).[4] The cellular mechanisms that determine how the delayed repolarization of ventricular cells (reflected by a prolongation of AP duration) leads to TdP are still unknown.[5] Nevertheless, it is widely accepted that increased inward or decreased outward currents lead to AP prolongation, followed by QT interval prolongation, TdP, and eventually syncope, which can result in sudden cardiac death.[5–7]

## ORIGIN OF CARDIAC CURRENT ALTERATIONS LEADING TO ACTION POTENTIAL AND QT INTERVAL PROLONGATION

Congenital (mostly genetic) and acquired causes for alterations of cardiac ionic currents that can lead to the prolongation of AP duration represent 2 distinct categories.[8] Over the past 20 years, thousands of mutations have been found in genes coding for either the cardiac channel pore-forming subunits or for ion channel regulatory proteins. These disorders are commonly known as genetic cardiac channelopathies.[8,9]

Congenital long QT syndrome (LQTS) is among these cardiac channelopathies that plays an

The group of H. Abriel is supported by a grant from the Swiss National Science Foundation (310030_147060).
The author has nothing to disclose.
Department of Clinical Research, University of Bern, Murtenstrasse, 35, Bern 3010, Switzerland
*E-mail address:* Hugues.Abriel@dkf.unibe.ch

Card Electrophysiol Clin 6 (2014) 777–783
http://dx.doi.org/10.1016/j.ccep.2014.08.006
1877-9182/14/$ – see front matter 

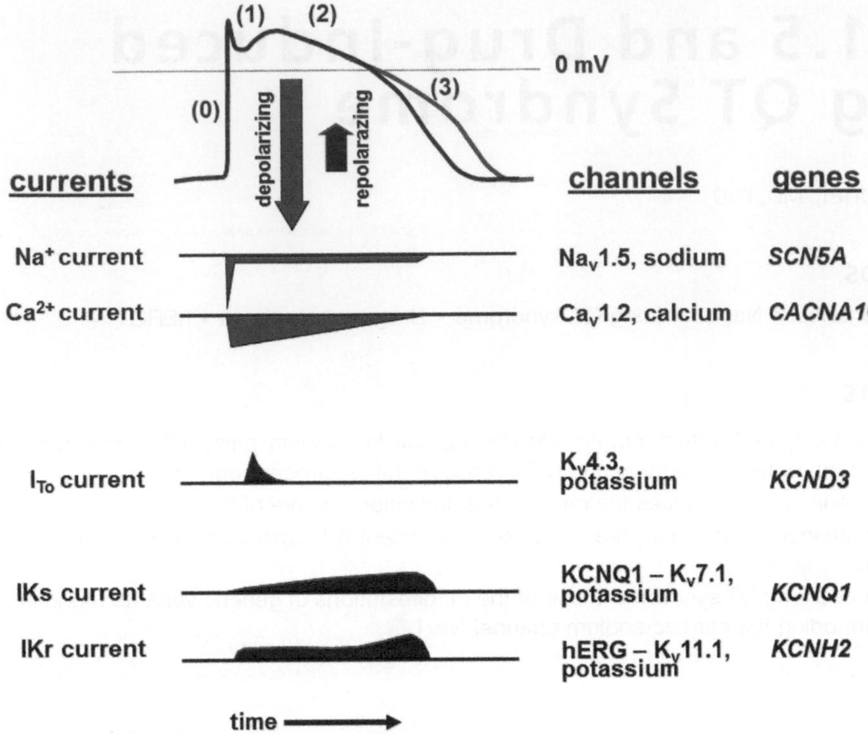


**Fig. 1.** Main depolarizing (*red*) and repolarizing (*blue*) current involved in the generation of the cardiac action potential (AP) of ventricular cells. The shapes representing the different currents are aligned with their approximated time of action during the cardiac AP. Phase 0 (upstroke depolarization) is caused by the rapid activation of voltage-gated sodium channels $Na_V1.5$ encoded by the gene *SCN5A*. These $Na_V1.5$ channels inactivate very rapidly after activation. This inactivation is almost complete, allowing for only small physiologic late $I_{Na}$ during the plateau phase 2. Any increase of this late $I_{Na}$ may reduce the repolarization reserve and can be pro-arrhythmogenic (see text). The first repolarization phase 1 (notch) is owing to the transient outward potassium current $I_{to}$. The plateau phase 2 is primarily maintained by an inward calcium current flowing through $Ca_V1.2$ voltage-gated channels, which then slowly inactivate. Repolarization of the AP (phase 3) is obtained through the concerted action of three outward delayed currents: $I_{Ks}$ (slow), $I_{Kr}$ (rapid), and $I_{K1}$. The main pore-forming subunits are KCNQ1 for $I_{Ks}$ (or $K_V7.1$), hERG for $I_{Kr}$ (or $K_V11.1$), and $K_{ir}2.1$ for $I_{K1}$. AP duration prolongation (*red line*) can be caused by either a reduction in the repolarizing current (*blue arrow*) or an increase in the depolarizing current (*red arrow*).

important clinical role.[10] The first genes that were discovered to be mutated in patients with such inherited arrhythmias were found in congenital LQTS families.[11,12] To date, more than 10 different genes coding for either ion channel subunits or ion channel interacting proteins have been linked to LQTS. The prolongation of the AP duration of ventricular cells may be caused by either loss-of-function mutations in the genes coding for potassium channel subunits or gain-of-function mutations in genes coding for sodium (*SCN5A*) or calcium (*CACNA1C*) ion channel subunits (see **Fig. 1**). In some cases, for example, the cardiac sodium channel $Na_V1.5$ multiprotein complex,[13] mutations have also been found in genes coding for proteins, for example, α1-syntrophin[14,15] and caveolin-3,[16] which regulate various ion channels (reviewed in the article by Kyle and Makielski elsewhere in this issue). Most of the mutations found in *SCN5A* that cause LQTS have been shown to alter the fast inactivation process of the sodium channel $Na_V1.5$ by either enhancing the reopening of the channels after inactivation or by increasing the likelihood that these channels enter into "bursting" mode (reviewed in Moreno and Clancy[17]), which increases the late cardiac $I_{Na}$ that is small under normal physiologic conditions (see **Fig. 1**).[18,19] LQTS associated with *SCN5A* mutations, LQTS type 3, is found in only approximately 10% of patients with LQTS. It is, however, more severe and more difficult to treat than other genetic forms (see the article by Ruan and colleagues elsewhere in this issue). Rare mutations in genes coding for interacting proteins (reviewed by Kyle and Makielski elsewhere in this issue) also increase the late $I_{Na}$, which can consequently lead to

LQTS. The mechanisms underlying the increase caused by mutations in $Na_v1.5$ interacting proteins are not completely understood. Computational studies[20] have shown that small increases, less than 50%, of the late $I_{Na}$ may significantly alter the repolarization phase of cardiac cells and increase the QT interval on computed pseudo ECG (**Fig. 2**). Importantly, the increase in the QT interval duration is not linear (see **Fig. 2**). Above a certain threshold, the QT interval is more prolonged with a comparable increase in the late $I_{Na}$.

In addition to genetic causes, several pathologic conditions may also increase the late $I_{Na}$ of $Na_v1.5$.[17,21] Cardiac ischemia and chronic heart failure are the most common pathologies known to lead to an increase in the late $I_{Na}$ (reviewed by Antzelevitch and associates[21]). During heart failure, the increased expression and activity of the

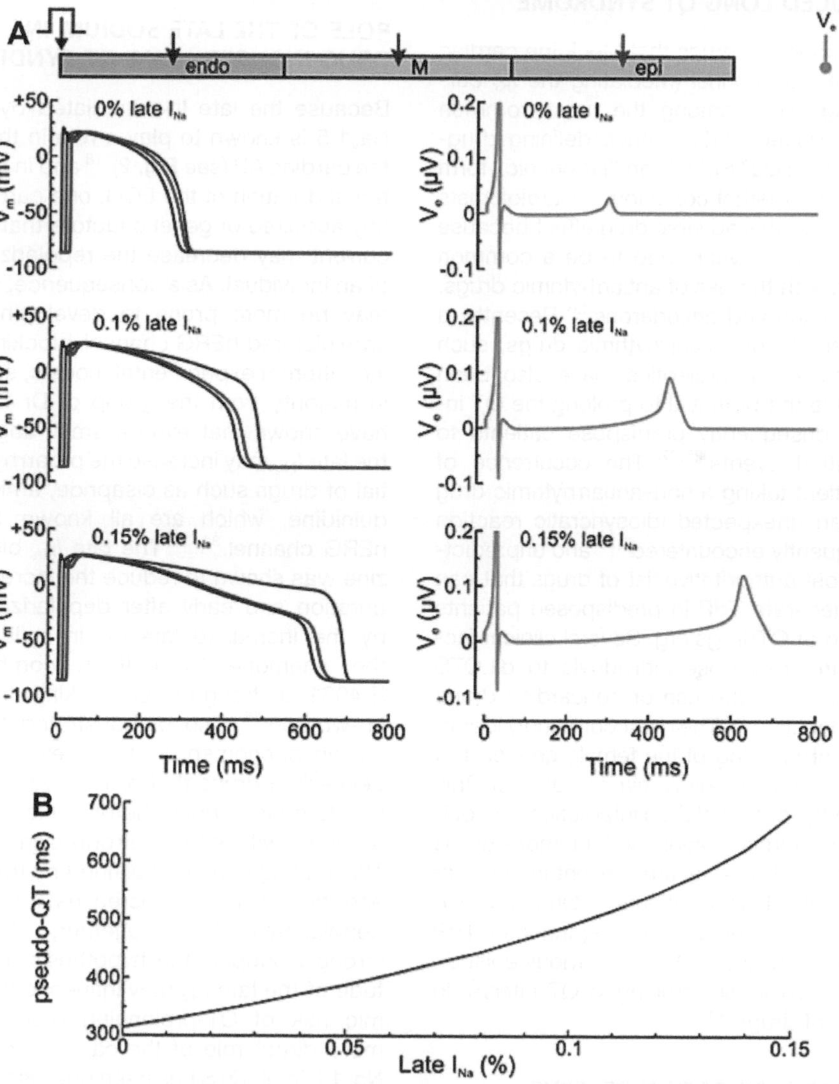


**Fig. 2.** Simulated transmural conduction of the cardiac action potential (AP) and the influence of the late $I_{Na}$ on AP duration and corresponding pseudo-ECGs. (*A*) The schematic on the top represents a computer simulation of a transmural cable, summarizing the ventricular free wall with endocardial (*endo, blue*), mid myocardial (*M, purple*), and epicardial cells (*epi, red*); see Sottas and colleagues[20] for methods. APs registered in the middle of the endocardial, mid myocardial, and epicardial segments (*left*), and reconstructed pseudo-ECGs (*right*) for 0%, 0.1%, and 0.15% late $I_{Na}$, respectively. (*B*) QT interval in the pseudo-ECG as a function of the increasing late $I_{Na}$. The increase of the QT interval duration is not linear (see text). (*Adapted from* Sottas V, Rougier JS, Jousset F, et al. Characterization of 2 genetic variants of $Na_v$ 1.5-arginine 689 found in patients with cardiac arrhythmias. J Cardiovasc Electrophysiol 2013;24(9):1037–46; with permission.)

calcium-calmodulin–activated protein kinase, CaMKIIδ, may lead to the hyperphosphorylation of $Na_v1.5$ and thus increased late $I_{Na}$.[22] The increased late $I_{Na}$ seen with cardiac ischemia and heart failure may play a predominant role in arrhythmia generation in patients, although further investigation is required to confirm this hypothesis. For this reason, late $I_{Na}$-blocking drugs, such as ranolazine, are currently being investigated for antiarrhythmic use in the clinical setting.[23]

## DRUG-INDUCED LONG QT SYNDROME

The administration of drugs that block the cardiac potassium hERG channel (mediating the $I_{Kr}$ current, see **Fig. 1**) is among the most common causes of acquired LQTS, hence defining drug-induced LQTS (diLQTS),[4,7,24] an "iatrogenic" form of this potentially lethal condition.[25] Cardiologists are well aware of this adverse drug effect because it was shown many years ago to be a common complication with the use of antiarrhythmic drugs, such as quinidine and amiodarone.[26] Recently, a large number of non–antiarrhythmic drugs, such as antibiotics and neuroleptics, have also been shown to have the potential to prolong the QT interval and consequently predispose patients to TdP and lethal events.[25,27] The occurrence of TdP in a patient taking a non–antiarrhythmic drug represents an unexpected idiosyncratic reaction that is infrequently encountered[7,25] and unpredictable. The most authoritative list of drugs that can potentially generate TdP in predisposed patients can be found at QTdrugs.org. Several clinical factors that can predispose individuals to diLQTS and TdP related to the use of noncardiac drugs have been identified.[28] The most commonly identified risk factor is being of the female gender, but heart disease and hypokalemia are also on this list. Importantly, potential drug interactions associated with the administration of 2 or more drugs prolonging the QT interval are present in approximately 40% of diLQTS patients.[28] Only approximately 20% of patients with drug-induced TdP have a family history of LQTS, a previous episode of TdP or an obviously prolonged QT interval in the absence of drugs.[28]

## CARDIAC REPOLARIZATION RESERVE

There is great variability in patients' responses to drugs that block the hERG channel, which can, in turn, prolong the QT interval.[7] This variability mainly originates from differences in pharmacokinetic and/or pharmacodynamic parameters between individuals. The concept of a cardiac "repolarization reserve" for a given patient was proposed by Dr D. Roden,[29,30] and is described as follows[29]: The "loss of one component (such as $I_{Kr}$) ordinarily will not lead to failure of repolarization (i.e., marked QT prolongation); as a corollary, individuals with subclinical lesions in other components of the system, say $I_{Ks}$ or calcium current, may display no QT change until $I_{Kr}$ block is superimposed." In other words, every individual has her/his own unique cardiac "repolarization reserve," and will tolerate differently any insults that contribute to the reduction of this reserve.

## ROLE OF THE LATE SODIUM IN DRUG-INDUCED LONG QT SYNDROME

Because the late INa mediated by the channel $Na_v1.5$ is known to play a role in the duration of the cardiac AP (see **Fig. 2**),[18] and in turn the QT interval duration of the ECG, one can propose that any acquired or genetic factors that increase this current may decrease the repolarization reserve of an individual. As a consequence, such patients may be more prone to developing TdP when administered hERG channel–blocking drugs. Using different experimental models, several studies in majority from the group of Dr L. Bellardinelli have shown that even a small augmentation of the late $I_{Na}$ may increase the proarrhythmic potential of drugs such as cisapride, amiodarone, and quinidine, which are all known to block the hERG channel.[31–33] The late $I_{Na}$ blocker ranolazine was shown to reduce the increase of the AP duration and early after depolarizations caused by the increased late $I_{Na}$ in cells treated with the anemone toxin II in combination with E-4031, a strong hERG-blocking drug.[34] Wu and co-workers[19] also demonstrated that the well-known phenomenon of the reverse use dependence[35] of drugs that prolong AP duration could be attenuated when the physiologic late $I_{Na}$ was reduced with either tetrodotoxin or ranolazine. This finding can be explained by the fact that the endogenous late $I_{Na}$ increases at a slower rate of depolarization.[19] Altogether, these results strongly support the hypothesis that the amplitude of the late $I_{Na}$ may influence the proarrhythmic risk of QT-prolonging drugs. Recently, a more direct role of the cardiac sodium channel $Na_v1.5$ in diLQTS has been proposed by the group of Dr D. Roden.[36] Chronic incubation of mouse cardiomyocytes with several classical diLQTS drugs, such as dofetilide, D-sotalol, and erythromycin, was shown to directly increase the late $I_{Na}$ via inhibition of one of cardiac phosphatidylinositol-3 kinases.[36] This study[36] illustrates that the molecular mechanisms underlying diLQTS may be more complex that initially thought.

## ROLE OF GENETIC VARIANTS IN *SCN5A* IN DRUG-INDUCED LONG QT SYNDROME

Most articles in this issue of *Cardiac Electrophysiology Clinics* address distinct pathologic phenotypes that have been linked to genetic variants in *SCN5A*. Based on the experimental data presented herein, it is conceivable that any variant that interferes with the fast inactivation of the Na$_V$1.5 channel may reduce the repolarization reserve of the individual carrying it. Even small increases in the late $I_{Na}$, including those that have a negligible effect on the AP duration and QT interval, may favor significant AP prolongation and arrhythmogenicity when exposed to hERG channel–blocking drugs. Illustrating this concept, the variant S1103Y in *SCN5A*, found with an allelic frequency of approximately 13% in African Americans,[37] has been shown to increase the late $I_{Na}$ by a factor of approximately 1.4.[38] This S1103Y variant has been associated with an increased risk for arrhythmias in patients with hypokalemia and those administered hERG-blocking drugs such as amiodarone.[38] Computational studies (reproduced in **Fig. 3**)[38] have illustrated that simulated APs obtained from cardiac cells with the S1103Y variant were more likely to generate arrhythmogenic early after depolarization when increasing $I_{Kr}$ block, thus simulating the administration of a hERG channel–blocking drug. Two studies[39,40] demonstrated the overrepresentation of this not-so-rare S1103Y *SCN5A* variant

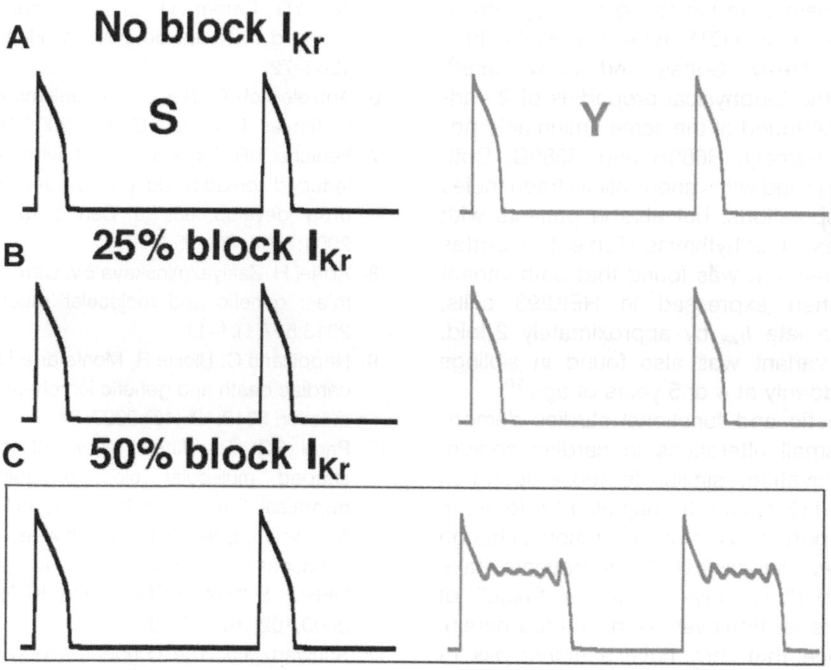

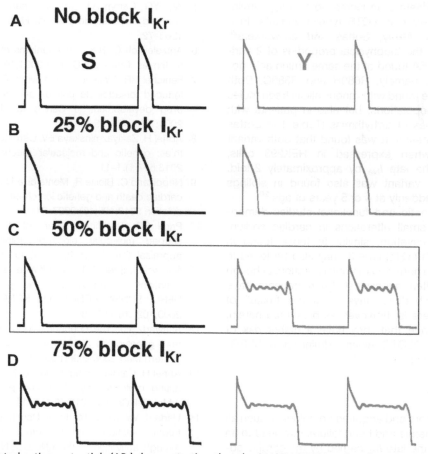


**Fig. 3.** Simulated action potentials (APs) demonstrating that the S1103Y *SCN5A* variant increases the susceptibility for developing arrhythmias. Simulated ventricular APs (see Splawski and associates[38] for methods) incorporating the biophysical properties of the S1103 (wild-type variant) and Y1103 (rare) variants are presented for 0% (*A*), 25% (*B*), 50% (*C*), and 75% (*D*) hERG channel (mediating the $I_{Kr}$ current) block. Both S1103- and Y1103-containing cells exhibit normal phenotypes under 0% and 25% of hERG block. When 50% of hERG channels are blocked (*C*), the Y1103 variant demonstrates abnormal repolarization with early after depolarizations. With 75% block (*D*), both S1103 and Y1103 show similar abnormal cellular repolarizations. (*From* Splawski I, Timothy KW, Tateyama M, et al. Variant of *SCN5A* sodium channel implicated in risk of cardiac arrhythmia. Science 2002;297(5585):1333–6; with permission.)

in sudden infant death syndrome cases, and it was recently reported[41] that African-American S1103Y carriers with heart failure and implanted with defibrillators presented with more arrhythmic events. Interestingly, when the intracellular pH was rendered more acidic, the S1103Y variant generated a late $I_{Na}$ that was markedly increased (~5% of the peak $I_{Na}$), suggesting that it may confer increased susceptibility to arrhythmias during cardiac ischemia.

The role of *SCN5A* in diLQTS was also demonstrated in a study[42] investigating the role of the L1825P variant found in one proband with TdP after the administration of cisapride, a gastroprokinetic drug with a high affinity for the hERG channel. The variant-induced biophysical alterations were studied in HEK293 cells[42] and, among other disturbances, the L1825P $Na_v1.5$ channels were shown to generate an increased late $I_{Na}$, similar to that observed in LQTS type 3 variants. In a more recent study, Sottas and co-workers[20] investigated the biophysical properties of 2 variants of *SCN5A* found at the same amino acid position R689, namely, R689H and R689C. Both variants were found with various allelic frequencies in control populations, but also in patients with different types of arrhythmias (Table 1 in Sottas and associates[20]). It was found that both variant channels, when expressed in HEK293 cells, increased the late $I_{Na}$ by approximately 2-fold. The R689H variant was also found in siblings who died suddenly at 4 or 5 years of age.[20]

These genetic and functional studies demonstrate that small alterations in cardiac sodium channel inactivation, similar to those found in patients with LQTS type 3, may also be found in patients with normal QT interval duration, although they are often subclinical. Such patients have been described to have a "forme fruste" of LQTS.[43] There is, however, as presented herein, good evidence that they have a higher risk of developing diLQTS when administered hERG-blocking drugs.

## SUMMARY

Genetic factors and acquired pathologies, such as cardiac ischemia and heart failure, may lead to an increase in the late $I_{Na}$ carried by the cardiac sodium channel $Na_v1.5$. As a result cardiac AP repolarization is delayed, which in turn reduces the cardiac repolarization reserve of afflicted patients. Such patients have been shown to be more susceptible to symptomatic diLQTS, which is one of the manifestations of genetic variants is found in the gene *SCN5A* encoding the cardiac sodium channel $Na_v1.5$.

## ACKNOWLEDGMENTS

The author thanks Dr A. Felley for her useful comments on this article.

## REFERENCES

1. Weidmann S. Effect of current flow on the membrane potential of cardiac muscle. J Physiol 1951; 115:227–36.
2. Kass RS. Genetically induced reduction in small currents has major impact. Circulation 1997;96(6): 1720–1.
3. Giudicessi JR, Ackerman MJ. Genotype- and phenotype-guided management of congenital long QT syndrome. Curr Probl Cardiol 2013;38(10):417–55.
4. Viskin S. Long QT syndromes and torsade de pointes. Lancet 1999;354(9190):1625–33.
5. Yap YG, Camm AJ. Drug induced QT prolongation and torsades de pointes. Heart 2003;89(11): 1363–72.
6. Antzelevitch C. Basic mechanisms of reentrant arrhythmias. Curr Opin Cardiol 2001;16(1):1–7.
7. Fenichel RR, Malik M, Antzelevitch C, et al. Drug-induced torsades de pointes and implications for drug development. J Cardiovasc Electrophysiol 2004;15(4):475–95.
8. Abriel H, Zaklyazminskaya EV. Cardiac channelopathies: genetic and molecular mechanisms. Gene 2013;517(1):1–11.
9. Napolitano C, Bloise R, Monteforte N, et al. Sudden cardiac death and genetic ion channelopathies. Circulation 2012;125(16):2027–34.
10. Priori SG. The fifteen years of discoveries that shaped molecular electrophysiology: time for appraisal. Circ Res 2010;107(4):451–6.
11. Splawski I, Shen J, Timothy KW, et al. Spectrum of mutations in long-QT syndrome genes. KVLQT1, HERG, SCN5A, KCNE1, and KCNE2. Circulation 2000;102(10):1178–85.
12. Schwartz PJ. The congenital long QT syndromes from genotype to phenotype: clinical implications. J Intern Med 2006;259(1):39–47.
13. Abriel H. Cardiac sodium channel Nav1.5 and interacting proteins: physiology and pathophysiology. J Mol Cell Cardiol 2010;48(1):2–11.
14. Ueda K, Valdivia C, Medeiros-Domingo A, et al. Syntrophin mutation associated with long QT syndrome through activation of the nNOS-SCN5A macromolecular complex. Proc Natl Acad Sci U S A 2008; 105(27):9355–60.
15. Wu G, Ai T, Kim JJ, et al. Alpha-1-syntrophin mutation and the long QT syndrome: a disease of sodium channel disruption. Circ Arrhythm Electrophysiol 2008;1(3):1193–201.
16. Vatta M, Ackerman MJ, Ye B, et al. Mutant caveolin-3 induces persistent late sodium current and is

associated with long-QT syndrome. Circulation 2006;114(20):2104–12.
17. Moreno JD, Clancy CE. Pathophysiology of the cardiac late Na current and its potential as a drug target. J Mol Cell Cardiol 2011;52(3):608–19.
18. Coraboeuf E, Deroubaix E, Coulombe A. Effect of tetrodotoxin on action potentials of the conducting system in the dog heart. Am J Physiol Heart Circ Physiol 1979;236(4):H561–7.
19. Wu L, Ma J, Li H, et al. Late sodium current contributes to the reverse rate-dependent effect of IKr inhibition on ventricular repolarization. Circulation 2011; 123(16):1713–20.
20. Sottas V, Rougier JS, Jousset F, et al. Characterization of 2 genetic variants of Nav1.5-arginine 689 found in patients with cardiac arrhythmias. J Cardiovasc Electrophysiol 2013;24(9):1037–46.
21. Antzelevitch C, Nesterenko V, Shryock JC, et al. The role of late I Na in development of cardiac arrhythmias. Handb Exp Pharmacol 2014;221:137–68.
22. Wagner S, Ruff HM, Weber SL, et al. Reactive oxygen species-activated Ca/Calmodulin Kinase II {delta} is required for late INa augmentation leading to cellular Na and Ca overload. Circ Res 2011; 108(5):555–65.
23. Maier LS, Layug B, Karwatowska-Prokopczuk E, et al. RAnoLazIne for the treatment of diastolic heart failure in patients with preserved ejection fraction: the RALI-DHF proof-of-concept study. JACC Heart Fail 2013;1(2):115–22.
24. Roden DM. Drug-induced prolongation of the QT interval. N Engl J Med 2004;350(10):1013–22.
25. Abriel H, Schläpfer J, Keller DI, et al. Molecular and clinical determinants of drug-induced long QT syndrome: an iatrogenic channelopathy. Swiss Med Wkly 2004;134(47–48):685–94.
26. Tartini R, Kappenberger L, Steinbrunn W, et al. Dangerous interaction between amiodarone and quinidine. Lancet 1982;1(8285):1327–9.
27. Kannankeril PJ, Roden DM. Drug-induced long QT and torsade de pointes: recent advances. Curr Opin Cardiol 2007;22(1):39–43.
28. Zeltser D, Justo D, Halkin A, et al. Torsade de pointes due to noncardiac drugs: most patients have easily identifiable risk factors. Medicine (Baltimore) 2003;82(4):282–90.
29. Roden DM. Repolarization reserve: a moving target. Circulation 2008;118(10):981–2.
30. Roden DM, Abraham RL. Refining repolarization reserve. Heart Rhythm 2011;8(11):1756–7.
31. Wu L, Shryock JC, Song Y, et al. An increase in late sodium current potentiates the proarrhythmic activities of low-risk QT-prolonging drugs in female rabbit hearts. J Pharmacol Exp Ther 2006;316(2):718–26.
32. Wu L, Rajamani S, Shryock JC, et al. Augmentation of late sodium current unmasks the proarrhythmic effects of amiodarone. Cardiovasc Res 2008;77(3): 481–8.
33. Wu L, Guo D, Li H, et al. Role of late sodium current in modulating the proarrhythmic and antiarrhythmic effects of quinidine. Heart Rhythm 2008;5(12): 1726–34.
34. Song Y, Shryock JC, Wu L, et al. Antagonism by ranolazine of the pro-arrhythmic effects of increasing late INa in guinea pig ventricular myocytes. J Cardiovasc Pharmacol 2004;44(2):192–9.
35. Hondeghem LM, Snyders DJ. Class III antiarrhythmic agents have a lot of potential but a long way to go. Reduced effectiveness and dangers of reverse use dependence. Circulation 1990;81(2): 686–90.
36. Yang T, Chun YW, Stroud DM, et al. Screening for acute IKr block is insufficient to detect torsades de pointes liability: role of late sodium current. Circulation 2014;130(3):224–34.
37. Ackerman MJ, Splawski I, Makielski JC, et al. Spectrum and prevalence of cardiac sodium channel variants among black, white, Asian, and Hispanic individuals: implications for arrhythmogenic susceptibility and Brugada/long QT syndrome genetic testing. Heart Rhythm 2004;1(5):600–7.
38. Splawski I, Timothy KW, Tateyama M, et al. Variant of SCN5A sodium channel implicated in risk of cardiac arrhythmia. Science 2002;297(5585):1333–6.
39. Plant LD, Bowers PN, Liu Q, et al. A common cardiac sodium channel variant associated with sudden infant death in African Americans, SCN5A S1103Y. J Clin Invest 2006;116(2):430–5.
40. Van Norstrand DW, Tester DJ, Ackerman MJ. Overrepresentation of the proarrhythmic, sudden death predisposing sodium channel polymorphism S1103Y in a population-based cohort of African-American sudden infant death syndrome. Heart Rhythm 2008;5(5):712–5.
41. Sun AY, Koontz JI, Shah SH, et al. The S1103Y cardiac sodium channel variant is associated with ICD events in African Americans with heart failure and reduced ejection fraction. Circ Cardiovasc Genet 2011;4(2):163–8.
42. Makita N, Horie M, Nakamura T, et al. Drug-induced long-QT syndrome associated with a subclinical SCN5A mutation. Circulation 2002;106(10): 1269–74.
43. Napolitano C, Schwartz PJ, Brown AM, et al. Evidence for a cardiac ion channel mutation underlying drug-induced QT prolongation and life-threatening arrhythmias. J Cardiovasc Electrophysiol 2000; 11(6):691–6.

# Disease Caused by Mutations in $Na_V$-β Subunit Genes

Argelia Medeiros-Domingo, MD, PhD[a,*], Carmen R. Valdivia, MD[b]

**KEYWORDS**

- Sodium channel β subunits • Sudden cardiac death • Epilepsy • Channelopathies
- Long QT syndrome • Atrial fibrillation • Brugada syndrome

**KEY POINTS**

- $Na_V$-β subunits associate with the $Na_V$-α or pore-forming subunit of the voltage-dependent sodium channel and play critical roles in channel expression, voltage dependence of the channel gating, cell adhesion, signal transduction, and channel pharmacology.
- Five $Na_V$-β subunits have been identified in humans, all of them implicated in many primary arrhythmia syndromes that cause sudden death or neurologic disorders, including long QT syndrome, Brugada syndrome, cardiac conduction disorders, idiopathic ventricular fibrillation, epilepsy, neurodegenerative diseases, and neuropsychiatric disorders.

## INTRODUCTION

Voltage-gated sodium channels ($Na_V$-α) are transmembrane proteins crucial for action potential generation, duration, and propagation in excitable cells. They contain 4 homologous domains, each containing 6 transmembrane segments. The pore-forming $Na_V$-α associates with 2 or more $Na_V$-β subunits, which are small single-segment transmembrane proteins that mediate multiple signaling pathways and are found to be essential for life (**Fig. 1**).[1,2]

$Na_V$-β subunits interact with all known voltage-gated sodium channel isoforms, altering their expression and function.[3–6] Recent studies have found that $Na_V$-β subunits are also capable of shaping the channel pharmacology with crucial therapeutic implications.[2,7,8] Five $Na_V$-β subunits have been identified in humans: β1, β1b, β2, β3, and β4, encoded by *SCN1B*, *SCN2B*, *SCN3B*, and *SCN4B* genes, respectively. All $Na_V$-β subunits share similar topology (**Fig. 2**) consisting of a large extracellular domain (N terminal) immunoglobinlike fold related to the L1 family of cell-adhesion molecules, a single transmembrane region, and a small intracellular domain (C terminal). β1 and β3 interact with the α subunit in a noncovalently form and share high homology (~50%), whereas β2 and β4 associate with $Na_V$-α via disulfide bonds and share only 20% homology; this interaction is potentially performed through the extracellular loop of domain IV, transmembrane segment 6 of $Na_V$-α.[9,10] It is interesting that β subunits do not share homology with their counterparts of calcium and potassium channels.[11] The β1b subunit is a splice variant of the β1 subunit via alternative intron 3 retention. The retained intron encodes a novel extracellular, a transmembrane, and an intracellular region sharing little homology with the β1 (see **Fig. 1**).[12]

An emergent property of $Na_V$-β subunits is that they are able to modulate other ion channels

The authors have nothing to disclose.

[a] Department of Cardiac Electrophysiology, University Hospital of Bern, Freiburgstrasse 10, Bern 3010, Switzerland; [b] Center for Arrhythmia Research, North Campus Research Complex, University of Michigan, 2nd floor, Buildings 20 and 26, 2800 Plymouth Road, Ann Arbor, MI 48109-2800, USA
* Corresponding author.
*E-mail address:* Argelia.medeiros@insel.ch

Card Electrophysiol Clin 6 (2014) 785–795
http://dx.doi.org/10.1016/j.ccep.2014.08.008
1877-9182/14/$ – see front matter 

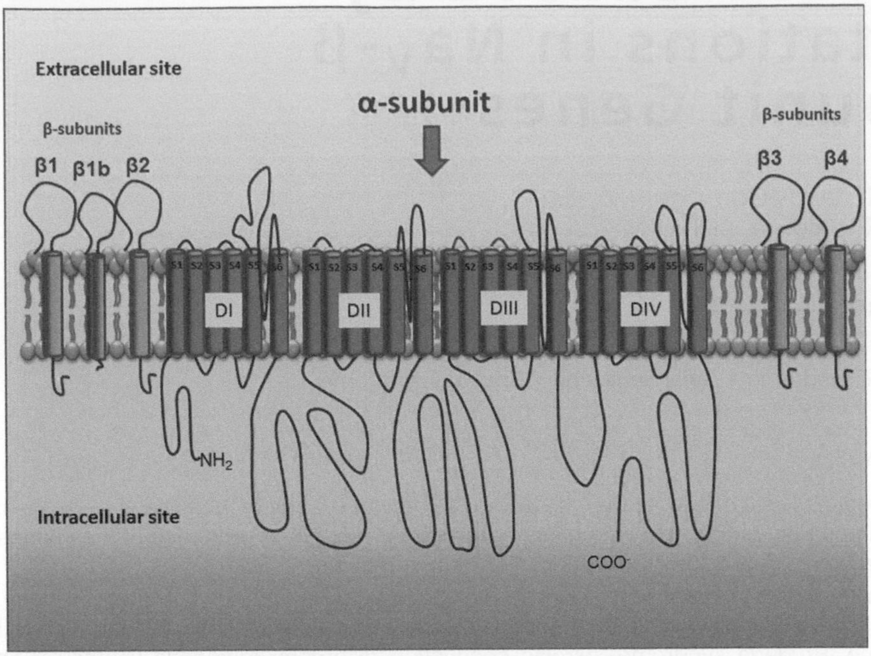


**Fig. 1.** Voltage-gated sodium channel. The $Na_V$-α subunits contain 4 functional domains (DI to DIV), each comprising 6 transmembral segments. S4 constitutes the voltage sensor and S5-S6 the pore-forming region. The $Na_V$-β subunits are single transmembrane proteins that associate with the $Na_V$-α subunits and play critical roles in channel expression, voltage dependence of the channel gating, cell adhesion, and signal transduction.

besides sodium channel isoforms. A physiologic role for $Na_V$-β1 in the functioning of neuronal Kv4.2-encoded $I_A$ channels, a major constituent of A-type ($I_A$) potassium currents and a key regulator of neuronal membrane excitability, has been reported.[13] Silencing of $Na_v$-β1 produced a reduction in KChIP2 mRNA (voltage-gated potassium [Kv] channel-interacting proteins) and protein and Kv4.x proteins resulting in remarkably decreased $I_{Na}$ and $I_{to}$.[14] Functional studies have also found that $Na_v$-β1 is able to interact and modify the gating properties of the potassium channel $I_{to}$ encoded by *KCND3*.[15] These broad spectrums of interaction and regulatory functions of the $Na_V$-β subunits explain their impact as disease-causing genes implicated in several neurologic and cardiac channelopathies. **Table 1** provides a brief overview of the $Na_V$-β subunit–associated diseases.

## CARDIAC DISEASES AND $NA_V$-β SUBUNITS

### *Long QT Syndrome*

Congenital long QT syndrome (LQTS) is characterized by abnormal ventricular repolarization caused by longer action potential duration, which is translated in the surface electrocardiogram (ECG) as prolonged QT intervals. Patients with LQTS exhibit ventricular arrhythmias manifested by syncope, seizures, or sudden cardiac death. Only 75% of patients with LQTS phenotype will have a clear pathogenic mutation, 90% of them localize to the potassium channels, $IK_S$, $IK_R$, or cardiac sodium channel $Na_V$1.5, encoded by *KCNQ1*, *KCNH2*, and *SCN5A*, respectively. The remaining 10% of mutations are located in auxiliary subunits or other proteins of the ion channel macromolecular complex. Mutations in *SCN5A* cause a "gain-of-function" phenotype characterized by an increase of the late sodium current (INaL). INaL may contribute to triggering arrhythmia in 2 ways: by delaying repolarization, resulting in early after-depolarizations and by spontaneous calcium release in sodium–calcium overload conditions, triggering delayed after-depolarization.[16] Because $Na_V$-β subunits closely regulate all sodium channel isoforms, they have been obvious candidates for LQTS phenotype. This was supported by early observation in mouse models; the *SCN1B* null mice presented with an increase in INaL and also exhibited prolonged QT intervals.[17] Actually, the first cardiac disease associated with $Na_V$-β subunits was LQTS.[18] The phenotype reported was typical for a sodium channel gain-of-function mutation, characterized by very long QT intervals (>700 ms), 2:1 intermittent atrioventricular block at a very young age (in this case diagnosed at birth [**Fig. 3**A]), and a molecular phenotype with clear increase in INaL (see **Fig. 3**B, C). The phenotype

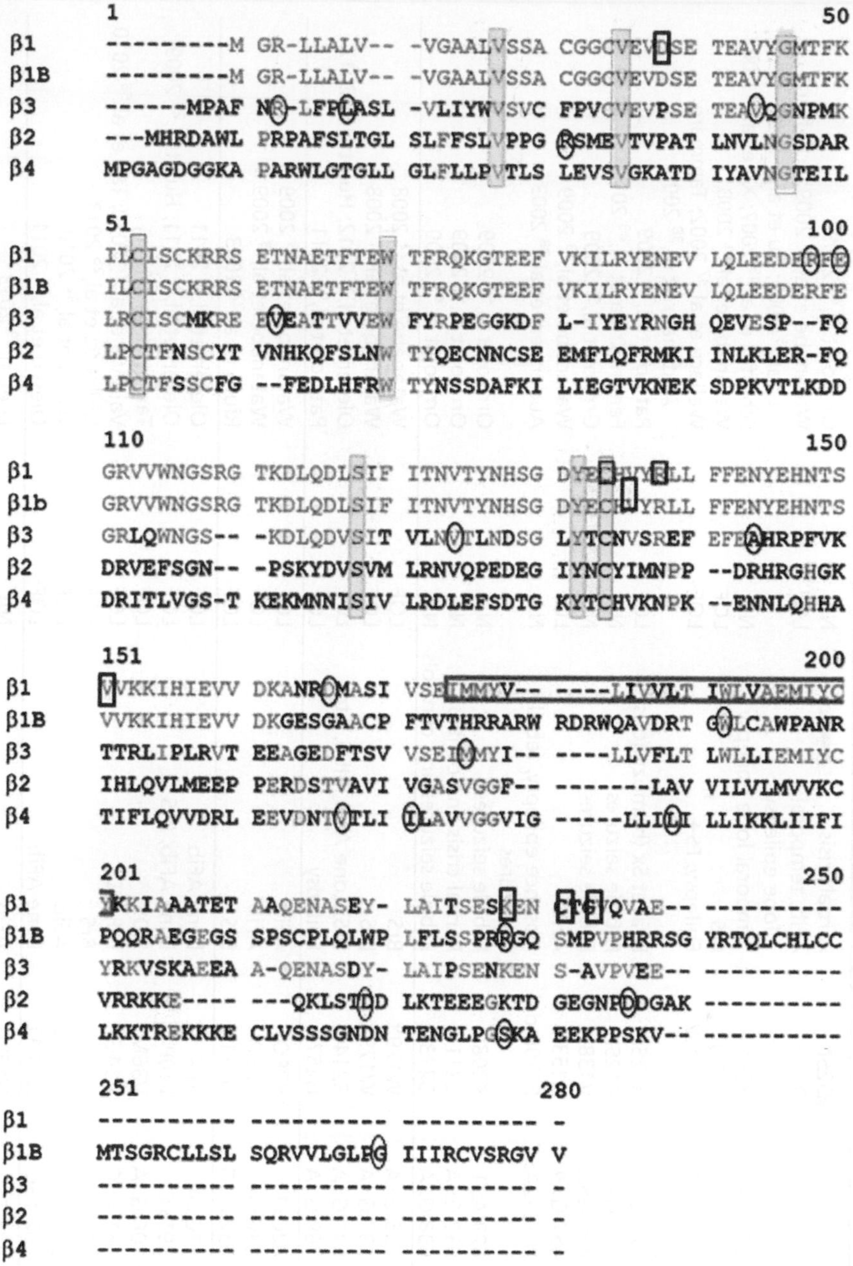


**Fig. 2.** Comparison of SCNB1-4 amino acid sequences. Human heart accession numbers β1(NM_001037.4), β1b (NM_199037.3), β2 (NM_004588.4), β3NM_001040151.1, and β4 (NM_001142348.1) were aligned using the Bioedit Clustalw multiple alignment software. β1 and β1b are splice variants of the same gene and share almost identical sequence, whereas β1 and β3 share 50% homology (*blue*). β2 and β4 share less that 20% sequence (*red*). Yellow columns show identical amino acids in the 5 subunits. Horizontal box shows the predicted transmembrane region of β1. Circles and squares show the single point mutations associated to arrhythmia syndrome or neurologic disorders, respectively.

of LQTS or gain of function of the cardiac sodium channel has been reported only in *SCN4B* mutations, whereas other NaV-β subunits have not been implicated in this phenotype. Mutations in *SCN4B* are considered a rare cause of LQTS.

## *Brugada Syndrome*

Brugada syndrome (BrS) is characterized by ST-segment elevation in right precordial leads (V1 to V3) unrelated to ischemia, electrolyte disturbances, or obvious structural heart disease[19] in

**Table 1**
**$Na_V$-β subunit–associated diseases**

| Gene | Protein | Chromosome | Base Change | AA Change | Phenotype | Functional Characterization | Reference |
|---|---|---|---|---|---|---|---|
| *SCN1B* | $Na_V$-β1 | 19q13.12 | 73G>A | D25N | Partial crisis | NA | Orrico et al,[44] 2009 |
| | | | 254 G>A | R85H | AFib, temporal lobe epilepsy | LOF | Watanabe et al,[33] 2009; Scheffer et al,[45] 2007; Xu et al,[67] 2007 |
| | | | 252 C>T | R85C | Temporal lobe epilepsy | NA | Scheffer et al,[45] 2007; Xu et al,[67] 2007 |
| | | | 259 G>C | E87Q | BrS | LOF | Watanabe et al,[21] 2008 |
| | | | 363 C>G | C121W | Epilepsy, FS+ | LOF | Wallace et al,[37] 2002; Tammaro; Audenaer et al,[38] 2003 |
| | | | 373 C>T | R125C | Dravet Sx (homozygous) | LOF | Patino et al,[39] 2009 |
| | | | 374 G>T | R125L | Febrile seizures | NA | Fendri-Kriaa et al,[43] 2011 |
| | | | 412 G>A | V138I | Febrile seizures | NA | Orrico et al,[44] 2009 |
| | | | 457 G>A | D153N | AFib | LOF | Watanabe et al,[33] 2009 |
| | | | IVS2 -2A>C | E170Fsdel | Absence epilepsy, febrile seizures | NA | Audenaert et al,[38] 2003 |
| | | | 623 A>T | K208I | Febrile seizures | NA | Orrico et al,[44] 2009 |
| | | | 632 G>A | C211Y | Partial crisis and controls | NA | Orrico et al,[44] 2009 |
| | | | 638 G>A | G213D | Febrile seizures and controls | NA | Orrico et al,[44] 2009 |
| *SCN1Bb* | $Na_V$-β1b | 19q13.12 | 536 G>A | W179X | BrS | LOF | Watanabe et al,[21] 2008 |
| | | | 537 G>A | W179X | BrS | LOF | Watanabe et al,[21] 2008 |
| | | | 641 G>A | R214Q | BrS, Lone AFib, SIDS, Ctrls | LOF | Olesen et al,[35] 2012; Hu et al,[15] 2012 |
| | | | 769 G>A | G257R | Epilepsy | LOF | Patino et al,[68] 2011 |
| *SCN2B* | $Na_V$-β2 | 11q23.3 | 82C>T | R28Q | AFib | LOF | Watanabe et al,[33] 2009 |
| | | | 83G>A | R28W | AFib | LOF | Watanabe et al,[33] 2009 |
| | | | 632 A>G | D211G | BrS | LOF | Riuró et al,[22] 2013 |
| *SCN3B* | $Na_V$-β3 | 11q23.3 | 17G>A | R6K | Lone AFib | LOF | Olesen et al,[34] 2011 |
| | | | 29T>C | L10P | Lone AFib, BrS | LOF | Olesen et al,[34] 2011; Hu et al,[23] 2009 |
| | | | 106 G>A | V36M | SIDS | LOF | Tan et al,[56] 2010 |
| | | | 161 A>C | V54G | IVF, SIDS | LOF | Valdivia et al,[27] 2010; Tan et al,[56] 2010 |
| | | | 328 G>A | V110I | BrS | LOF | Ishikawa et al,[25] 2013 |
| | | | 389 C>T | A130V | AFib | LOF | Wang et al,[32] 2010 |
| | | | 482 T>C | M161T | Lone AFib | LOF | Olesen et al,[34] 2011 |
| *SCN4B* | $Na_V$-β4 | 11q23.3 | 485 T>G | V162G | AFib | NA | Li et al,[69] 2013 |
| | | | 496 A>C | I166L | AFib | NA | Li et al,[69] 2013 |
| | | | 535 C>T | L179F | LQTS | GOF | Medeiros et al,[18] 2007 |

*Abbreviations:* AFib, atrial fibrillation; FS, febrile seizures; GOF, gain of function; IVF, idiopathic ventricular fibrillation; LOF, loss of function; NA, not available; SIDS, sudden infant death syndrome.

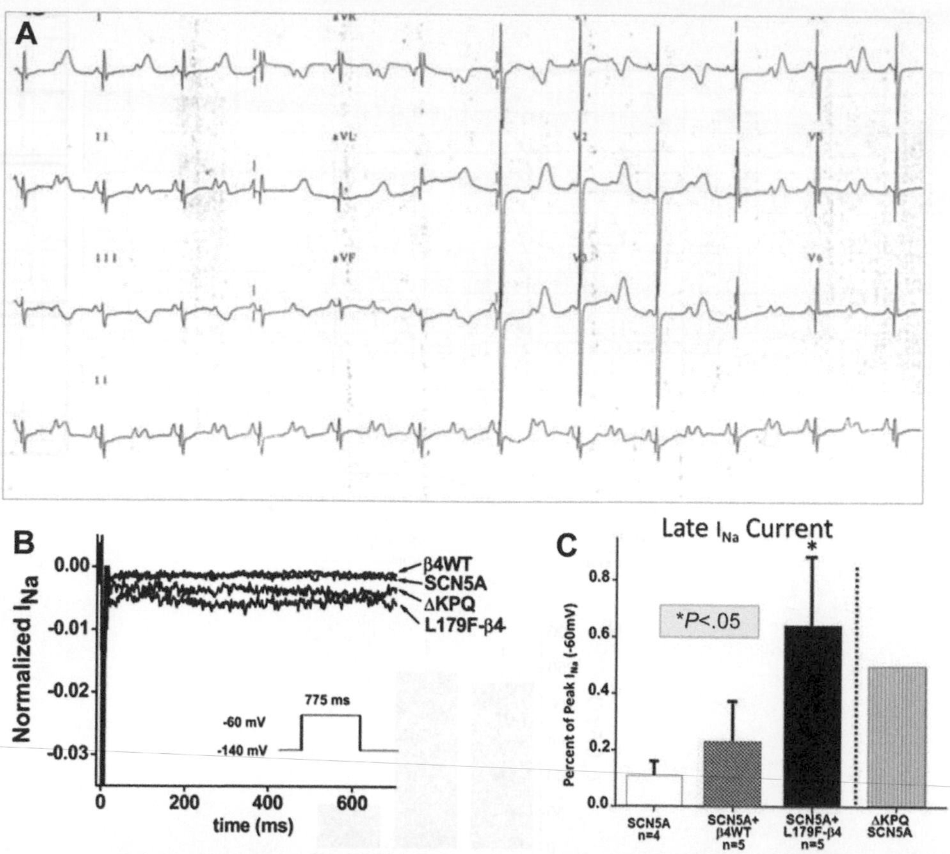


**Fig. 3.** $Na_V$-β subunits and long QT syndrome. (*A*) Twelve-lead ECG from a 3-year-old patient with L179F-β4 mutation showing 2:1 AV block and very long QT intervals greater than 700 ms (normal <460 ms). (*B*) Functional studies in HEK-293 cells showing the normalized persistent late sodium current elicited by the L179F-β4 mutant, comparable with the late sodium current obtained with the well-known LQTS mutation ΔKPQ. (*C*) Functional study results showing the average of persistent late sodium current obtained by the expression of SCN5A alone, SCN5A+ β4 wild type, SCN5A+ L179F-β4, and SCN5A-ΔKPQ as prototype of LQTS mutation. L179F-β4 led to a significant increase in late sodium current. (*From* Medeiros-Domingo A, Kaku T, Tester DJ, et al. Scn4b-encoded sodium channel beta4 subunit in congenital long-qt syndrome. Circulation 2007;116:139; with permission.)

association with syncope or sudden cardiac death. These ECG changes are usually intermittent, with the first symptoms usually appearing in the third or fourth decade of life; BrS is actually a rare finding during childhood.[20] When a patient with Brugada features in the ECG is asymptomatic, it is called only BrS-like ECG and not BrS. These patients may be asymptomatic throughout their life and, in the absence of symptoms, a BrS-like ECG is considered to confer a low risk of sudden death. To date, 18 genes have been implicated in BrS, but most affected individuals (about one-third) will have a mutation in the cardiac sodium channel $Na_V1.5$, encoded by *SCN5A*. In consequence, $Na_V$-β subunit genes have also been good candidates for BrS and have recently been implicated in this syndrome, particularly *SCN1B*,[21] *SCN2B*,[22] and *SCN3B*.[23–25] Mutations in $Na_V$-β subunit genes elicited a loss of function of INa (**Fig. 4**), providing an arrhythmogenic mechanism consistent with those previously described for *SCN5A* mutations causing BrS. It has been reported that a $Na_V$-β1-SNP is associated with the development of Brugada syndrome in Japanese patients with BrS-like ECG pattern.[26]

## *Idiopathic Ventricular Fibrillation*

Idiopathic ventricular fibrillation (IVF) is characterized by ventricular arrhythmias and sudden cardiac death in the absence of structural heart disease or recognizable channelopathy phenotype. Patients are usually young (<40 years) and present with syncope or cardiac arrest caused by ventricular arrhythmias. Frequently, the ECG of these patients exhibit an early ventricular repolarization pattern characterized by "J-waves" and ST segment elevation in the inferolateral leads of

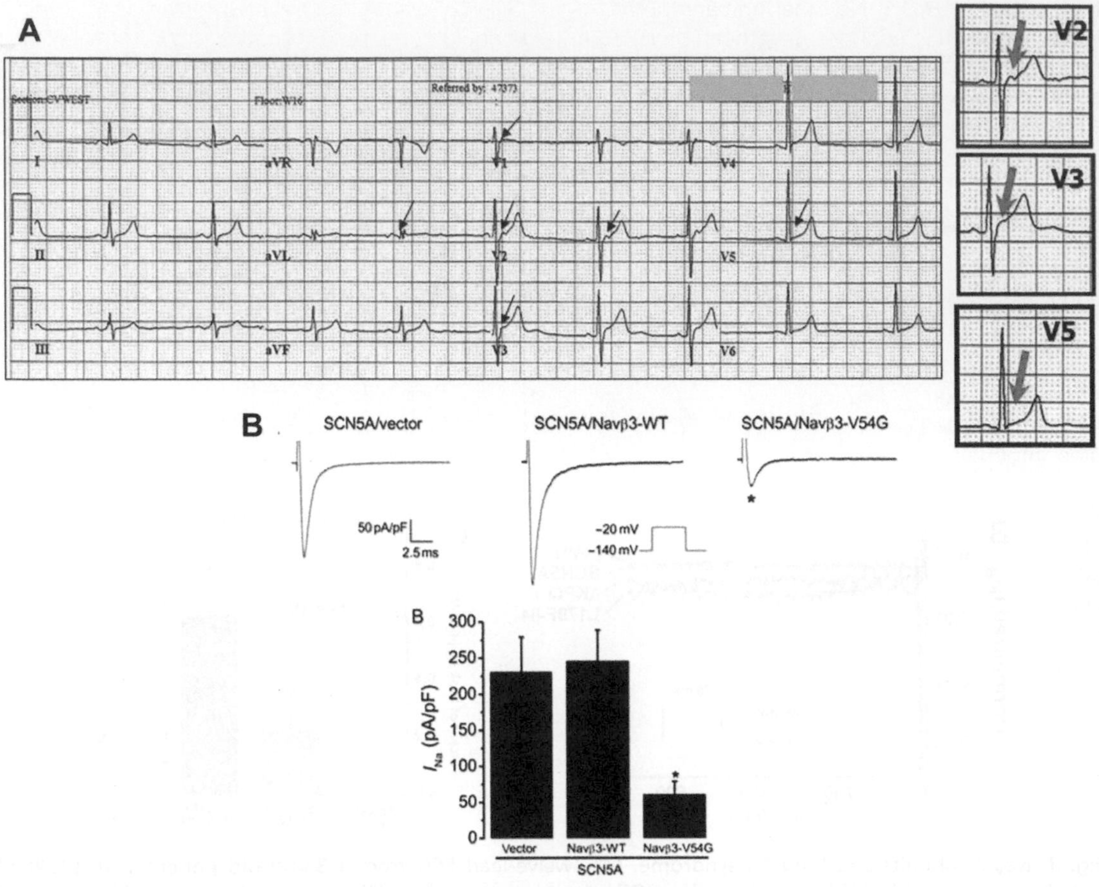


**Fig. 4.** $Na_V$-β subunits and idiopathic ventricular fibrillation. (*A*) 12-lead ECG of an 18-year-old patient who had sudden cardiac death while exercising. There is J point elevation in precordial leads (*arrow*). Genetic test found a V54G-β3 mutation. (*B*) V54G-β3 was engineered by site-directed mutagenesis and expressed in HEK-293 cells. Patch-clamp experiments exhibit a significant (*star*) loss of function phenotype elicited by the V54G-β3 mutant compared with SCN5A alone or SCN5A+ β3 wild type. (*From* Valdivia CR, Medeiros-Domingo A, Ye B, et al. Loss-of-function mutation of the scn3b-encoded sodium channel {beta}3 subunit associated with a case of idiopathic ventricular fibrillation. Cardiovasc Res 2010;86:394–5; with permission.)

the ECG. Importantly, this pattern is common in young males and athletes, thus, it is useful as a retrospective marker when symptoms develop but cannot be used as a predictive or diagnostic ECG marker in asymptomatic individuals. To date, 7 genes have been implicated in IVF, including the cardiac isoform of sodium channel (*SCN5A*) and its regulatory subunit, *SCN3B*.[27] The *SCN3B* knockout mice exhibit shorter action potential duration, shorter ventricular effective refractory periods, and monomorphic and polymorphic ventricular tachycardia.[28] In humans, a novel mutation in *SCN3B* was reported in a young man who developed sudden death during exercise. Functional studies found a loss of function phenotype in the cardiac sodium channel, and the patient exhibited the typical early repolarization pattern in the ECG (see **Fig. 4**). It is possible that BrS and IVF belong to the same spectrum of a single disease; in fact, at the molecular level, they share some of the mechanisms or gene mutations. Loss-of-function mutations in *SCN5A* may be associated with both IVF and BrS and loss-of-function mutations in $Na_V$-β3 subunit have been reported as well in IVF and BrS.

## *Cardiac Conduction Disorders*

Cardiac conduction disease (CCD) is characterized by prolongation in the P wave, PR, QRS intervals or bundle branch block with or without ST segment elevation or QT prolongation. Inheritable CCD has been attributed to loss of function mutation in *SCN5A*.[29] Thus, although sodium channel-interacting proteins represent logical candidate genes for the CCD phenotype, only loss-of-function mutations in *SCN1B* have been associated with cardiac conduction disorders in the context of BrS.[21] No other primary mutations in $Na_V$-interacting subunits have been reported in humans with cardiac conduction disorders, despite the fact that several studies in mice found a crucial role of these proteins in the cardiac conduction system. SCN3B-knockout mice exhibit important intracardiac conduction abnormalities,[30] and, interestingly, in the SCN5A-1798insD mutant mice, differential expression of β4 was found to contribute to strain-dependent conduction defect.[31]

### *Atrial Fibrillation*

Atrial fibrillation (AFib) is the most common arrhythmia in the general population and contributes importantly to morbidity and mortality. It is characterized by a rapid and chaotic activation of the atrial myocardium. AFib is caused by genetic and environmental factors.[32,33] The genetic component of AFib is broad, and several ion channel genes and ion channel interacting proteins have been linked to this condition. Mutations in *SCN1B*, *SCN1Bb*, *SCN2B*, and *SCN3B*[32] have been reported in AFib. Overall, functional studies found loss-of-function phenotype in vitro.[33–35] Recently, 2 mutations in *SCN4B* transmitted in an autosomal dominant pattern and co-segregated with the disease have been reported[34]; both mutations were predicted to be disease causing; however, functional studies were not conducted.

Some patients exhibit atrial fibrillation alone or with mixed phenotype.[32,34] BrS has been reported in AFib cases with mutations in *SCN1B* or *SCN2B*.[33]

## NEUROLOGIC DISEASES AND $NA_V$-β SUBUNITS

### *Epilepsy, Febrile Seizures, and Dravet Syndrome*

Epilepsy is a chronic neurologic disorder characterized by recurrent seizures that involve high-frequency neuronal action potentials requiring voltage-gated sodium channels. The *SCN2B* SNP rs602594 has been associated with epilepsy.[36] Generalized epilepsy with febrile seizures plus (GEFS+) is a clinically and genetically heterogeneous syndrome with childhood onset, characterized by febrile seizures (FS) and a variety of afebrile epileptic seizure types. Mutations in *SCN1B* have been described in GEFS+[37] in a family with early-onset, absence epilepsy. The mutation in *SCN1B* identified was a deletion of 5 amino acids in the extracellular immunoglobulinlike domain of β1 and potential loss of function.[38]

Dravet syndrome represents a severe and intractable pediatric epileptic encephalopathy. Functional deletion or homozygous mutations of *SCN1B* results in Dravet syndrome.[39,40] Animal models have found that *SCN1B* deletion may contribute to the development of hyperexcitability[41] through defective neuronal proliferation, migration, and pathfinding; moreover, *SCN1B* null nociceptive neurons are hyperexcitable.[42]

Missense mutations in *SCN1B* have also been reported in febrile seizures phenotype, partial crisis, and temporal lobe epilepsy.[43–45]

The SCN3B null model has severe arrhythmogenic phenotype; yet, these mice display normal neurologic phenotype, most likely because of a compensatory mechanism by SCN1B. In patients with temporal lobe epilepsy, the expression of β3 in the hippocampus is extensively downregulated; however, the functional consequences of this observation are unknown.[46]

In general, mutations in SCNB genes render neurons hyperexcitable, mainly by 2 different mechanisms: by impaired $Na_V$-α regulation and by cell adhesion interactions.

### *Pain Sensation*

Changes in β1 and β2 expression have been implicated in altered pain sensation. In peripheral nerve axons, missense mutations in *SCN1B* reduce the number of functional Na(+) channels at the node of Ranvier.[47] The spared nerve injury model of neuropathic pain results in increased β2 expression in rat sensory neurons.[48] *SCN2B* null mice are found to be more sensitive to noxious thermal stimuli than wild type, suggesting that β2 expression may play an important role in neuropathic pain sensation.[49]

### *Neurodegenerative Disease*

Multiple sclerosis is a central nervous system disease caused by demyelination and axonal degeneration. The *SCN2B* null mutation is neuroprotective in the experimental allergic encephalomyelitis mouse model of multiple sclerosis.[50] In addition, levels of *SCN4B* are reduced in mouse models of Huntington's disease before onset of motor symptoms, and a similar reduction has also been reported in patients.[51]

### *Sudden Unexplained Death in Epilepsy*

Childhood-onset epilepsy is associated with a substantial risk of epilepsy-related mortality,[52] which appears to be 20 times higher in patients with epilepsy compared with the general population. A significant body of literature suggests the prominent role of cardiac arrhythmias in the pathogenesis of sudden unexplained death in epilepsy. Long-standing epilepsy can cause physiologic and anatomic autonomic instability resulting in life-threatening arrhythmias. Tachyarrhythmias, bradyarrhythmias, and asystole are commonly seen during the ictal, interictal, and postictal phases in epilepsy patients. It is unclear if these rhythm disturbances need attention, as some of them may be benign findings.

Interestingly, in a Dravet syndrome model, the SCN1A-R1407X knock-in mice, exhibited a cardiac phenotype characterized by increased excitability, action potential duration prolongation, and triggered activity, suggesting that altered cardiac electrical function in Dravet syndrome may contribute to increased susceptibility for arrhythmogenesis and sudden unexplained death in epilepsy[53]; however, this link is not proven yet with the $Na_V$-β subunits.

## SUDDEN INFANT DEATH SYNDROME AND $NA_V$-β SUBUNITS

Sudden infant death syndrome (SIDS) is the sudden and unexpected death of an infant before 1 year of age that is not predicted by medical history and remains unexplained after thorough investigation, including autopsy and detailed death scene investigation.[54] SIDS is the leading cause of death in the first 6 months after birth in the industrialized world. The genetic contribution of SIDS has been investigated extensively. It is known that approximately 10% of SIDS cases may stem from potentially lethal cardiac channelopathies.[55] Nearly half of them have been reported to be cardiac sodium channel mutations. The analyses of the main 4 $Na_V$-β subunit genes found that 3% of the SIDS victims might host a mutation in $Na_V$-β subunits. To date, only 2 of the 5 $Na_V$-β subunits have been implicated in SIDS, loss of function mutations in *SCN3B*, and gain of function mutations in *SCN4B*.[56] A functional polymorphism R214Q in the splice variant *SCN1Bb* has been reported in SIDS and control cases and might play a role as modifier of the substrate responsible for SIDS.[15]

## CANCER AND $NA_V$-β SUBUNITS

Several voltage-gated sodium channels and all main $Na_V$-β subunits have been found to be expressed in cancer cells. In metastatic breast cancer, along with the pore-forming α subunit $Na_V1.5$, the β1 subunit is abundant and regulates cellular adhesion and migration of metastatic breast cancer cell lines.[57] These observations have important prognostic implications for breast cancer progression. $Na_V$-β subunit transcripts and voltage-gated Na(+) channels are also expressed in lung cancer cells and are associated with an increased invasiveness capacity.[58] In prostate cancer as well all main $Na_V$-β subunits have been found at much higher levels in strong versus weakly metastatic cells.[59]

## SUMMARY

It has been 30 years since the purification of the first $Na_V$-β subunits,[60] $Na_V$-β1 and $Na_V$-β2. Since their first description, it was evident that they interact closely with the voltage-gated sodium channels. Currently, it is clear that $Na_V$-β subunit genes not only have remarkable effects on voltage-gated sodium channels, but also regulate other voltage-gated potassium channels. Mutations in $Na_V$-β subunit genes result in a variety of human neurologic diseases and primary arrhythmia syndromes associated with sudden death, and their differential expression by some cancer cells during metastasis is shown to have important prognostic implications.

Most $Na_V$-β subunit mutations result mainly in INa loss-of-function phenotype, but some mutations result in INa gain-of-function phenotype providing the molecular basis for LQTS.

It is intriguing that the same mutation in $Na_V$-β subunits exhibits a predominant cardiac or neurologic phenotype. This finding may be partially explained by the fact that the $Na_V$-β subunits have selected interaction with specific sodium channel isoforms, and $Na_V$-α isoforms exhibit differential expression across the different tissues.[61–63] Additionally, other sodium channel interacting protein variations might be able to augment or attenuate the clinical phenotype.[64–66] Moreover, interaction of $Na_V$-β subunits with the main α subunit isoform depends on other conditions as shown recently with β2, which modulates $Na_V1.5$ mainly in the presence of sialic acids, whereas modulation of $Na_V1.2$ by β2 is sialic acid independent.[61] All these conditions might contribute to the development of the phenotype in $Na_V$-β subunit mutations.

## REFERENCES


1. Patino GA, Isom LL. Electrophysiology and beyond: multiple roles of na+ channel beta subunits in development and disease. Neurosci Lett 2010; 486:53–9.
2. Gilchrist J, Das S, Van Petegem F, et al. Crystallographic insights into sodium-channel modulation by the beta4 subunit. Proc Natl Acad Sci U S A 2013;110:E5016–24.
3. Isom LL, De Jongh KS, Patton DE, et al. Primary structure and functional expression of the beta 1

subunit of the rat brain sodium channel. Science 1992;256:839–42.
4. Laedermann CJ, Syam N, Pertin M, et al. Beta1- and beta3- voltage-gated sodium channel subunits modulate cell surface expression and glycosylation of nav1.7 in hek293 cells. Front Cell Neurosci 2013; 7:137.
5. Baroni D, Picco C, Barbieri R, et al. Antisense-mediated post-transcriptional silencing of scn1b gene modulates sodium channel functional expression. Biol Cell 2014;106:13–29.
6. Aman TK, Grieco-Calub TM, Chen C, et al. Regulation of persistent na current by interactions between beta subunits of voltage-gated na channels. J Neurosci 2009;29:2027–42.
7. Uebachs M, Albus C, Opitz T, et al. Loss of beta1 accessory na+ channel subunits causes failure of carbamazepine, but not of lacosamide, in blocking high-frequency firing via differential effects on persistent na+ currents. Epilepsia 2012;53:1959–67.
8. Doeser A, Soares-da-Silva P, Beck H, et al. The effects of eslicarbazepine on persistent na(+) current and the role of the na(+) channel beta subunits. Epilepsy Res 2014;108:202–11.
9. Makita N, Bennett PB, George AL Jr. Molecular determinants of beta 1 subunit-induced gating modulation in voltage-dependent na+ channels. J Neurosci 1996;16:7117–27.
10. Yu FH, Westenbroek RE, Silos-Santiago I, et al. Sodium channel beta4, a new disulfide-linked auxiliary subunit with similarity to beta2. J Neurosci 2003; 23:7577–85.
11. Isom LL, De Jongh KS, Catterall WA. Auxiliary subunits of voltage-gated ion channels. Neuron 1994;12:1183–94.
12. Qin N, D'Andrea MR, Lubin ML, et al. Molecular cloning and functional expression of the human sodium channel beta1b subunit, a novel splicing variant of the beta1 subunit. Eur J Biochem 2003; 270:4762–70.
13. Marionneau C, Carrasquillo Y, Norris AJ, et al. The sodium channel accessory subunit navbeta1 regulates neuronal excitability through modulation of repolarizing voltage-gated k(+) channels. J Neurosci 2012;32:5716–27.
14. Deschenes I, Armoundas AA, Jones SP, et al. Post-transcriptional gene silencing of kchip2 and navbeta1 in neonatal rat cardiac myocytes reveals a functional association between na and ito currents. J Mol Cell Cardiol 2008;45:336–46.
15. Hu D, Barajas-Martinez H, Medeiros-Domingo A, et al. A novel rare variant in scn1bb linked to brugada syndrome and sids by combined modulation of na(v)1.5 and k(v)4.3 channel currents. Heart Rhythm 2012;9:760–9.
16. Moreno JD, Yang PC, Bankston JR, et al. Ranolazine for congenital and acquired late ina-linked arrhythmias: in silico pharmacological screening. Circ Res 2013;113:e50–61.
17. Lopez-Santiago LF, Meadows LS, Ernst SJ, et al. Sodium channel scn1b null mice exhibit prolonged qt and rr intervals. J Mol Cell Cardiol 2007;43:636–47.
18. Medeiros-Domingo A, Kaku T, Tester DJ, et al. Scn4b-encoded sodium channel beta4 subunit in congenital long-qt syndrome. Circulation 2007; 116:134–42.
19. Wilde AA, Antzelevitch C, Borggrefe M, et al. Proposed diagnostic criteria for the brugada syndrome: consensus report. Circulation 2002;106: 2514–9.
20. Probst V, Denjoy I, Meregalli PG, et al. Clinical aspects and prognosis of brugada syndrome in children. Circulation 2007;115:2042–8.
21. Watanabe H, Koopmann TT, Le Scouarnec S, et al. Sodium channel beta1 subunit mutations associated with brugada syndrome and cardiac conduction disease in humans. J Clin Invest 2008;118: 2260–8.
22. Riuro H, Beltran-Alvarez P, Tarradas A, et al. A missense mutation in the sodium channel beta2 subunit reveals scn2b as a new candidate gene for brugada syndrome. Hum Mutat 2013;34:961–6.
23. Hu D, Barajas-Martinez H, Burashnikov E, et al. A mutation in the beta 3 subunit of the cardiac sodium channel associated with brugada ecg phenotype. Circ Cardiovasc Genet 2009;2:270–8.
24. Kurakami K, Ishii K. Is a novel scn3b mutation commonly found in scn5a-negative brugada syndrome patients? Circ J 2013;77:900–1.
25. Ishikawa T, Takahashi N, Ohno S, et al. Novel scn3b mutation associated with brugada syndrome affects intracellular trafficking and function of nav1.5. Circ J 2013;77:959–67.
26. Ogawa R, Kishi R, Takagi A, et al. A novel microsatellite polymorphism of sodium channel beta1-subunit gene (scn1b) may underlie abnormal cardiac excitation manifested by coved-type st-elevation compatible with brugada syndrome in Japanese. Int J Clin Pharmacol Ther 2010;48: 109–19.
27. Valdivia CR, Medeiros-Domingo A, Ye B, et al. Loss-of-function mutation of the scn3b-encoded sodium channel {beta}3 subunit associated with a case of idiopathic ventricular fibrillation. Cardiovasc Res 2010;86:392–400.
28. Hakim P, Gurung IS, Pedersen TH, et al. Scn3b knockout mice exhibit abnormal ventricular electrophysiological properties. Prog Biophys Mol Biol 2008;98:251–66.
29. Papadatos GA, Wallerstein PM, Head CE, et al. Slowed conduction and ventricular tachycardia after targeted disruption of the cardiac sodium channel gene scn5a. Proc Natl Acad Sci U S A 2002;99: 6210–5.

30. Hakim P, Brice N, Thresher R, et al. Scn3b knockout mice exhibit abnormal sino-atrial and cardiac conduction properties. Acta Physiol (Oxf) 2010;198:47–59.
31. George AL Jr. Genetic modulation of impaired cardiac conduction: sodium channel beta4 subunit missing in action. Circ Res 2009;104:1238–9.
32. Wang P, Yang Q, Wu X, et al. Functional dominant-negative mutation of sodium channel subunit gene scn3b associated with atrial fibrillation in a chinese geneid population. Biochem Biophys Res Commun 2010;398:98–104.
33. Watanabe H, Darbar D, Kaiser DW, et al. Mutations in sodium channel beta1- and beta2-subunits associated with atrial fibrillation. Circ Arrhythm Electrophysiol 2009;2:268–75.
34. Olesen MS, Jespersen T, Nielsen JB, et al. Mutations in sodium channel beta-subunit scn3b are associated with early-onset lone atrial fibrillation. Cardiovasc Res 2011;89:786–93.
35. Olesen MS, Holst AG, Svendsen JH, et al. Scn1bb r214q found in 3 patients: 1 with brugada syndrome and 2 with lone atrial fibrillation. Heart Rhythm 2012;9:770–3.
36. Baum L, Haerian BS, Ng HK, et al. Case-control association study of polymorphisms in the voltage-gated sodium channel genes scn1a, scn2a, scn3a, scn1b, and scn2b and epilepsy. Hum Genet 2013;133(5):651–9.
37. Wallace RH, Scheffer IE, Parasivam G, et al. Generalized epilepsy with febrile seizures plus: mutation of the sodium channel subunit scn1b. Neurology 2002;58:1426–9.
38. Audenaert D, Claes L, Ceulemans B, et al. A deletion in scn1b is associated with febrile seizures and early-onset absence epilepsy. Neurology 2003;61: 854–6.
39. Patino GA, Claes LR, Lopez-Santiago LF, et al. A functional null mutation of scn1b in a patient with dravet syndrome. J Neurosci 2009;29:10764–78.
40. Ogiwara I, Nakayama T, Yamagata T, et al. A homozygous mutation of voltage-gated sodium channel beta(i) gene scn1b in a patient with dravet syndrome. Epilepsia 2012;53:e200–3.
41. Brackenbury WJ, Yuan Y, O'Malley HA, et al. Abnormal neuronal patterning occurs during early postnatal brain development of scn1b-null mice and precedes hyperexcitability. Proc Natl Acad Sci U S A 2013;110:1089–94.
42. Lopez-Santiago LF, Brackenbury WJ, Chen C, et al. Na+ channel scn1b gene regulates dorsal root ganglion nociceptor excitability in vivo. J Biol Chem 2011;286:22913–23.
43. Fendri-Kriaa N, Kammoun F, Salem IH, et al. New mutation c.374c>t and a putative disease-associated haplotype within scn1b gene in tunisian families with febrile seizures. Eur J Neurol 2011;18:695–702.
44. Orrico A, Galli L, Grosso S, et al. Mutational analysis of the scn1a, scn1b and gabrg2 genes in 150 italian patients with idiopathic childhood epilepsies. Clin Genet 2009;75:579–81.
45. Scheffer IE, Harkin LA, Grinton BE, et al. Temporal lobe epilepsy and gefs+ phenotypes associated with scn1b mutations. Brain 2007;130:100–9.
46. van Gassen KL, de Wit M, van Kempen M, et al. Hippocampal nabeta3 expression in patients with temporal lobe epilepsy. Epilepsia 2009;50: 957–62.
47. Kiernan MC, Krishnan AV, Lin CS, et al. Mutation in the na+ channel subunit scn1b produces paradoxical changes in peripheral nerve excitability. Brain 2005;128:1841–6.
48. Pertin M, Ji RR, Berta T, et al. Upregulation of the voltage-gated sodium channel beta2 subunit in neuropathic pain models: characterization of expression in injured and non-injured primary sensory neurons. J Neurosci 2005;25:10970–80.
49. Lopez-Santiago LF, Pertin M, Morisod X, et al. Sodium channel beta2 subunits regulate tetrodotoxin-sensitive sodium channels in small dorsal root ganglion neurons and modulate the response to pain. J Neurosci 2006;26:7984–94.
50. O'Malley HA, Shreiner AB, Chen GH, et al. Loss of na+ channel beta2 subunits is neuroprotective in a mouse model of multiple sclerosis. Mol Cell Neurosci 2009;40:143–55.
51. Oyama F, Miyazaki H, Sakamoto N, et al. Sodium channel beta4 subunit: down-regulation and possible involvement in neuritic degeneration in huntington's disease transgenic mice. J Neurochem 2006; 98:518–29.
52. Sillanpaa M, Shinnar S. Sudep and other causes of mortality in childhood-onset epilepsy. Epilepsy Behav 2013;28:249–55.
53. Auerbach DS, Jones J, Clawson BC, et al. Altered cardiac electrophysiology and sudep in a model of dravet syndrome. PLoS One 2013;8:e77843.
54. Moon RY. Sids and other sleep-related infant deaths: expansion of recommendations for a safe infant sleeping environment. Pediatrics 2011;128: 1030–9.
55. Van Norstrand DW, Ackerman MJ. Genomic risk factors in sudden infant death syndrome. Genome Med 2010;2:86.
56. Tan BH, Pundi KN, Van Norstrand DW, et al. Sudden infant death syndrome-associated mutations in the sodium channel beta subunits. Heart Rhythm 2010;7:771–8.
57. Chioni AM, Brackenbury WJ, Calhoun JD, et al. A novel adhesion molecule in human breast cancer cells: voltage-gated na+ channel beta1 subunit. Int J Biochem Cell Biol 2009;41:1216–27.
58. Roger S, Rollin J, Barascu A, et al. Voltage-gated sodium channels potentiate the invasive capacities

of human non-small-cell lung cancer cell lines. Int J Biochem Cell Biol 2007;39:774–86.
59. Diss JK, Fraser SP, Walker MM, et al. Beta-subunits of voltage-gated sodium channels in human prostate cancer: quantitative in vitro and in vivo analyses of mrna expression. Prostate Cancer Prostatic Dis 2008;11:325–33.
60. Hartshorne RP, Catterall WA. The sodium channel from rat brain. Purification and subunit composition. J Biol Chem 1984;259:1667–75.
61. Johnson D, Bennett ES. Isoform-specific effects of the beta2 subunit on voltage-gated sodium channel gating. J Biol Chem 2006;281:25875–81.
62. Maier SK, Westenbroek RE, Yamanushi TT, et al. An unexpected requirement for brain-type sodium channels for control of heart rate in the mouse sinoatrial node. Proc Natl Acad Sci U S A 2003;100:3507–12.
63. Maier SK, Westenbroek RE, McCormick KA, et al. Distinct subcellular localization of different sodium channel alpha and beta subunits in single ventricular myocytes from mouse heart. Circulation 2004;109:1421–7.
64. Ueda K, Valdivia C, Medeiros-Domingo A, et al. Syntrophin mutation associated with long qt syndrome through activation of the nnos-scn5a macromolecular complex. Proc Natl Acad Sci U S A 2008;105: 9355–60.
65. Hu RM, Tan BH, Orland KM, et al. Digenic inheritance novel mutations in scn5a and snta1 increase late i(na) contributing to lqt syndrome. Am J Physiol Heart Circ Physiol 2013;304:H994–1001.
66. Milstein ML, Musa H, Balbuena DP, et al. Dynamic reciprocity of sodium and potassium channel expression in a macromolecular complex controls cardiac excitability and arrhythmia. Proc Natl Acad Sci U S A 2012;109:E2134–43.
67. Xu R, Thomas EA, Gazina EV, et al. Generalized epilepsy with febrile seizures plus-associated sodium channel beta1 subunit mutations severely reduce beta subunit-mediated modulation of sodium channel function. Neuroscience 2007;148:164–74.
68. Patino GA, Brackenbury WJ, Bao Y, et al. Voltage-gated Na+ channel beta1B: a secreted cell adhesion molecule involved in human epilepsy. J Neurosci 2011;31:14577–91.
69. Li RG, Wang Q, Xu YJ. Mutations of the SCN4B-encoded sodium channel beta4 subunit in familial atrial fibrillation. Int J Mol Med 2013;32:144–50.

# Diseases Caused by Mutations in $Na_v1.5$ Interacting Proteins

John W. Kyle, PhD, Jonathan C. Makielski, MD*

**KEYWORDS**

• Arrhythmia • Macromolecular complex • Long QT syndrome • Brugada syndrome
• Sudden infant death syndrome • Cardiomyopathy • Late sodium current • SCN5a

**KEY POINTS**

- Sodium current, which underlies cardiac excitability, flows through a pore protein $Na_v1.5$, which is part of a larger complex of interacting proteins.
- Mutations in 7 $Na_v1.5$ interacting proteins have been associated with dysfunctional sodium current and inherited cardiac diseases.
- The mechanisms by which mutations in interacting proteins cause specific dysfunction involve targeting/trafficking and phosphorylation/nitrosylation of the $Na_v1.5$ complex.
- Mutations in as yet unidentified interacting proteins may account for cardiac disease for which a genetic basis is not yet known.

## CLINICAL IMPORTANCE

In this review, we summarize current understanding of cardiac diseases caused by mutations in proteins that interact with the cardiac sodium channel $Na_v1.5$. $Na_v1.5$ is encoded by the gene *SCN5A* and forms the pore through which flows the majority of sodium current ($I_{Na}$). More than 30 sodium channel interacting proteins (SCIPs) have been identified (**Table 1**).[1,2] Excluding the 4 β-subunits, which are covered in the article elsewhere in this issue by Isom LL and colleagues, mutations in 7 additional SCIPs have been associated with cardiac diseases (**Table 2**). These diseases include inherited arrhythmia syndromes, such as long QT syndrome (LQTS), Brugada syndrome (BrS), and atrial fibrillation, as well as inherited cardiomyopathy. We also include sudden infant death syndrome (SIDS) as a disease where deaths may be presumed to have a cardiac cause and where approximately 10% have been associated with channelopathies.[3] Mutations in SCIPs are a rare cause of inherited arrhythmia (<1% of LQTS and BrS), but they account for approximately 5% of SIDS overall[3] or one half of the SIDS cases associated with channelopathies. Mutations in *SNTA1* alone represent approximately 25% of SIDS-associated channelopathies (approximately 2.5% of SIDS overall). Despite the overall rarity, the study of these mutations has provided insight into the regulation of $I_{Na}$ and the pathophysiology of arrhythmia in common acquired cardiac diseases, such as ischemia and heart failure. In addition, an important percentage of BrS and SIDS remain without a linked genotype and SCIPs, both known (see **Table 1**) or as yet unidentified, could account for the etiology of an important percentage of these syndromes.

## DEFINITION OF SODIUM CHANNEL INTERACTING PROTEINS AND THE SODIUM CHANNEL COMPLEX

SCIPs are defined as proteins that co-localize with $Na_v1.5$ as part of a sodium channel complex (SCC)

Disclosure Statement: No conflicts to disclose.
Division of Cardiovascular Medicine, Department of Medicine, University of Wisconsin, 8407 WIMR II, 1111 Highland Avenue, Madison, WI 53705, USA
* Corresponding author.
*E-mail address:* jcm@medicine.wisc.edu

Card Electrophysiol Clin 6 (2014) 797–809
http://dx.doi.org/10.1016/j.ccep.2014.08.007
1877-9182/14/$ – see front matter 

**Table 1**
**$Na_v1.5$ interacting proteins (SCIPs)**

| Protein | Gene | Size (aa) | Evidence for $Na_v1.5$ Association | Effect on $I_{Na}$ |
|---|---|---|---|---|
| 14-3-3η | *Ywhah* | 246 | Co-IP[64] | (↓)RecR, (−) SSI[64] |
| α-Actinin 2 | *Actn2* | 894 | Co-IP[65] | (↑)$I_{Na}$ Peak[65] |
| Ankyrin G | *Ank3* | 4377 | Co-IP[66,67] | (↑)Surface Density, (↑)$I_{Na}$ Peak[66,67] |
| α1-Syntrophin | *Snta1* | 505 | GST-PD, Co-IP[18,19,23] | Regulate $I_{Na}$ late[18,19,23] |
| β1, β1b | *Scn1b* | β1 218<br>β1b 268 | Co-IP[68] | Kinetics conflicting<br>(↓)$I_{Na}$ late[69,70]<br>(↑)RecR[71]<br>(↑)$I_{Na}$ peak[72,73] |
| β2 | *Scn2b* | 215 | Co-IP[68] | Sialylation status,[74] (↑)late current[75] |
| β3 | *Scn3b* | 215 | Co-IP[76] | (↑)$I_{Na}$, (↑)RecR[77] (+) SSI, (↑)RefractPer.,[78] |
| β4 | *Scn4b* | 228 | Co-IP[79] | (↑) AP upstroke velocity, (+) SSI[80] |
| β4 Spectrin | *Sptbn4* | 2564 | Co-IP[81] | (↑)$I_{Na}$ peak, (+) SSI via Phos.@ S571[81] |
| Calmodulin | *Calm1* | 152 | GST-PD[82]<br>NMR[83] | (+)SSI[84,85] |
| CaMKinase II isoform 3 | *Camk2d* | 510 | Co-IP[81] | (−) SSI, Phos. @ S571S, 516, T594, (↑)$I_{Na}$ Late[86] |
| Caveolin-3 | *Cav3* | 151 | Co-IP[32] | (↓)$I_{Na}$ late[29,30,32] |
| Connexin 40 | *Gja5* | 358 | Co-loc[87] | ? |
| Connexin 43 | *Gja1* | 382 | Co-IP[88] | (↑)$I_{Na}$ peak[89] |
| Desmoglein 2 | *Dsg2* | 1118 | Co-IP[90] | (↑)$I_{Na}$ peak[90] |
| Dystrophin | *Dmd* | 3685 | Co-IP[91] | (↑)$I_{Na}$ peak[91] |
| Fibroblast growth factor FGF12B, 13 | *Fgf12*<br>*Fgf13* | 181 | Co-IP[92] | (+) SSI, (↑) RecR[92] |
| λ2 syntrophin | *Sntg2* | 539 | GST-PD[93] | (+) Activ[93] |
| GPD1L | *Gpd1l* | 351 | GST-PD[37] | (↑)$I_{Na}$ by phosphorylation[37] 80 or ROS[39] |
| MOG1 | *Rangrf* | 218 | GST-PD, co-IP[44] | (↑)Surface density, (↑)$I_{Na}$ peak[44] |
| Nedd4-2 | *Nedd4l* | 975 | GST-PD[8] | (↑)$I_{Na}$ peak[8] |
| nNOS | *Nos1* | 1434 | GST-PD,Co-IP[19] | (↑)$I_{Na}$ late,[19] (↑)$I_{Na}$ peak[22,23] |
| Plakophilin-2 | *Pkp2* | 881 | Co-IP[54] | (↑)$I_{Na}$ peak, (+) SSI[56] |
| PMCA4b | *Atp2b4* | 1241 | GST-PD,Co-IP[19,20] | (↓)$I_{Na}$ late[19] |
| SAP97 | *Dlg1* | 904 | Co-IP[10] | (↑)$I_{Na}$ peak[10] |
| SLMAP | *Slmap* | 828 | [a,59] | (↑)$I_{Na}$ peak[59] |
| Telethonin | *Tcap* | 167 | Co-IP[13] | (−) Activ[13] |
| PTPH1 | *Ptpn3* | 913 | GST-PD[94] | (−) SSI[94] |
| Utrophin | *Utrn* | 3433 | Co-IP[91] | (↓)$I_{Na}$ peak[91] |
| Zasp | *Ldb3* | 727 | GST-PD[63] | (↑)$I_{Na}$ peak[63] |

*Abbreviations:* (↓), decrease in; (↑), increase in; (+), depolarizing shift; (−), hyperpolarizing shift; Activ, activation; Co-IP, co-immunoprecipitation; GST-PD, pull-down with a GST fusion protein; $I_{Na}$ late, late sodium current or persistent current; $I_{Na}$ peak, peak sodium current; RecR, recovery rate; RefractPer., refractory period; ROS, reactive oxygen species; SSI, steady state inactivation.

[a] SLMAP has not yet been shown to associate with $Na_v1.5$.

*Adapted from* Adsit GS, Vaidyanathan R, Galler CM, et al. Channelopathies from mutations in the cardiac sodium channel protein complex. J Mol Cell Cardiol 2013;61:34–43.

and where a physical association has been shown by co-immunoprecipitation, glutathione-s-transferase–fusion protein pull down, or other binding assay, such as yeast-2 hybrid assay. SCIPs have been variously called and classified as accessory proteins, auxiliary proteins, associated proteins, anchoring proteins, β-subunits, scaffolding proteins, adaptor proteins, and regulatory

**Table 2**
**Sodium channel interacting protein (SCIP) with disease-causing mutations that have been shown to affect $I_{Na}$**

| SCIP | Gene Name | Common Name | Chromosome | MW kDa | Splice Variants | Disease | Disease Mutations |
|---|---|---|---|---|---|---|---|
| SNTA1 | *SNTA1* | α1-Syntrophin | 20q11.2 | 54 | 1 | LQT12[19,25]<br>SIDS[23] | A257G, A261V, 390V<br>T262P, T372M, G460S |
| CAV3 | *CAV3* | Caveolin-3 | 3p25 | 17 | 1 | LQT9[29]<br>SIDS[30] | A85T, F97C, S141R<br>V14L, T78M, L79R |
| GPD11 | *GPD1L* | Glycerol -3-Phoshphate dehydrogenase 1-Like | 3p22.3 | 38 | 1 | BrS[12,38]<br>SIDS[36,37] | A280V<br>E83K, I124V, R273C |
| MOG1 | *RANGRF* | MOG1 | 17p13.1 | 20 | 4 | BrS[46]<br>AF[47] | E83D<br>**E61X** |
| PKP2 | *PKP2* | Plakophillin-2 | 12p11 | 97 | 2 | BrS[56] | S183N, M365V, R635Q<br>**T526A** |
| ZASP | *LDB3* | Z-band alternatively spliced PDZ motif protein | 10q23.2 | 77 | 7 | LVNC[61,63] | D117N (isoform2) |
| SLMAP | *SLMAP* | Sarcolemma membrane-associated protein | 3p21.2 | 95 | 8 | BrS[59] | V269I, E710A |
| $Na_V1.5$ | *SCN5A* | Cardiac sodium channel | 3p21 | 227 | 6 | LQT3, BrS, SIDS, CM, and others | >400 |

Bolded mutations reported to be associated with >1 syndrome.
Information on splice variants can be found at the Uniprot web site, specifically for SNTA1: http://www.uniprot.org/uniprot/Q13424, CAV3: http://www.uniprot.org/uniprot/P56539, GPD1L: http://www.uniprot.org/uniprot/Q8N335, MOG1: http://www.uniprot.org/uniprot/Q9HD47, PKP2: http://www.uniprot.org/uniprot/Q13835, SLMAP: http://www.uniprot.org/uniprot/Q14BN4, ZASP: http://www.uniprot.org/uniprot/O75112.
*Abbreviations:* AF, atrial fibrillation; BrS, Brugada syndrome; CM, cardiomyopathy; LQT, long QT; LVNC, left ventricular noncompaction; SIDS, sudden infant death syndrome.

proteins.[2,4–6] Each term has intuitive implications for structure or function, but the terms are not usually rigorously defined and classifications may overlap. Co-localization may occur through direct interaction with $Na_V1.5$ or indirectly through other SCIPs. For example, both α1-syntrophin and ankyrin-G serve to connect SCIPs to $Na_V1.5$ and are called adapter or scaffolding proteins. In many cases, the sites of physical interaction are known, and most SCIPs have also been shown to affect $I_{Na}$ function. On the other hand, some proteins affect $I_{Na}$ or "interact functionally," but have not been shown to be physically associated with the SCC and do not meet this formal definition of an SCIP. For example, protein kinase C (PKC) affects $Na_V1.5$ density,[7] but has not been shown to be associated with the SCC. A broader definition of SCIPs might include proteins such as chaperones that associate during trafficking to the membrane or tags for recycling/degradation, such as ubiquitin,[8] but for this review we use the narrower definition. Another issue with the definition is that, through the cytoskeleton and scaffolding proteins, the SCC may be attached more distantly to many other complexes in the cell. As the field evolves, more precise definitions of "interacting" based on proximity, time, location, and function will emerge.

Although more than 30 SCIPs have been identified (see **Table 1**), they are not present in every complex at all times. Indeed, 2 distinct "pools" of SSCs have been identified in cardiac myocytes, one at the lateral membrane associated with SNTA1 and a second at the intercalated disc with SAP97/plakophilin-2 (PKP2).[9,10] Also, the dynamic nature of the SCC is not known; are the components "permanent" for the approximately 35 hour half-life[11] of the channel at the cell surface, or are they transient over some time period?

## MUTATIONS, DISEASE, AND CAUSALITY

When a mutation is identified in a patient with a particular disease, perhaps the strongest evidence of causality is the strength of genetic linkage analysis. As an example, glycerol phosphate dehydrogenase 1 like (GPD1L) was discovered through a strong genetic linkage to the BrS phenotype[12]; however, most mutations in SCIPs do not have this level of genetic linkage evidence for causality. Absence of a mutation in "control" populations and high conservation of the residue across species provides additional genetic evidence for causality. Plausible pathogenicity of a candidate disease mutation is often built on the functional importance of the mutation by studies at the molecular and cellular levels. The mechanisms by which $I_{Na}$ dysfunction causes clinical syndromes is covered in detail in other articles in this issue, but can be briefly conceptualized as a gain of function where $I_{Na}$, particularly late $I_{Na}$ corresponding with phases 2 and 3 of the action potential, is increased, or as "loss of function," where $I_{Na}$, particularly peak or early $I_{Na}$, corresponding with phases 0 and 1 of the action potential, is decreased.

## SCOPE OF THIS REVIEW

We feature 5 SCIPs that meet this definition and also include sarcolemma membrane-associated protein (SLMAP) and Z-band alternatively spliced PDZ motif protein (ZASP) as 2 more putative SCIPs (see **Table 2**; **Fig. 1**) that have evidence of causation of a cardiac disease through changes in $I_{Na}$. SCIPs that are not considered include mutations in the SCIP telethonin associated with irritable bowel syndrome,[13] but not associated with cardiac disease, which is the scope of this review. A mutation within $Na_v1.5$ disrupted association with the SCIP ankyrin-G in BrS patients,[14] but this is not included because no disease-causing mutations in ankyrin-G itself have been yet identified. Mutations (D130G and F142L) in the SCIP calmodulin (CALM1; see **Table 1**) were discovered in infants with long QT arrhythmia[15]; both showed decreased sensitivity to calcium, but the effects on $I_{Na}$ are not yet established.

## SNTA1 AND LONG QT SYNDROME/SUDDEN INFANT DEATH SYNDROME

SNTA1 or α1-syntrophin is a 54 kDa cytoplasmic membrane-associated adaptor protein that is a member of the multigene syntrophin family and is coded for by the *SNTA1* gene.[16] Syntrophins contain 3 protein interacting domains: (1) A PDZ domain (postsynaptic density protein-95/disc large/zona occludens-1), (2) a plextrin homology (PH) domain, one of which is split by the PDZ domain in SNTA1, and (3) a syntrophin unique domain (see **Fig. 1**A). SNTA1 also contains a second intact PH domain after the split PH domain. SNTA1 serves as an adaptor to link proteins with signaling molecules, such as neuronal nitric oxide synthase (nNOS) or calmodulin, or even other adaptor proteins, such as dystrophin.[16] An adaptor protein itself does not possess intrinsic activity, but localization of bound signaling molecules to the microenvironment provides specificity.[17] The PDZ domain on SNTA1 interacts with a PDZ binding domain on the last 3 amino acids of the *C*-terminus of $Na_v1.5$ as shown by pull down of SNTA1 by a GST fusion protein containing 66 amino acids of the $Na_v1.5$ *C*-terminus (**Fig. 2**).[18] When the last 3 amino acids (SIV) of the $Na_v1.5$ *C*-terminus were deleted syntrophins and dystrophins were no longer pulled down.

A screen for mutations in SNTA1 in a cohort of 50 unrelated LQTS patients negative for 11 established LQTS genes yielded a missense mutation (A390V-SNTA) in an 18-year-old man with syncope.[19] Previous work on nNOS in brain established a physical association between SNTA1, nNOS, and the plasma membrane calcium adenosine triphosphatase subtype 4b calcium pump (PMCA4b).[20] Other studies in heart established that PMCA4b inhibited nNOS.[21] SNTA1 also associated with $Na_v1.5$ in heart,[18] and together these studies raised the possibility that SNTA1 was part of an SCC in heart with SNTA1 connecting nNOS and PMCA4b to $Na_v1.5$ (see **Fig. 2**). Confirmation of a $Na_v1.5$/SNTA1/nNOS/PMCA4b complex was demonstrated in transfected HEK cells where GST–$Na_v1.5$ *C*-terminal fusion constructs pulled down wild-type (WT)-SNTA1, nNOS, and PMCA4b. When A390V-SNTA1 was coexpressed instead of WT-SNTA1, the association with PMCA4b was lost.[19] The A390V mutation is within the second PH2 domain in SNTA1 (see **Figs. 1**A and **2**) and is thought to be the stronger of 2 association sites between PMCA4b and SNTA1, the weaker association being between a PDZ domain on the *C*-terminus tail of PMCA4b and the PDZ domain within the split PH1 domain on SNTA1.[16] The loss of association of PMCA4b with A390V-SNTA1 resulted in increased *S*-nitrosylation of $Na_v1.5$ and increased late $I_{Na}$, and both increases were prevented by the addition of NG-monomethyl-L-arginine, an arginine analog and specific inhibitor of nNOS.[19] These results support the idea that late $I_{Na}$ was increased secondary to *S*-nitrosylation of $Na_v1.5$ caused by A390V-SNTA1 disruption of association of the nNOS inhibitor PMCA4b (see **Fig. 2**).

A screen of 39 LQTS patients negative for mutations in known LQTS susceptibility genes identified a single missense mutation in SNTA1 (A257G-SNTA1) in 3 unrelated patients.[22] A257G is in a highly conserved region of SNTA1 and it was not found in controls. Expression studies with A257G-SNTA1 showed increased peak $I_{Na}$ but no change in late $I_{Na}$. Kinetic effects with coexpression of A257G-SNTA1 included a negative shift of 7 to 10 mV in steady-state activation. Computer modeling supported the role of A257G-SNTA1 in triggering arrhythmia.[22] It should be noted that the expression studies did not include nNOS or PMCA4b, which were shown[19] to be required for increased late $I_{Na}$ with A390V-SNTA1, and this could explain why no disproportionate increase in late $I_{Na}$ was observed. Together, these studies[19,22] established SNTA1 as a cause of LQTS and was designated LQT12.

SNTA1 was screened for mutations in 282 SIDS cases and 6 rare missense mutations (G54R, P56S, T262P, S287R, T372M, and G460S) were found in 8 cases that were absent in 800 controls.[23]

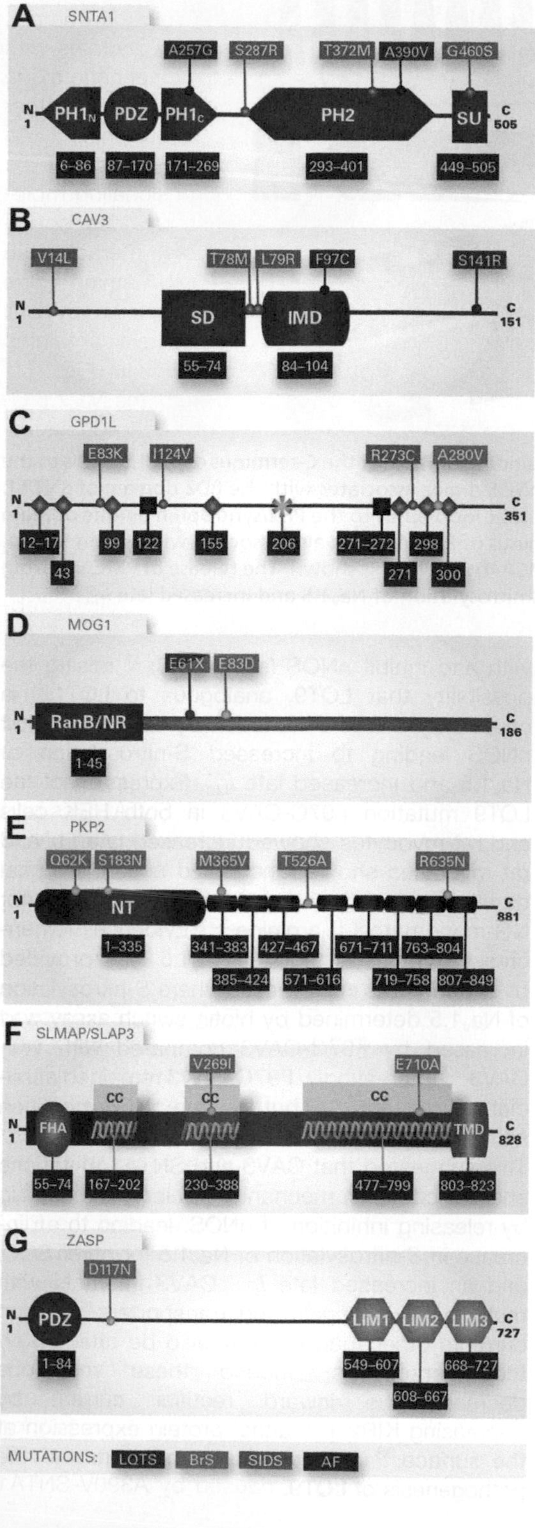


**Fig. 1.** Sodium channel interacting proteins (SCIPs) diagrams showing locations of mutations causing $Na_v1.5$-related cardiac disease and select functional domains. The *N*- and *C*-termini are indicated as *N* and *C* with the amino acid number beneath. The amino acids corresponding to each domain are shown below (amino acid range for domains are assigned based on http://www.uniprot.org/). Disease-causing mutations are indicated at the top of each panel with the box color coded for diseases long QT syndrome (LQTS), Brugada syndrome (BrS), sudden infant death syndrome (SIDS), and atrial fibrillation (AF) as noted at the figure bottom, with references for these mutations given in **Table 2**. (*A*) SNTA1: Two parts of the split PH domain are shown as $PH1_N$ and $PH1_C$ with the PDZ domain located between them. PH2 is the second PH domain and syntrophin unique domain is the syntrophin unique domain (http://www.uniprot.org/uniprot/Q13424). (*B*). CAV3: SD is the CAV3 scaffold domain and *IMD* is the intramembrane domain. http://www.uniprot.org/uniprot/P56539 (*C*) GPD1L: NAD binding sites are indicated as *diamonds*, substrate binding regions are *red boxes*, and the active site is indicated as *asterisk* (http://www.uniprot.org/uniprot/Q8N335). (*D*) MOG1: RanBD/NR is the Ran-binding/GTP release domain[42] (http://www.uniprot.org/uniprot/Q9HD47). (*E*) PKP2: The *N*-terminal domain is marked *NT* and the 8 armadillo repeats are indicated as *red boxes* (http://www.uniprot.org/uniprot/Q13835). (*F*) SLMAP: The long cytoplasmic *N*-terminus with a forkhead-associated domain is marked *FHA*, coiled-coiled leucine zipper domains labeled *CC* are shown as coils, and a transmembrane domain is labeled *TMD*. (http://www.uniprot.org/uniprot/Q14BN4). (*G*) ZASP: The PDZ domain at the *N*-terminal end is marked *PDZ* and the 3 Lim zinc binding domains labeled *Lim1*, *Lim2*, and *Lim3* (http://www.uniprot.org/uniprot/O75112).

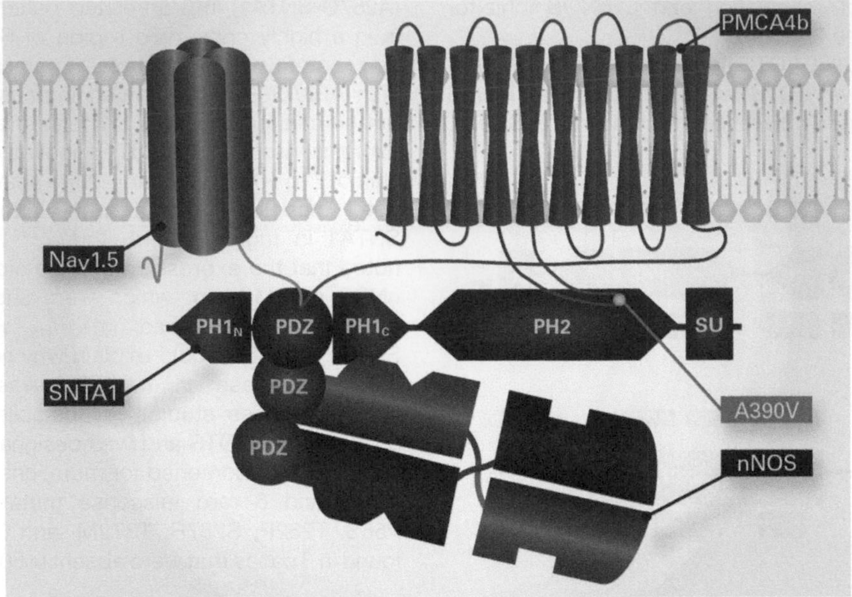


**Fig. 2.** The $Na_v1.5$/SNTA1/nNOS/PMCA4b complex. The PDZ binding domain at the *C*-terminus of $Na_v1.5$ binds to the PDZ domain of SNTA1. One of the PDZ domains from the nNOS dimer associates with the PDZ domain of SNTA1. PMCA4b interacts with SNTA1 at 2 locations, the 4-5 cytoplasmic loop binds to the PH2/syntrophin unique domain region of SNTA1 and the PDZ binding domain in the *C*-terminus of PMCA4b can also associate with PDZ in SNTA1. The A390V-SNTA1 BrS mutation that disrupts binding of PMCA4b to SNTA1 is shown. The release of PMCA4b from the complex results in upregulation of nNOS and increased nitrosylation of $Na_v1.5$ and increased late $I_{Na}$.

When these were co-expressed with $Na_v1.5$, PMCA4b, and nNOS the results for S287R, T372M, and G460S were similar to A390V-SNTA showing increased late $I_{Na}$ that was blocked by nNOS inhibitors, thereby establishing mutations in SNTA1 as a plausible cause of SIDS. Missense mutations in both SNTA1 and $Na_v1.5$ (A261V-SNTA and R800L-$Na_v1.5$) were found in a 3-generation family with LQTS.[24] Co-expression of both mutations showed increased late $I_{Na}$ that was the sum of each mutation expressed alone, suggesting additive effects to produce the phenotype. In another example of interaction, the P74L-SNTA1 polymorphism mitigated the deleterious effect of the LQT12 A257G-SNTA1 mutation.[25]

## *Caveolin-3 and Long QT Syndrome/Sudden Infant Death Syndrome*

Caveolin-3 (CAV3) is a small, approximately 17-kDa integral membrane protein highly expressed in skeletal muscle and heart.[26–28] CAV3 is a member of a family of caveolins that are the major proteins of caveolae, cholesterol-enriched invaginations of the sarcolemma (**Fig. 3**). CAV3 mutations (see **Fig. 1**B) were identified in LQTS (classified as LQT9)[29] and SIDS,[30] and showed increased late $I_{Na}$ when co-expressed with $Na_v1.5$. CAV3 has also been shown to associate with and inhibit nNOS (see **Fig. 3**),[31] raising the possibility that LQT9, analogous to LQT12, is caused by a loss of function by CAV3 to inhibit nNOS leading to increased *S*-nitrosylation of $Na_v1.5$ and increased late $I_{Na}$. Expression of the LQT9 mutation F97C-CAV3 in both HEK cells and rat myocytes showed increased late $I_{Na}$ and rat myocytes showed increased action potential duration that were abrogated by the NOS inhibitor NG-monomethyl-L-arginine.[32] Evidence for increased *S*-nitrosylation of $Na_v1.5$ was provided by experiments in HEK cells where *S*-nitrosylation of $Na_v1.5$ determined by biotin switch assay was increased by F97C-CAV3 compared with WT-CAV3.[32] Interestingly, F97C-CAV3 remained associated with the SCC but lost the nNOS inhibition activity as determined by enzymatic assay.[32] This suggested that CAV3 and SNTA1 mutations share a common mechanism to increase late $I_{Na}$ by releasing inhibition of nNOS, leading to an increase in *S*-nitrosylation of $Na_v1.5$ (or other SCC) and an increased late $I_{Na}$. CAV3 interacts with multiple ion channels and transporters, and ion currents other than $I_{Na}$ may also be affected by these mutations. Indeed these mutations decrease the inward rectifier current by decreasing KIR2.1 channel protein expression at the surface,[33] and this likely contributes to the pathogenesis of LQT9.

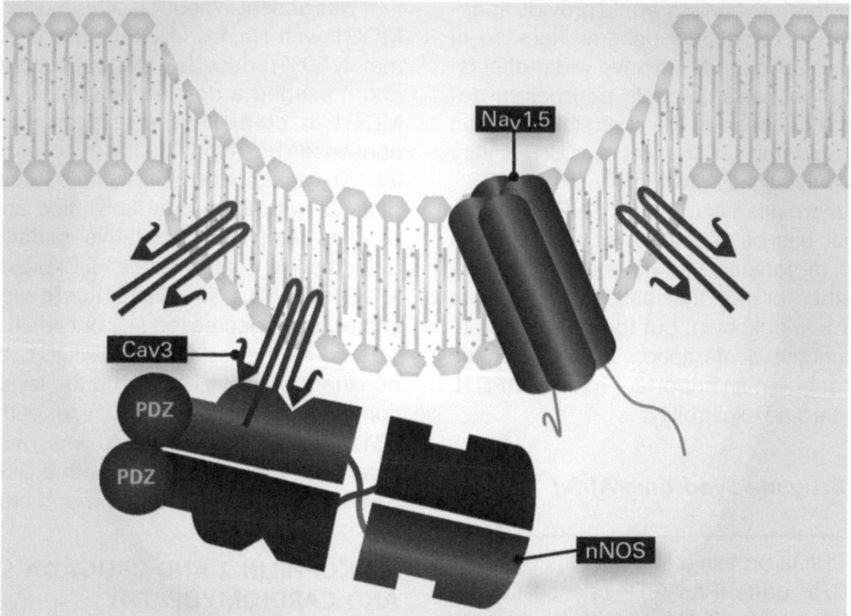


**Fig. 3.** The CAV3/nNOS/Na$_v$1.5 complex in caveolae. The triangles on CAV3 represents amino acids 62–72 and are homologous to the CAV1 region that has been shown to bind to and inhibit endothelial nitric oxide synthase (eNOS) activity.[95] The binding site on nNOS shown is located at W681 and W683 and is based on the homologous site on eNOS.[95]

## GLYCEROL PHOSPHATE DEHYDROGENASE 1 LIKE AND BRUGADA SYNDROME

GPD1L is a 38-kDa protein (see **Fig. 1**C) with very high homology to human cytoplasmic GPD1,[34] an enzyme that catalyzes the reversible reaction converting dihydroxyacetone phosphate to glycerol 3-phosphate with the subsequent oxidation of nicotinamide adenine dinucleotide phosphate to nicotinamide adenine dinucleotide (NAD)$^+$. cGDP1 is an NAD-dependent cytosolic enzyme that is an important link between the glycolytic pathway and triglyceride synthesis. GPD1L was unknown as a human protein until the mutation A280V-GPD1L was implicated in BrS by linkage analysis and gene walking in a large family.[35] This BrS mutation[12] and 3 novel SIDS-associated GPDL1 mutations (E83K, I124V, and R273C)[36] decreased $I_{Na}$ by greater than 50% when the mutant GPD1L cDNAs were transfected into HEK cells expressing Na$_v$1.5.[12,36] The SIDS mutations transfected in mouse myocytes[36] also increased late $I_{Na}$. In heterologous expression systems, GPD1L co-localized with Na$_v$1.5 and was shown to be associated with Na$_v$1.5 by co-immunoprecipitation, and Na$_v$1.5 was pulled down by GST-GPD1L (both WT and GPD1L mutants),[37] establishing GPD1L as an SCIP. GPD1L was localized at the cell surface[12] and the A280V mutant decreased cell surface expression approximately 30%,[12] but the mechanism for the decrease was unknown. How does a defect in an enzyme that is presumably involved in metabolic pathways specifically target Na$_v$1.5? Two different but not mutually exclusive mechanisms have been proposed. One hypothesis[37] has the A280V-GPD1L mutation leading to an increased concentration of glycerol-3-phosphate, which would increase other substrates in the pathway to diacyl-glycerol. The diacyl-glycerol concentration would increase primarily in the area near the Na$_v$1.5/GPD1L SCC and upregulate PKC, which is known to decrease $I_{Na}$ by direct channel phosphorylation at S1503.[7] In support of this hypothesis, E83K-SNTA1 and A280V-SNTA1 decreased both $I_{Na}$ and cell surface expression of Na$_v$1.5, and these decreases were abrogated both by pharmacologic blockers of the PKC-related pathway and also by co-expression with the PKC phosphorylation-deficient Na$_v$1.5 mutant S1503A.[37] This mechanism could account for specificity by co-localization of GPD1L and intermediates with Na$_v$1.5 substrate and direct phosphorylation of Na$_v$1.5. Another proposed mechanism has the mutant increase nicotinamide adenine dinucleotide phosphate and, through PKC effects on mitochondria, to increase reactive oxygen species, which then decreases $I_{Na}$ by unspecified mechanisms.[38,39] It is not clear, however, how this mechanism would provide specificity for $Na_V1.5$, because a general increase in reactive oxygen species would have wider effects. Either or both mechanisms could be operant depending on the direction of the reversible reaction that GPD1L regulates. GPD1L causing BrS is very rare[40] and is only slightly more common in SIDS,[3] but of wider interest is linkage of an SNP upstream of GPD1L that has been associated with sudden cardiac death in patients with coronary artery disease.[41] Whether or not this association occurs through $Na_V1.5$ is unknown, but the localization to $Na_V1.5$, the functional interaction, and the genetic associations suggest an important role for GPD1L in regulating cardiac excitability.

### *MOG1 and Brugada Syndrome/Atrial Fibrillation*

MOG1 is a 20-kDa protein (see **Fig. 1**D) coded for by the *RANGRF* gene (Ran GTP release factor). The yeast homolog, scMOG1, is primarily located in the nucleus and acts as a Ran GTP release factor regulating nuclear import and export of proteins. Human MOG1 binds to both yeast and human Ran, has a GTP release activity that has been mapped to the first 45 amino acids (see **Fig. 1**D),[42] and can partially rescue the growth defect in yeast cells lacking scMOG1, showing that it retains some of the activity of the yeast homologue.[43] MOG1 was identified as an SCIP in human heart by a yeast 2-hybrid screen using a human heart cDNA library as prey[44] and the second intracellular loop of Nav1.5 between repeats II–III as bait.[44] Although MOG1 is mostly found in the nucleus, it also co-localizes with $Na_V1.5$ at the intercalated disc.[44] $Na_V1.5$ and MOG1 co-immunoprecipitation and GST pull-down assays confirmed the association between the $Na_V1.5$ cytoplasmic loop II and in vitro translated MOG1. The GST pull-down assay using in vitro translated proteins is notable because it demonstrates a direct interaction without the need for intermediates to link MOG1 to $Na_V1.5$, although the precise interaction sites are not known. Co-expression of $Na_V1.5$ and MOG1 in HEK cells increased $I_{Na}$ 2-fold without affecting steady-state activation, steady-state inactivation, or recovery from inactivation. Similarly, overexpression of MOG1 in mouse neonatal cardiomyocytes increased $I_{Na}$ with no change in single channel conductance, suggesting that the increased $I_{Na}$ was caused by an increase in channel number at the cell surface. Knock down of MOG1 by small interfering RNA (siRNA) in neonatal mouse cardiomyocytes decreased $I_{Na}$.[45]

A screen of 246 BrS patients[46] yielded a missense mutation (E83D-MOG1) in a female patient with BrS that was absent in controls. Co-expression of E83D-MOG1 with $Na_V1.5$ in HEK cells caused approximately 50% reduced $I_{Na}$ without a change in kinetics, and it exerted a dominant-negative effect on WT-MOG1 in co-expression experiments. The E61X nonsense mutation causing a premature stop (E61X) was reported in 4 patients in a screen of 197 patients with lone atrial fibrillation and in 1 of 23 patients with BrS,[47] but this mutation was also detected in 2 control subjects. Expression of E61X-MOG1 with $Na_V1.5$ in CHO-K1 cells showed approximately 50% decreased $I_{Na}$, but when E61X-MOG1 was co-expressed with WT-MOG1, there was no dominant-negative effect and the levels of $I_{Na}$ were comparable with controls. The pathogenicity of E61X was further questioned when it was detected in an asymptomatic patient with a BrS ECG and in 5 other asymptomatic family members.[48]

## PLAKOPHILIN-2 AND BRUGADA SYNDROME AND CARDIOMYOPATHY

PKP2 is a 98-kDa protein and a member of a family of desmosomal proteins localized primarily at the intercalated disc in cardiomyocytes. PKP2 has a 335 amino acid *N*-terminus that is the site of interaction with binding partners (see **Fig. 1**E).[49,50] There are 8 to 9 armadillo repeats, a signature feature of the family, and a characteristic bend occurs between armadillo repeats 5 and 6, followed by a short *C*-terminus.[49,50] PKP2 is a scaffolding protein that, with other desmosomal proteins, forms a bridge between cadherens and intermediate filaments. Mutations in PKP2 have been linked to familial arrhythmogenic cardiomyopathy (AC), also called arrhythmogenic right ventricular cardiomyopathy.[51] As with heart failure[52] and other cardiac diseases, $Na_V1.5$ is often reduced in AC.[53] In autopsy samples from 5 AC patients and 5 normal controls, immunohistochemistry at the intercalated discs showed that levels of $Na_V1.5$, Cx43 and plakoglobin were reduced in most patients (65%–74%), whereas PKP2 was not affected unless there was a PKP2 mutation.[53] These results show that levels of expression of $Na_V1.5$ at the intercalated disc can be reduced independent of PKP2. Evidence that PKP2 is an SCIP was first provided in siRNA knock down experiments of PKP2 in rat cardiomyocytes,[54] where PKP2 protein was reduced and $I_{Na}$ reduced approximately 50% with no apparent loss of total $Na_V1.5$ protein. This suggested a redistribution of $Na_V1.5$ from the cell surface to intracellular locations. Evidence for association between PKP2 and $Na_V1.5$ was provided by pull down of $Na_V1.5$ by a GST fusion construct containing the *N*-terminus of PKP2.[54] The kinetics of $Na_V1.5$ were altered after siRNA knock down of PKP2 with a negative shift in steady-state inactivation and slower recovery from inactivation.[54] Optical mapping showed a slowing of conduction,[55] suggesting PKP2 as a potential causative agent in BrS. Subsequently, a screen of 200 BrS patients without evidence of AC and negative for mutations in other genes linked with BrS, yielded 5 PKP2 missense mutations (Q62K, S183N, M365V, T526A, and R635Q; see **Fig. 1**E).[56] $I_{Na}$ and the number of $Na_v1.5$ channels found at the intercalated disc were decreased when PKP2 mutants were expressed in a rat atrial cell line (HL1 cells), human embryonic stem cell–derived cardiomyocytes, or in induced pluripotent stem cells derived cardiomyocytes from an AC patient. A dominant-negative effect was absent when WT and mutant PKP2 were co-expressed. In contrast with PKP2 siRNA knock down studies in cardiomyocytes, sodium channel kinetics were not affected.[56] Single channel properties were also unaffected and taken together with immunohistochemical data are consistent with a reduction of $Na_v1.5$ protein at the intercalated discs.[56] These data support a role for PKP2 in targeting and transport of $Na_v1.5$ to the intercalated disc[56] as recently reviewed.[57]

## SARCOLEMMA MEMBRANE-ASSOCIATED PROTEIN AND BRUGADA SYNDROME

SLMAP (or SLAP) is a 95-kDa protein that is localized to the sarcolemma and t-tubules near the sarcoplasmic reticulum. SLMAP3, the longest of 3 alternatively splice forms (37, 46, and 74 kDa, respectively) is predominant in heart (see **Fig. 1**F).[58] SLMAP and ZASP are recently identified disease-causing SCIPs included in this review despite falling outside the strict definition of a disease-causing SCIP put forth earlier. A screen of 190 unrelated BrS patients identified 2 missense mutations (V269I and E710A) in SLMAP.[59] Both mutations decreased $I_{Na}$ and also cell surface expression of both SLMAP and $Na_v1.5$ in HEK cells, with no change in $I_{Na}$ gating kinetics. SLMAP and $Na_v1.5$, failed to co-immunoprecipitate, suggesting that SLMAP may not be a tightly associated part of the SCC.[59] SLMAP may play a role in targeting of $Na_v1.5$ and is a candidate for further study as a BrS-linked gene, but it has not yet been firmly established as an SCIP.

## Z-BAND ALTERNATIVELY SPLICED PDZ MOTIF PROTEIN AND DILATED CARDIOMYOPATHY/ LEFT VENTRICULAR NONCOMPACTION SYNDROME

ZASP is encoded by the gene *LDB3Z4* (Lim Domain-Binding Protein 3) and is a member of a group of 10 genes that code for proteins that contain both PDZ and multiple LIM domains (see **Fig. 1**G).[60] Multiple alternative spliced forms of ZASP exist and the protein coded by longest transcript is 77 kDa (see **Table 2**). All alternatively spliced forms of ZASP have an *N*-terminal PDZ domain but some forms lack the *C*-terminal Lim domains (see **Table 2**). LIM domains contain a cysteine-rich consensus Zinc-finger sequence and are protein interaction domains.[60] Mutations in ZASP have been identified in patients with dilated cardiomyopathy and left ventricular noncompaction[61] and cardiac-specific loss of the murine ZASP homologue results in a severe dilated cardiomyopathy and premature death.[62] In addition to a role in stabilizing the sarcomere structure, ZASP can act as an adaptor protein as, for example, to bridge alpha-actinin-2 through its *N*-terminal PDZ domain with PKC or PKA through its *C*-terminal LIM domains[5] or to bridge the L-type calcium channel through its *C*-terminal PDZ-binding motif with PKA through the LIM-binding domain.[5] Mutations in ZASP have been associated with myofibrillar myopathy and dilated cardiomyopathy.[61] D117N-ZASP, a mutation reported previously,[61] was found in a patient with left ventricular noncompaction syndrome[63] and, when co-expressed with $Na_v1.5$ in HEK293 cells and in rat neonatal myocytes, it caused an approximately 30% reduction in $I_{Na}$. Steady-state activation was shifted +9 mV in HEK cells and +15 mV in myoctes and inactivation was shifted by +4 mV in HEK cells and +10 mV in myocytes, and recovery from inactivation was slowed.[63] Computer modeling supported the hypothesis that the reduction in $I_{Na}$ mediated by ZASP-D117N would generate arrhythmias. Association with Nav1.5 was demonstrated by co-immunoprecipitation using purified ZASP (or D117N- ZASP) produced in *Escherichia coli* mixed with homogenates from $Na_v1.5$ transfected HEK cells or myocytes.[63] The reported association of ZASP with $Na_v1.5$[63] and subsequently with L-type calcium channels[5] acts as a reminder that SCIPs can be promiscuous (see also Cav3) and the pathogenesis may be complex.

## SUMMARY

SCIPs serve multiple functions, including targeting of the SCC to the sarcolemma and regulating function through such mechanisms as posttranslational modification (phosphorylation and nitrosylation). Specificity to $Na_v1.5$ and $I_{Na}$ can be achieved by directly interacting with the $Na_v1.5$ channel protein, but also by localizing signaling pathway components to the local milieu.[17] When this regulation is disturbed by mutations in SCIPs, the resulting dysregulation of $I_{Na}$ can be a mechanism for diseases such as inherited arrhythmia syndromes and SIDS. Although at present mutations in SCIPs are a relatively rare cause of cardiac disease, they are prime candidates to account for BrS syndrome and other inherited arrhythmia syndromes, as well as SIDS and cardiomyopathies, where genetic causes are suspected but not yet demonstrated. At a more basic level, understanding the mechanisms of how mutations in SCIPs cause disease may give insight into the etiology and treatment options of the more common acquired cardiac diseases, including the contribution of subtle genetic variations as susceptibility variants to cardiac disease.

## ACKNOWLEDGMENTS

The authors thank Maeve Makielski for figure artwork.

## REFERENCES

1. Adsit GS, Vaidyanathan R, Galler CM, et al. Channelopathies from mutations in the cardiac sodium channel protein complex. J Mol Cell Cardiol 2013; 61:34–43.
2. Abriel H. Cardiac sodium channel Na(v)1.5 and interacting proteins: physiology and pathophysiology. J Mol Cell Cardiol 2010;48(1):2–11.
3. Makielski JC. Sudden infant death syndrome. In: Zipes DP, Jalife J, editors. Cardiac electrophysiology: from cell to bedside. 6th edition. Philadelphia: Elsevier; 2014. p. 975–80.
4. Isom LL, De Jongh KH, Catterall WA. Auxiliary subunits of voltage-gated ion channels. Neuron 1994; 12:1183–94.
5. Lin C, Guo X, Lange S, et al. Cypher/ZASP is a novel A-kinase anchoring protein. J Biol Chem 2013;288(41):29403–13.
6. Vaidyanathan R, Makielski JC. Scaffolding proteins and ion channel diseases. In: Zipes DP, Jalife J, editors. Cardiac electrophysiology: from cell to bedside. 6th edition. Philadelphia: Elsevier; 2014. p. 229–34.
7. Murray KT, Hu NN, Daw JR, et al. Functional effects of protein kinase C activation on the human cardiac Na+ channel. Circ Res 1997;80(3):370–6.
8. van Bemmelen MX, Rougier JS, Gavillet B, et al. Cardiac voltage-gated sodium channel Nav1.5 is regulated by Nedd4-2 mediated ubiquitination. Circ Res 2004;95(3):284–91.
9. Shy D, Gillet L, Abriel H. Cardiac sodium channel NaV1.5 distribution in myocytes via interacting proteins: the multiple pool model. Biochim Biophys Acta 2013;1833(4):886–94.
10. Petitprez S, Zmoos AF, Ogrodnik J, et al. SAP97 and dystrophin macromolecular complexes determine two pools of cardiac sodium channels Nav1.5 in cardiomyocytes. Circ Res 2011;108(3): 294–304.
11. Maltsev VA, Kyle JW, Mishra S, et al. Molecular identity of the late sodium current in adult dog cardiomyocytes identified by Nav1.5 antisense inhibition. Am J Physiol Heart Circ Physiol 2008;295(2): H667–76.
12. London B, Michalec M, Mehdi H, et al. Mutation in glycerol-3-phosphate dehydrogenase 1 like gene (GPD1-L) decreases cardiac Na+ current and causes inherited arrhythmias. Circulation 2007; 116(20):2260–8.
13. Mazzone A, Strege PR, Tester DJ, et al. A mutation in telethonin alters nav1.5 function. J Biol Chem 2008;283(24):16537–44.
14. Mohler PJ, Rivolta I, Napolitano C, et al. Nav1.5 E1053K mutation causing Brugada syndrome blocks binding to ankyrin-G and expression of Nav1.5 on the surface of cardiomyocytes. Proc Natl Acad Sci U S A 2004;101(50):17533–8.
15. Crotti L, Johnson CN, Graf E, et al. Calmodulin mutations associated with recurrent cardiac arrest in infants. Circulation 2013;127(9):1009–17.
16. Bhat HF, Adams ME, Khanday FA. Syntrophin proteins as Santa Claus: role(s) in cell signal transduction. Cell Mol Life Sci 2013;70(14):2533–54.
17. Barouch LA, Harrison RW, Skaf MW, et al. Nitric oxide regulates the heart by spatial confinement of nitric oxide synthase isoforms. Nature 2002; 416(6878):337–9.
18. Gavillet B, Rougier JS, Domenighetti AA, et al. Cardiac sodium channel Nav1.5 is regulated by a multiprotein complex composed of syntrophins and dystrophin. Circ Res 2006;99(4):407–14.
19. Ueda K, Valdivia C, Medeiros-Domingo A, et al. Syntrophin mutation associated with long QT syndrome through activation of the nNOS-SCN5A macromolecular complex. Proc Natl Acad Sci U S A 2008;105(27):9355–60.
20. Williams JC, Armesilla AL, Mohamed TM, et al. The sarcolemmal calcium pump, alpha-1 syntrophin, and neuronal nitric-oxide synthase are parts of a macromolecular protein complex. J Biol Chem 2006;281(33):23341–8.
21. Oceandy D, Cartwright EJ, Emerson M, et al. Neuronal nitric oxide synthase signaling in the heart is regulated by the sarcolemmal calcium pump 4b. Circulation 2007;115(4):483–92.
22. Wu G, Ai T, Kim JJ, et al. alpha-1-syntrophin mutation and the long-QT syndrome: a disease of sodium channel disruption. Circ Arrhythm Electrophysiol 2008;1(3):193–201.
23. Cheng J, Van Norstrand DW, Medeiros-Domingo A, et al. Alpha1-syntrophin mutations identified in

sudden infant death syndrome cause an increase in late cardiac sodium current. Circ Arrhythm Electrophysiol 2009;2(6):667–76.

24. Hu RM, Tan BH, Orland KM, et al. Digenic inheritance novel mutations in SCN5a and SNTA1 increase late I(Na) contributing to LQT syndrome. Am J Physiol Heart Circ Physiol 2013;304(7):H994–1001.
25. Cheng J, Norstrand DW, Medeiros-Domingo A, et al. LQTS-associated mutation A257G in alpha1-syntrophin interacts with the intragenic variant P74L to modify its biophysical phenotype. Cardiogenetics 2011;1(10):55–9.
26. Balijepalli RC, Kamp TJ. Caveolae, ion channels and cardiac arrhythmias. Prog Biophys Mol Biol 2008;98(2–3):149–60.
27. Li S, Galbiati F, Volonte D, et al. Mutational analysis of caveolin-induced vesicle formation. Expression of caveolin-1 recruits caveolin-2 to caveolae membranes. FEBS Lett 1998;434(1–2):127–34.
28. McNally EM, de Sa ME, Duggan DJ, et al. Caveolin-3 in muscular dystrophy. Hum Mol Genet 1998; 7(5):871–7.
29. Vatta M, Ackerman MJ, Ye B, et al. Mutant caveolin-3 induces persistent late sodium current and is associated with long-QT syndrome. Circulation 2006;114(20):2104–12.
30. Cronk LB, Ye B, Kaku T, et al. Novel mechanism for sudden infant death syndrome: persistent late sodium current secondary to mutations in caveolin-3. Heart Rhythm 2007;4(2):161–6.
31. Venema VJ, Ju H, Zou R, et al. Interaction of neuronal nitric-oxide synthase with caveolin-3 in skeletal muscle. Identification of a novel caveolin scaffolding/inhibitory domain. J Biol Chem 1997; 272(45):28187–90.
32. Cheng J, Valdivia CR, Vaidyanathan R, et al. Caveolin-3 suppresses late sodium current by inhibiting nNOS-dependent S-nitrosylation of SCN5A. J Mol Cell Cardiol 2013;61:102–10.
33. Vaidyanathan R, Vega AL, Song C, et al. The interaction of caveolin 3 with the inward rectifier channel Kir2.1; physiology and pathology related to LQT9. J Biol Chem 2013;288(24):17472–80.
34. Ou X, Ji C, Han X, et al. Crystal structures of human glycerol 3-phosphate dehydrogenase 1 (GPD1). J Mol Biol 2006;357(3):858–69.
35. Weiss R, Barmada MM, Nguyen T, et al. Clinical and molecular heterogeneity in the Brugada syndrome: a novel gene locus on chromosome 3. Circulation 2002;105(6):707–13.
36. Van Norstrand DW, Valdivia CR, Tester DJ, et al. Molecular and functional characterization of novel glycerol-3-phosphate dehydrogenase 1 like gene (GPD1-L) mutations in sudden infant death syndrome. Circulation 2007;116(20):2253–9.
37. Valdivia CR, Ueda K, Ackerman MJ, et al. GPD1L links redox state to cardiac excitability by PKC-dependent phosphorylation of the sodium channel SCN5A. Am J Physiol Heart Circ Physiol 2009; 297(4):H1446–52.
38. Liu M, Sanyal S, Gao G, et al. Cardiac Na+ current regulation by pyridine nucleotides. Circ Res 2009; 105(8):737–45.
39. Liu M, Liu H, Dudley SC Jr. Reactive oxygen species originating from mitochondria regulate the cardiac sodium channel. Circ Res 2010;107(8):967–74.
40. Makiyama T, Akao M, Haruna Y, et al. Mutation analysis of the glycerol-3 phosphate dehydrogenase-1 like (GPD1L) gene in Japanese patients with Brugada syndrome. Circ J 2008;72(10):1705–6.
41. Westaway SK, Reinier K, Huertas-Vazquez A, et al. Common variants in CASQ2, GPD1L, and NOS1AP are significantly associated with risk of sudden death in patients with coronary artery disease. Circ Cardiovasc Genet 2011;4(4):397–402.
42. Steggerda SM, Paschal BM. Identification of a conserved loop in Mog1 that releases GTP from Ran. Traffic 2001;2(11):804–11.
43. Marfatia KA, Harreman MT, Fanara P, et al. Identification and characterization of the human MOG1 gene. Gene 2001;266(1–2):45–56.
44. Wu L, Yong SL, Fan C, et al. Identification of a new co-factor, MOG1, required for the full function of cardiac sodium channel Nav 1.5. J Biol Chem 2008;283(11):6968–78.
45. Chakrabarti S, Wu X, Yang Z, et al. MOG1 rescues defective trafficking of Na(v)1.5 mutations in Brugada syndrome and sick sinus syndrome. Circ Arrhythm Electrophysiol 2013;6(2):392–401.
46. Kattygnarath D, Maugenre S, Neyroud N, et al. MOG1: a new susceptibility gene for Brugada syndrome. Circ Cardiovasc Genet 2011;4(3):261–8.
47. Olesen MS, Jensen NF, Holst AG, et al. A novel nonsense variant in Nav1.5 cofactor MOG1 eliminates its sodium current increasing effect and may increase the risk of arrhythmias. Can J Cardiol 2011;27(4):523.
48. Campuzano O, Berne P, Selga E, et al. Brugada syndrome and p.E61X_RANGRF. Cardiol J 2014; 21(2):121–7.
49. Bass-Zubek AE, Godsel LM, Delmar M, et al. Plakophilins: multifunctional scaffolds for adhesion and signaling. Curr Opin Cell Biol 2009;21(5):708–16.
50. Kowalczyk AP, Green KJ. Structure, function, and regulation of desmosomes. Prog Mol Biol Transl Sci 2013;116:95–118.
51. van Tintelen JP, Entius MM, Bhuiyan ZA, et al. Plakophilin-2 mutations are the major determinant of familial arrhythmogenic right ventricular dysplasia/cardiomyopathy. Circulation 2006;113(13):1650–8.
52. Valdivia CR, Chu WW, Pu JL, et al. Increased late sodium current in myocytes from a canine heart failure model and from failing human heart. J Mol Cell Cardiol 2005;38(3):475–83.

53. Noorman M, Hakim S, Kessler E, et al. Remodeling of the cardiac sodium channel, connexin43, and plakoglobin at the intercalated disk in patients with arrhythmogenic cardiomyopathy. Heart Rhythm 2013;10(3):412–9.
54. Sato PY, Musa H, Coombs W, et al. Loss of plakophilin-2 expression leads to decreased sodium current and slower conduction velocity in cultured cardiac myocytes. Circ Res 2009;105(6):523–6.
55. Cerrone M, Noorman M, Lin X, et al. Sodium current deficit and arrhythmogenesis in a murine model of plakophilin-2 haploinsufficiency. Cardiovasc Res 2012;95(4):460–8.
56. Cerrone M, Lin X, Zhang M, et al. Missense mutations in plakophilin-2 cause sodium current deficit and associate with a Brugada syndrome phenotype. Circulation 2014;129(10):1092–103.
57. Cerrone M, Delmar M. Desmosomes and the sodium channel complex: Implications for arrhythmogenic cardiomyopathy and Brugada syndrome. Trends Cardiovasc Med 2014;24(5):184–90.
58. Wielowieyski PA, Sevinc S, Guzzo R, et al. Alternative splicing, expression, and genomic structure of the 3' region of the gene encoding the sarcolemmal-associated proteins (SLAPs) defines a novel class of coiled-coil tail-anchored membrane proteins. J Biol Chem 2000;275(49):38474–81.
59. Ishikawa T, Sato A, Marcou CA, et al. A novel disease gene for Brugada syndrome: sarcolemmal membrane-associated protein gene mutations impair intracellular trafficking of hNav1.5. Circ Arrhythm Electrophysiol 2012;5(6):1098–107.
60. te Velthuis AJ, Isogai T, Gerrits L, et al. Insights into the molecular evolution of the PDZ/LIM family and identification of a novel conserved protein motif. PLoS One 2007;2(2):e189.
61. Vatta M, Mohapatra B, Jimenez S, et al. Mutations in Cypher/ZASP in patients with dilated cardiomyopathy and left ventricular non-compaction. J Am Coll Cardiol 2003;42(11):2014–27.
62. Zheng M, Cheng H, Banerjee I, et al. ALP/Enigma PDZ-LIM domain proteins in the heart. J Mol Cell Biol 2010;2(2):96–102.
63. Xi Y, Ai T, De Lange E, et al. Loss of function of hNav1.5 by a ZASP1 mutation associated with intraventricular conduction disturbances in left ventricular noncompaction. Circ Arrhythm Electrophysiol 2012;5(5):1017–26.
64. Allouis M, Le Bouffant F, Wilders R, et al. 14-3-3 is a regulator of the cardiac voltage-gated sodium channel Nav1.5. Circ Res 2006;98(12):1538–46.
65. Ziane R, Huang H, Moghadaszadeh B, et al. Cell membrane expression of cardiac sodium channel Na(v)1.5 is modulated by alpha-actinin-2 interaction. Biochemistry 2010;49(1):166–78.
66. Mohler PJ, Wehrens XH. Mechanisms of human arrhythmia syndromes: abnormal cardiac macromolecular interactions. Physiology (Bethesda) 2007;22:342–50.
67. Lowe JS, Palygin O, Bhasin N, et al. Voltage-gated Nav channel targeting in the heart requires an ankyrin-G dependent cellular pathway. J Cell Biol 2008;180(1):173–86.
68. Dhar Malhotra J, Chen C, Rivolta I, et al. Characterization of sodium channel alpha- and beta-subunits in rat and mouse cardiac myocytes. Circulation 2001;103(9):1303–10.
69. Valdivia CR, Nagatomo T, Makielski JC. Late currents affect kinetics for heart and skeletal Na channel α and β1 subunits expressed in HEK293 cells. J Mol Cell Cardiol 2002;34(8):1029–39.
70. Maltsev VA, Kyle JW, Undrovinas A. Late Na+ current produced by human cardiac Na+ channel isoform Nav1.5 is modulated by its beta1 subunit. J Physiol Sci 2009;59(3):217–25.
71. Herfst LJ, Potet F, Bezzina CR, et al. Na+ channel mutation leading to loss of function and non-progressive cardiac conduction defects. J Mol Cell Cardiol 2003;35(5):549–57.
72. Nuss HB, Chiamvimonvat N, Perez-Garcia MT, et al. Functional association of the β1 subunit with human cardiac (hH1) and rat skeletal muscle (μ1) sodium channel α subunits expressed in Xenopus oocytes. J Gen Physiol 1995;106(6):1171–91.
73. Lopez-Santiago LF, Meadows LS, Ernst SJ, et al. Sodium channel Scn1b null mice exhibit prolonged QT and RR intervals. J Mol Cell Cardiol 2007;43(5):636–47.
74. Johnson D, Bennett ES. Isoform-specific effects of the beta2 subunit on voltage-gated sodium channel gating. J Biol Chem 2006;281(36):25875–81.
75. Mishra S, Undrovinas NA, Maltsev VA, et al. Post-transcriptional silencing of SCN1B and SCN2B genes modulates late sodium current in cardiac myocytes from normal dogs and dogs with chronic heart failure. Am J Physiol Heart Circ Physiol 2011;301(4):H1596–605.
76. Hakim P, Brice N, Thresher R, et al. Scn3b knockout mice exhibit abnormal sino-atrial and cardiac conduction properties. Acta Physiol (Oxf) 2010;198(1):47–59.
77. Fahmi AI, Patel M, Stevens EB, et al. The sodium channel beta-subunit SCN3b modulates the kinetics of SCN5a and is expressed heterogeneously in sheep heart. J Physiol 2001;537(Pt 3):693–700.
78. Hakim P, Gurung IS, Pedersen TH, et al. Scn3b knockout mice exhibit abnormal ventricular electrophysiological properties. Prog Biophys Mol Biol 2008;98(2–3):251–66.
79. Medeiros-Domingo A, Kaku T, Tester DJ, et al. SCN4B-encoded sodium channel {beta}4 subunit in congenital long-QT syndrome. Circulation 2007;116:136–42.
80. Remme CA, Scicluna BP, Verkerk AO, et al. Genetically determinod differences in sodium current

characteristics modulate conduction disease severity in mice with cardiac sodium channelopathy. Circ Res 2009;104(11):1283–92.

81. Hund TJ, Koval OM, Li J, et al. A beta(IV)-spectrin/CaMKII signaling complex is essential for membrane excitability in mice. J Clin Invest 2010;120(10):3508–19.
82. Kim J, Ghosh S, Liu H, et al. Calmodulin mediates Ca2+ sensitivity of sodium channels. J Biol Chem 2004;279(43):45004–12.
83. Chagot B, Chazin WJ. Solution NMR structure of Apo-calmodulin in complex with the IQ motif of human cardiac sodium channel NaV1.5. J Mol Biol 2011;406(1):106–19.
84. Tan HL, Kupershmidt S, Zhang R, et al. A calcium sensor in the sodium channel modulates cardiac excitability. Nature 2002;415(6870):442–7.
85. Aiba T, Hesketh GG, Liu T, et al. Na+ channel regulation by Ca2+/calmodulin and Ca2+/calmodulin-dependent protein kinase II in guinea-pig ventricular myocytes. Cardiovasc Res 2010;85(3):454–63.
86. Koval OM, Snyder JS, Wolf RM, et al. Ca2+/calmodulin-dependent protein kinase II-based regulation of voltage-gated Na+ channel in cardiac disease. Circulation 2012;126(17):2084–94.
87. van der Velden HM, Jongsma HJ. Cardiac gap junctions and connexins: their role in atrial fibrillation and potential as therapeutic targets. Cardiovasc Res 2002;54(2):270–9.
88. Malhotra JD, Thyagarajan V, Chen C, et al. Tyrosine-phosphorylated and nonphosphorylated sodium channel beta1 subunits are differentially localized in cardiac myocytes. J Biol Chem 2004;279(39):40748–54.
89. Jansen JA, Noorman M, Musa H, et al. Reduced heterogeneous expression of Cx43 results in decreased Nav1.5 expression and reduced sodium current that accounts for arrhythmia vulnerability in conditional Cx43 knockout mice. Heart Rhythm 2012;9(4):600–7.
90. Rizzo S, Lodder EM, Verkerk AO, et al. Intercalated disc abnormalities, reduced Na(+) current density, and conduction slowing in desmoglein-2 mutant mice prior to cardiomyopathic changes. Cardiovasc Res 2012;95(4):409–18.
91. Albesa M, Ogrodnik J, Rougier JS, et al. Regulation of the cardiac sodium channel Nav1.5 by utrophin in dystrophin-deficient mice. Cardiovasc Res 2011;89(2):320–8.
92. Wang C, Hennessey JA, Kirkton RD, et al. Fibroblast growth factor homologous factor 13 regulates Na+ channels and conduction velocity in murine hearts. Circ Res 2011;109(7):775–82.
93. Ou YJ, Strege P, Miller SM, et al. Syntrophin gamma 2 regulates SCN5A Gating by a PDZ domain-mediated interaction. J Biol Chem 2003;278(3):1915–23.
94. Jespersen T, Gavillet B, van Bemmelen MX, et al. Cardiac sodium channel Na(v)1.5 interacts with and is regulated by the protein tyrosine phosphatase PTPH1. Biochem Biophys Res Commun 2006;348(4):1455–62.
95. Trane AE, Pavlov D, Sharma A, et al. Deciphering the binding of caveolin-1 to client protein endothelial nitric oxide synthase (eNOS): scaffolding subdomain identification, interaction modeling, and biological significance. J Biol Chem 2014;289(19):13273–83.

# Use of Drugs in Long QT Syndrome Type 3 and Brugada Syndrome

Pieter G. Postema, MD, PhD[a,*],
Raymond L. Woosley, MD, PhD[b,c]

**KEYWORDS**

• Long QT syndrome • Brugada syndrome • Drugs • Arrhythmias • Sudden death

**KEY POINTS**

- *SCN5A* gene–related channelopathies, long QT syndrome, and Brugada syndrome are well known; both cardiovascular and noncardiovascular drugs can have detrimental effects in these disorders.
- The mechanisms by which these drugs can be dangerous, particularly through further reduction of $I_{Kr}$ and $I_{Na}$ for long QT syndrome and Brugada syndrome, respectively, are understood.
- Administration of drugs with possible untoward effects in these syndromes requires careful consideration and monitoring.
- Online databases are available to help the physician determine which drugs are potentially unsafe.

## INTRODUCTION

Congenital long QT syndrome and Brugada syndrome are entities associated with characteristic electrocardiographic abnormalities and an inherited propensity for ventricular arrhythmias and premature sudden death; both are estimated to have a prevalence of about 1 in 2000.[1–3] They belong to a larger family of entities that can be grouped under the heading "inheritable arrhythmia syndromes," which are also known as channelopathies. This term is based on the fact that in many of these patients a mutation is found in a gene encoding for a cardiac ion channel or its regulators and where the mutation alters the normal function of this ion channel. These cardiac ion channels are responsible for the electrical activation and recovery of the heart during each heartbeat because of their role in the transport of sodium, potassium, or calcium ions across the cardiac cell membranes resulting in their respective currents ($I$): $I_{Na}$, $I_K$, and $I_{Ca}$. Disruption of this delicate process can result in these syndromes and may lead to malignant arrhythmias and subsequently in cardiac arrest and sudden death. Importantly, these disastrous effects may become manifest at any time, from birth until advanced age, mostly depending on the severity of the mutation, the presence of other mutations or genetic variants, and numerous other factors (for a more complete review see, eg, Cerrone and colleagues[4]).

Genetic subtypes that are based on the specific gene that is mutated are known for both long QT syndrome and Brugada syndrome. For example, long QT syndrome type 1 and type 2 (**Fig. 1**) are based on mutations in the *KCNQ1* gene that reduce the slow component of the potassium-rectifying current $I_{Ks}$, and in the *KCNH2* gene that reduce the rapid component of the potassium-

Conflicts of Interest: None.
[a] Department of Cardiology, Heart Center, Academic Medical Center, Meibergdreef 9, Amsterdam 1105 AZ, The Netherlands; [b] Arizona Center for Education and Research on Therapeutics (AZCERT), 1822 E. Innovation Park Drive, Oro Valley, AZ 85755, USA; [c] University of Arizona, Sarver Heart Center, 1501 North Campbell Avenue, Tucson, AZ 85724, USA
* Corresponding author.
*E-mail address:* p.g.postema@cardiologie-amc.nl

Card Electrophysiol Clin 6 (2014) 811–817
http://dx.doi.org/10.1016/j.ccep.2014.08.004

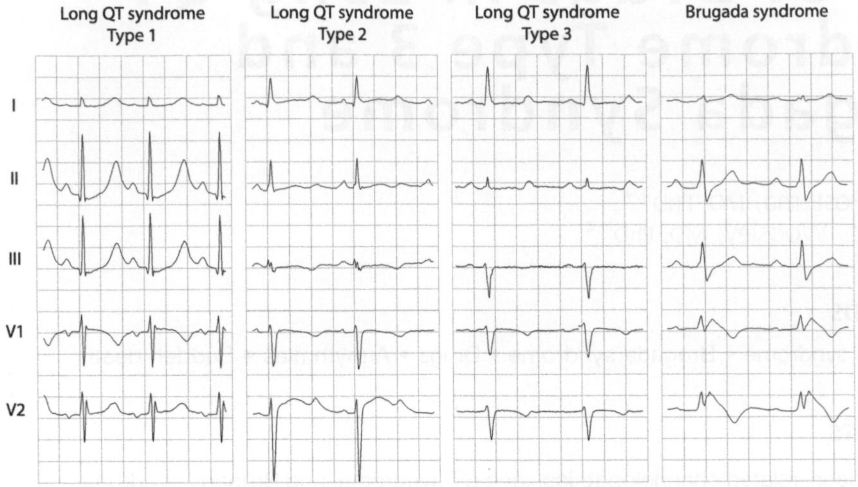


**Fig. 1.** Shown are examples of an ECG (leads I, II, III, V1, and V2) from patients with type 1, type 2, or type 3 long QT syndrome, and from a patient with Brugada syndrome, all in the absence of provoking drugs. Note the excessively prolonged QT intervals in the patients with long QT syndrome, with typical broad-based high amplitude T-waves in type 1 long QT syndrome, bifid T-waves in type 2 long QT syndrome, and late-onset T-waves in type 3 long QT syndrome. In the patient with Brugada syndrome, the coved-type ST elevation in V1 and V2 (known as type-1 Brugada ECG) is evident, as are other indicators of conduction slowing (prolonged PQ and QRS).

rectifying current $I_{Kr}$, respectively. In contrast, long QT syndrome type 3 (see **Fig. 1**) is caused by mutations in the *SCN5A* gene resulting in increased *persistent* inward sodium current $I_{Na}$. The *SCN5A* gene is also predominantly involved in Brugada syndrome but now mutations reduce the *fast* inward sodium current $I_{Na}$. This *SCN5A*-related form of Brugada syndrome has by some investigators been described as "type 1" Brugada syndrome,[5] not to be mistaken for the type-1 Brugada electrocardiographic pattern (ECG): the diagnostic ECG feature of Brugada syndrome (see **Fig. 1**). One should also realize that long QT syndrome and Brugada syndrome are not the only phenotypical expressions of *SCN5A* channelopathies. They also may result in conduction defects[6] or even in overlap syndromes, which may display many different phenotypes in combination.[7] Of importance, we know that many drugs can reduce cardiac $I_{Na}$, $I_K$, and/or $I_{Ca}$, making these drugs potentially lethal in patients with these syndromes whose ionic currents are already critically depressed.[8–10] In this article we particularly focus on the issue of safe drug use in the *SCN5A*-related channelopathies that result in long QT syndrome and Brugada syndrome.

## LONG QT TYPE 3

Type 3 long QT syndrome, 1 of 12 known types,[4] is also the third most prevalent type. Type 1 and type 2 each represent about 40%, whereas type 3 has a prevalence of about 5% to 10%.[11–13] All other types are less frequent or even rare. However, in the absence of genetic testing or a positive genetic test result, this genetic labeling cannot be performed. One should realize that even in the largest worldwide long QT syndrome registry, only 50% of the patients are positively genotyped.[14] This implies that genetic subtyping is not available in the other 50% of these patients. Even in experienced centers, the yield of genetic testing in long QT syndrome is only approximately 30% in isolated cases and up to approximately 80% in the presence of familial segregation of the phenotype.[13] It is intuitive that the number of patients who are positively genetically tested is much lower than 50% outside the registries or in those who are not seen in experienced arrhythmia centers with genetic testing as standard of care.

The most common characteristic of mutations resulting in long QT syndrome is its ability to reduce either $I_{Kr}$ or $I_{Ks}$. A reduction of the other major rectifying potassium current, $I_{K1}$, is not particularly related to lengthening of the QT interval.[15,16] However, in long QT syndrome type 3, it is an intensification of the persistent inward sodium current by a gain-of-function sodium channel mutation that causes prolongation of the action potential and the subsequent prolongation of the QT interval. Of note, recognizing prolongation of the QT interval may sometimes be difficult,[17] but suggestions to improve its recognition are available.[18,19]

As the inheritance in this syndrome is now, by definition, based on carrier status of a genetic defect, it is important to realize that the clinical phenotype (ie, prolongation of the QT interval) is not uniformly present. There are patients who have the same mutation that in their siblings causes prolonged QT intervals and cardiac arrhythmias, whereas they themselves have normal QT intervals and do not experience any untoward events caused by the long QT syndrome mutation. This intriguing feature is named "incomplete penetrance" and has been seen in all inheritable cardiac arrhythmia syndromes.[20,21] Still, whenever a patient who has a normal baseline ECG but also has a 50% chance of inheritance of a mutation associated with the long QT syndrome, provocation testing either by brisk standing or an exercise test, or by the use of provocative drugs like epinephrine/adrenaline, and Holter monitoring is recommended to evaluate whether repolarization reserve is impaired.[22–25]

Although we are learning more and more about the pivotal elements that result in the penetrance of a clinical phenotype of long QT syndrome,[26] this still remains an important area of further research. It is also important to realize that there are silent mutation carriers (ie, those without a prolonged QT interval but who may show excessive sensitivity to certain QT prolonging drugs and therefore cannot be considered to also have a low risk of drug toxicity).

## BRUGADA SYNDROME

In contrast to long QT syndrome, where experienced centers report that mutations can be identified in 30% to 80% of cases, in Brugada syndrome the positive yield of genetic testing is only approximately 20% in isolated cases and up to approximately 45% in families with known inheritance.[13] When mutations are uncovered, they are mostly observed in the *SCN5A* gene (>75%), but also may be found in the calcium channel gene and only rarely in other genes.[5,27] One may even argue that the scientific reliability of many of the reports of mutations in rare genes that have been putatively associated with Brugada syndrome is weak, as there is, for example, often no evidence of segregation with the phenotype.[28]

In Brugada syndrome the pathogenicity of most mutations is created by a decrease in the fast inward sodium current $I_{Na}$. Whether this decrease in $I_{Na}$ also results in repolarization abnormalities in addition to depolarization abnormalities is subject of ongoing research.[29] Either way, the presence of the characteristic type-1 Brugada ECG is often variable,[30,31] suggesting fluctuating electrophysiological properties. This variability of the ECG in Brugada syndrome is, in contrast to long QT syndrome, not considered to be a result of incomplete penetrance. Instead, incomplete penetrance in the Brugada syndrome is manifest in its variable reaction to strong sodium channel blocking drugs. It appears that not all patients with a sodium channel mutation in a given Brugada syndrome family will display the characteristic type-1 ECG on provocation with sodium channel blocking drugs.[32] The exact risk of a cardiac arrest when a patient with Brugada syndrome is given other cardiovascular or noncardiovascular drugs with cardiac sodium channel blocking effects is hard to predict, but some drugs are certainly more dangerous than others,[8] taking into consideration the patient-specific risk factors that should be accounted for.[10]

## OVERLAP SYNDROMES

As mentioned earlier, there are sodium channel mutations that may cause a mixture of associated phenotypes even within family members carrying the same mutation. The most prevalent overlap syndrome is the combination of conduction disorder and a Brugada phenotype.[33–35] The presence of this overlap syndrome is also intuitive, because both are expected results from a decrease in fast inward sodium current caused by loss-of-function sodium channel mutations.

The risk of cardiac arrhythmic events with the use of certain drugs in these patients will probably be similar to those of patients with Brugada syndrome. Therefore, it is generally advised that the same drugs should be avoided in either condition. However, there also are mutations that cause both a *decrease* in *fast* inward sodium current and also an *increase* in the *persistent* inward sodium current. These patients may thus display a conduction disease phenotype, Brugada syndrome phenotype or long QT syndrome type 3 phenotype or combinations thereof.[7,36–38] For these patients, the risk of drug-induced cardiac events will be partly determined by their phenotype, but will often involve restriction of drugs associated with untoward events in Brugada syndrome as well as drugs associated with untoward events in long QT syndrome.[10]

## MECHANISMS OF DRUG INTERACTION

In all types of long QT syndrome and Brugada syndrome, there are probably dominant pathways by which both cardiovascular and noncardiovascular drugs may cause the intermediate phenotype of either QT prolongation or the development of the type-1 Brugada ECG, and/or result in malignant ventricular arrhythmias, cardiac arrest, or sudden death. In long QT syndrome, the most important mechanism appears to be blockade of the rapid potassium-rectifying current $I_{Kr}$,[39] in Brugada syndrome it is the blockade of the fast inward sodium current $I_{Na}$.[40]

Although long QT syndrome type 3 is dependent on an increase of persistent inward sodium current, there are no drugs available, as far as we know, that further increase this current and would subsequently further prolong the QT interval and further increase the risk for arrhythmias. Most, if not all, of the chemicals with this action are toxins, like anthopleurin A, that would be eliminated during drug development.[41]

Therefore additional drug-induced prolongation of the action potential and the QT interval, with a subsequent increase in risk for arrhythmias, in type 3 long QT syndrome will be dependent on the destabilization of the other repolarizing currents, which works in concert with the already critically altered persistent sodium inward current. The 3 relevant outward currents in this perspective are the rapid potassium-rectifying current ($I_{Kr}$), the delayed potassium-rectifying current ($I_{Ks}$), and the inward rectifier potassium outward current ($I_{K1}$). As already mentioned, the most important of these 3 currents in respect to its possible detrimental action in long QT syndrome, is considered to be blockade of $I_{Kr}$,[9,39] although evidence is also accumulating for blockade of $I_{Ks}$.[42] Importantly, one should realize that both cardiovascular and noncardiovascular drugs have the ability to block cardiac ion channels. In long QT syndrome for example, antibiotics, psychotropic drugs, and drugs in many other classes are among the more than 140 drugs that may result in excessive QT prolongation and arrhythmias.[9,39] Still, at this moment we do not have clear data on a subset of drugs that would be more hazardous, or less hazardous, when used in a particular type of long QT syndrome.[9,10] However, there is evidence that the opposite is true, some beta-blockers are more effective in decreasing arrhythmic events in certain subtypes of long QT syndrome than other beta-blockers.[43] This knowledge base does suggest that unsafe drugs also can have differential effects in different subtypes of long QT syndrome, although evidence is lacking at this time. Nevertheless, it is intuitive that with a more dangerous phenotype (eg, in terms of QT prolongation and/or the presence of a history of arrhythmias or cardiac arrest), the more strictly one should avoid potentially dangerous drugs. In addition, there appear to be many more patient characteristics aside the specific mutation that may set a patient at risk for drug-induced arrhythmic events.[44] One must consider the gender of the patient, their drug metabolism capacity, and concomitant drugs taken, to name but a few.

In Brugada syndrome, it appears that the common pathway to an increase in risk for arrhythmic events is more homogeneous; almost all of these drugs cause blockade of the fast sodium inward current $I_{Na}$.[8,10] Also in Brugada syndrome, one should realize that both cardiovascular and noncardiovascular drugs might result in cardiac sodium channel blockade and subsequent untoward events. Specifically, psychotropic drugs are among the noncardiovascular drugs with cardiac $I_{Na}$ blocking effects and arrhythmias in Brugada syndrome.[8] Equivalent to long QT syndrome, there are currently no clear data available to suggest that different genetic subtypes of Brugada syndrome, based on different mutations, display more severe or less severe reactions to the different drugs. Again, there are specific patient characteristics that can be demonstrated that influence the risk profile and that can be used to make decisions regarding drug use.[4,10,45]

## DRUG LISTS ONLINE

At www.QTdrugs.org (also reached through www.CredibleMeds.org), one can find a comprehensive list of drugs that should be avoided in patients with long QT syndrome.[9,10] As mentioned earlier, there is, however, a paucity on data on the relative risk of drug use for the specific subtypes of patients with long QT syndrome. However, even if available, this would only be of limited value, because for at least 50% of patients with long QT syndrome patients, mutation has been identified or sought for. In analogy to www.QTdrugs.org, a Web site concerning the safe use of drugs also has been developed for Brugada syndrome: www.BrugadaDrugs.org. Also on this list, physicians and patients can find information on the relative safety of drugs in patients with Brugada syndrome. Both of these Web sites have been recommended in the latest consensus document on inheritable arrhythmia syndromes.[46] For both syndromes there is a paucity of data on alternative drugs that may indeed be used safely. This represents a gap in our current knowledge base that warrants further explorative efforts to be able to provide both an unsafe and a safe list of drugs.[10] Because the lists of drugs that have potential harm for patients with these syndromes are long and steadily increasing, the prescriber should check the lists regularly, subscribe to their update services, and/or develop clinical decision support systems that assist their safe prescribing of these drugs.[47]

## SENSIBLE TREATMENT BASED ON THE CARDIAC PHENOTYPE

For both syndromes, when a decision is made to administer a certain drug with probable unsafe characteristics to a patient, careful monitoring is advised. In some patients, this may require hospital admission for intensive ECG monitoring, whereas in other patients monitoring can be performed in an outpatient setting.[10,45,48] Intuitively, one should be more careful in patients with a higher risk profile (eg, in patients with a critical phenotype, previous adverse reactions to drugs, or previous life-threatening arrhythmias) than in patients without an arrhythmia history and a mild or absent phenotype. However, when a high-risk patient is already equipped with an implantable cardioverter defibrillator (ICD) because of his or her high risk, one may more easily consider administration of relatively contraindicated or moderate-risk drugs in an outpatient setting, in the absence of an extremely high-risk phenotype at that moment, because the patient will most probably be protected against sudden death. Although most comorbidities that may require drug administration will occur with advancing age, particularly in long QT syndrome, arrhythmias are more likely to occur in the young.[49] In these young patients, particularly antibiotics may be considered, which needs careful consideration and adequate safety monitoring. Still, also after the age of 40 years, a continued risk for events remains,[50] necessitating continued awareness for risk stratification use of safer alternatives if they are available. In Brugada syndrome, most arrhythmic events are clustered between the age of 30 and 50 years, which already is an age in which comorbidities may surface. Especially the intended use of antiarrhythmic drugs and psychotropic drugs should be carefully considered and will require judicious monitoring.[45]

Sensible use of drugs is thus warranted in these syndromes. For example, in the event of atrial fibrillation in long QT syndrome (although the risk of developing atrial fibrillation is certainly not especially high in these patients), one should definitely refrain from drugs like ibutilide, dofetilide, flecainide, sotalol, or amiodarone. In Brugada syndrome, there is a high risk for atrial fibrillation but administration of flecainide could be extremely dangerous, vernakalant is relatively contraindicated, and also amiodarone is preferably avoided. In contrast, ivabradine can probably be administered safely. Whether beta-blockers can be safely administered in Brugada syndrome is disputed, but there are some reports that propranolol may result in the occurrence of the intermediate phenotype (ie, the development of a type-1 Brugada syndrome ECG). There is currently no evidence that sotalol would be inappropriate in patients with Brugada syndrome.[45] Also quinidine for the treatment of atrial fibrillation in Brugada syndrome can most probably be very valuable. Of course, in patients with a pacemaker or ICD, the use of beta-blockers can be more readily considered. Some forms of long QT syndrome may be bradycardia dependent, particularly type 3. Although in type 3 long QT syndrome, beta-blockers will often have protective properties,[51] in some specific *SCN5A* mutations that cause an overlap syndrome, pacemakers are implanted to prevent bradycardia and sudden death.[7,52,53]

As for ventricular arrhythmias, in long QT syndrome, when there is insufficient protection with beta-blockers, one may well consider left stellectomy to decrease the risk for events.[46] In long QT syndrome type 3, mexiletine also may be considered.[54] In Brugada syndrome, there is increasing evidence that quinidine decreases the risk for events.[55–57] It is therefore extremely troublesome that the availability of quinidine is becoming limited and that patients are subjected to an increased risk of malignant and possibly fatal arrhythmias without this potentially life-saving drug.[55,56]

## SUMMARY

In long QT syndrome type 3 and Brugada syndrome, both cardiovascular and noncardiovascular drugs may have detrimental effects on the intermediate phenotype of QT prolongation and development of the type-1 Brugada ECG, and may subsequently result in potentially fatal arrhythmias. Cautious and considered use of drugs in these syndromes is thus warranted. In this review, we have intended to provide a knowledge base, considerations, and recommendations addressing this issue.

## REFERENCES

1. Van der Werf C, van Langen IM, Wilde AA. Sudden death in the young: what do we know about it and how to prevent? Circ Arrhythm Electrophysiol 2010; 3:96–104.
2. Schwartz PJ, Stramba-Badiale M, Crotti L, et al. Prevalence of the congenital long-QT syndrome. Circulation 2009;120:1761–7.
3. Postema PG. About Brugada syndrome and its prevalence. Europace 2012;14:925–8.
4. Cerrone M, Cummings S, Alansari T, et al. A clinical approach to inherited arrhythmias. Circ Cardiovasc Genet 2012;5:581–90.
5. Crotti L, Marcou CA, Tester DJ, et al. Spectrum and prevalence of mutations involving BrS1- through

BrS12-susceptibility genes in a cohort of unrelated patients referred for Brugada syndrome genetic testing: implications for genetic testing. J Am Coll Cardiol 2012;60:1410–8.

6. Tan HL, Bink-Boelkens MT, Bezzina CR, et al. A sodium-channel mutation causes isolated cardiac conduction disease. Nature 2001;409:1043–7.
7. Postema PG, van den Berg MP, van Tintelen JP, et al. Founder mutations in the Netherlands. SCN5a 1795insD, the first described arrhythmia overlap syndrome and one of the largest and best described characterised families worldwide. Neth Heart J 2009;17:422–8.
8. Postema PG, Wolpert C, Amin AS, et al. Drugs and Brugada syndrome patients: review of the literature, recommendations, and an up-to-date website (www.brugadadrugs.org). Heart Rhythm 2009;6:1335–41.
9. Woosley RL, Romero K. Assessing cardiovascular drug safety for clinical decision-making. Nature reviews. Cardiology 2013;10:330–7.
10. Postema PG, Neville J, de Jong JS, et al. Safe drug use in long QT syndrome and Brugada syndrome: comparison of website statistics. Europace 2013;15:1042–9.
11. Sauer AJ, Moss AJ, McNitt S, et al. Long QT syndrome in adults. J Am Coll Cardiol 2007;49:329–37.
12. Splawski I, Shen J, Timothy KW, et al. Spectrum of mutations in long-QT syndrome genes. KVLQT1, HERG, SCN5A, KCNE1, and KCNE2. Circulation 2000;102:1178–85.
13. Hofman N, Tan HL, Alders M, et al. Yield of molecular and clinical testing for arrhythmia syndromes: report of 15 years' experience. Circulation 2013;128:1513–21.
14. Spazzolini C, Mullally J, Moss AJ, et al. Clinical implications for patients with long QT syndrome who experience a cardiac event during infancy. J Am Coll Cardiol 2009;54:832–7.
15. Zhang L, Benson DW, Tristani-Firouzi M, et al. Electrocardiographic features in Andersen-Tawil syndrome patients with KCNJ2 mutations: characteristic T-U-wave patterns predict the KCNJ2 genotype. Circulation 2005;111:2720–6.
16. Postema PG, Ritsema van Eck HJ, Opthof T, et al. IK1 modulates the U-wave: insights in a 100 year old enigma. Heart Rhythm 2009;6:393–400.
17. Viskin S, Rosovski U, Sands AJ, et al. Inaccurate electrocardiographic interpretation of long QT: the majority of physicians cannot recognize a long QT when they see one. Heart Rhythm 2005;2:569–74.
18. Postema PG, de Jong JS, van der Bilt IA, et al. Accurate electrocardiographic assessment of the QT-interval: teach the tangent. Heart Rhythm 2008;5:1015–8.
19. Postema PG, Wilde AA. The measurement of the QT interval. Curr Cardiol Rev 2014;10(3):287–94.
20. Priori SG, Napolitano C, Gasparini M, et al. Clinical and genetic heterogeneity of right bundle branch block and ST-segment elevation syndrome: a prospective evaluation of 52 families. Circulation 2000;102:2509–15.
21. Priori SG, Napolitano C, Schwartz PJ. Low penetrance in the long-QT syndrome: clinical impact. Circulation 1999;99:529–33.
22. Viskin S, Postema PG, Bhuiyan ZA, et al. The response of the QT-interval to the brief tachycardia provoked by standing. A bedside test for diagnosing Long-QT syndrome. J Am Coll Cardiol 2010;55:1955–61.
23. Sy RW, van der Werf C, Chattha IS, et al. Derivation and validation of a simple exercise-based algorithm for prediction of genetic testing in relatives of LQTS probands. Circulation 2011;124:2187–94.
24. Adler A, van der Werf C, Postema PG, et al. The phenomenon of "QT stunning": the abnormal QT prolongation provoked by standing persists even as the heart rate returns to normal in patients with long QT syndrome. Heart Rhythm 2012;9:901–8.
25. Krahn AD, Healey JS, Chauhan V, et al. Systematic assessment of patients with unexplained cardiac arrest: Cardiac Arrest Survivors With Preserved Ejection Fraction Registry (CASPER). Circulation 2009;120:278–85.
26. Amin AS, Giudicessi JR, Tijsen AJ, et al. Variants in the 3' untranslated region of the KCNQ1-encoded Kv7.1 potassium channel modify disease severity in patients with type 1 long QT syndrome in an allele-specific manner. Eur Heart J 2012;33:714–23.
27. Bezzina CR, Barc J, Mizusawa Y, et al. Common variants at SCN5A-SCN10A and HEY2 are associated with Brugada syndrome, a rare disease with high risk of sudden cardiac death. Nat Genet 2013;45:1409.
28. Wilde AA, Ackerman MJ. Exercise extreme caution when calling rare genetic variants novel arrhythmia syndrome susceptibility mutations. Heart Rhythm 2010;7:1883–5.
29. Wilde AA, Postema PG, Di Diego JM, et al. The pathophysiological mechanism underlying Brugada syndrome. Depolarization versus repolarization. J Mol Cell Cardiol 2010;49:543–53.
30. Mizumaki K, Fujiki A, Tsuneda T, et al. Vagal activity modulates spontaneous augmentation of ST elevation in the daily life of patients with Brugada syndrome. J Cardiovasc Electrophysiol 2004;15:667–73.
31. Veltmann C, Schimpf R, Echternach C, et al. A prospective study on spontaneous fluctuations between diagnostic and non-diagnostic ECGs in Brugada syndrome: implications for correct phenotyping and risk stratification. Eur Heart J 2006;27:2544–54.
32. Probst V, Wilde AA, Barc J, et al. SCN5A mutations and the role of genetic background in the

pathophysiology of Brugada syndrome. Circ Cardiovasc Genet 2009;2:552–7.
33. Rossenbacker T, Carroll SJ, Liu H, et al. Novel pore mutation in SCN5A manifests as a spectrum of phenotypes ranging from atrial flutter, conduction disease, and Brugada syndrome to sudden cardiac death. Heart Rhythm 2004;1:610–5.
34. Chockalingam P, Rammeloo LA, Postema PG, et al. Fever-induced life-threatening arrhythmias in children harboring an SCN5A mutation. Pediatrics 2011;127:e239–44.
35. Watanabe H, Koopmann TT, Le Scouarnec S, et al. Sodium channel beta1 subunit mutations associated with Brugada syndrome and cardiac conduction disease in humans. J Clin Invest 2008;118:2260–8.
36. Bezzina C, Veldkamp MW, van den Berg MP, et al. A single Na(+) channel mutation causing both long-QT and Brugada syndromes. Circ Res 1999;85:1206–13.
37. Veldkamp MW, Viswanathan PC, Bezzina C, et al. Two distinct congenital arrhythmias evoked by a multidysfunctional Na(+) channel. Circ Res 2000;86:E91–7.
38. Makita N, Behr E, Shimizu W, et al. The E1784K mutation in SCN5A is associated with mixed clinical phenotype of type 3 long QT syndrome. J Clin Invest 2008;118:2219–29.
39. Roden DM. Drug-induced prolongation of the QT interval. N Engl J Med 2004;350:1013–22.
40. Brugada R, Brugada J, Antzelevitch C, et al. Sodium channel blockers identify risk for sudden death in patients with ST-segment elevation and right bundle branch block but structurally normal hearts. Circulation 2000;101:510–5.
41. Groome J, Lehmann-Horn F, Holzherr B. Open- and closed-state fast inactivation in sodium channels: differential effects of a site-3 anemone toxin. Channels (Austin) 2011;5:65–78.
42. Veerman CC, Verkerk AO, Blom MT, et al. Slow delayed rectifier potassium current blockade contributes importantly to drug-induced Long QT syndrome. Circ Arrhythm Electrophysiol 2013;6:1002–9.
43. Chockalingam P, Crotti L, Girardengo G, et al. Not all beta-blockers are equal in the management of long QT syndrome types 1 and 2: higher recurrence of events under metoprolol. J Am Coll Cardiol 2012;60:2092–9.
44. Zeltser D, Justo D, Halkin A, et al. Torsade de pointes due to noncardiac drugs: most patients have easily identifiable risk factors. Medicine (Baltimore) 2003;82:282–90.
45. Postema PG, Tan HL, Wilde AA. Ageing and Brugada syndrome: considerations and recommendations. J Geriatr Cardiol 2013;10:75–81.
46. Priori SG, Wilde AA, Horie M, et al. HRS/EHRA/APHRS expert consensus statement on the diagnosis and management of patients with inherited primary arrhythmia syndromes expert consensus statement on inherited primary arrhythmia syndromes. Heart Rhythm 2013;10:1932–63.
47. Haugaa KH, Bos JM, Tarrell RF, et al. Institution-wide QT alert system identifies patients with a high risk of mortality. Mayo Clin Proc 2013;88:315–25.
48. Van Gorp V, Danschutter D, Huyghens L, et al. Monitoring the safety of antiepileptic medication in a child with Brugada syndrome. Int J Cardiol 2010;145:e64–7.
49. Goldenberg I, Moss AJ, Peterson DR, et al. Risk factors for aborted cardiac arrest and sudden cardiac death in children with the congenital long-QT syndrome. Circulation 2008;117:2184–91.
50. Goldenberg I, Moss AJ, Bradley J, et al. Long-QT syndrome after age 40. Circulation 2008;117:2192–201.
51. Wilde AA, Kaufman ES, Shimizu W, et al. Sodium channel mutations, risk of cardiac events, and efficacy of beta-blocker therapy in type 3 Long QT syndrome [abstract]. Heart Rhythm 2012;9:S321.
52. Van den Berg MP, Haaksma J, Veeger NJ, et al. Diurnal variation of ventricular repolarization in a large family with LQT3-Brugada syndrome characterized by nocturnal sudden death. Heart Rhythm 2006;3:290–5.
53. Van den Berg MP, Wilde AA, Viersma JW, et al. Possible bradycardic mode of death and successful pacemaker treatment in a large family with features of long QT syndrome type 3 and Brugada syndrome. J Cardiovasc Electrophysiol 2001;12:630–6.
54. Schwartz PJ, Priori SG, Locati EH, et al. Long QT syndrome patients with mutations of the SCN5A and HERG genes have differential responses to Na+ channel blockade and to increases in heart rate. Implications for gene-specific therapy. Circulation 1995;92:3381–6.
55. Marquez MF, Bonny A, Hernandez-Castillo E, et al. Long-term efficacy of low doses of quinidine on malignant arrhythmias in Brugada syndrome with an implantable cardioverter-defibrillator: a case series and literature review. Heart Rhythm 2012;9(12):1995–2000.
56. Viskin S, Wilde AA, Guevara-Valdivia ME, et al. Quinidine, a life-saving medication for Brugada syndrome, is inaccessible in many countries. J Am Coll Cardiol 2013;61(23):2383–7.
57. Viskin S, Wilde AA, Tan HL, et al. Empiric quinidine therapy for asymptomatic Brugada syndrome: time for a prospective registry. Heart Rhythm 2009;6:401–4.

# Sodium Current Disorders
## Clinician's View

Yuka Mizusawa, MD, Hanno L. Tan, MD, PhD*

**KEYWORDS**

- Sodium current disorder • Brugada syndrome • Long QT syndrome • Sick sinus syndrome
- Cardiac conduction disturbance • Atrial fibrillation • Dilated cardiomyopathy

**KEY POINTS**

- The mechanism of sodium current disorders remains largely unknown and carriership of a mutation in one of the sodium channel–related genes has as yet no relevance for clinical decision making except for long QT syndrome type 3 (LQT3).
- Research has shown the complexity of sodium current disorders but has also implicated the involvement of common/rare gene variants or newly found sodium channel interacting proteins.
- Research findings have given possibilities for untangling the intricate mechanism of sodium current disorders.
- Further genetic and functional research on sodium current disorders may provide clinically relevant insights into sodium current disorders in the future.

## INTRODUCTION

The complexity of sodium current disorders was presented in several reports in the late 1990s. One article published in 1999 reported on a large Dutch family carrying a single familial mutation, *SCN5A* 1795insD. This mutation shows gain- and loss-of-function of sodium channel and leads to overlap syndrome manifesting several different phenotypes, such as Brugada syndrome (BrS), long QT syndrome (LQTS) type 3 (LQT3), and cardiac conduction disease (CCD).[1] With regard to structural disease, an *SCN5A* mutation was reported in 1996 in a family with dilated cardiomyopathy (DCM) and bradyarrhythmias and/or tachyarrhythmias.[2]

Extensive research has been performed to date to unravel the complexity of sodium current disorders (including overlap syndrome), which resulted in elucidation of part of their mechanisms. Yet, this new knowledge has brought us to an even more intricate world. For example, clinicians have come to realize that the sodium channel forms a macro molecular complex including sodium channel α- and β-subunits and interacting proteins. This is an exciting discovery, considering that genetic analysis encoding such proteins and their functional tests may provide further insight into sodium current disorders and may eventually lead to better risk stratification or treatments. As another exciting aspect, the advance of genotyping technology brought the possibility of sequencing the whole genome to find variants associated with a disease. This will certainly bring more clues of primary electrical disease, such as sodium current disorders. However, it means that many more steps in research are required before clinicians fully understand the whole picture of sodium current disorders.

Currently, much remains unknown with respect to the (patho)physiology of sodium current disorders, and mutation carriership in the sodium channel–related genes and related proteins

Disclosures: The authors have nothing to disclose.
Department of Cardiology, Heart Center, Academic Medical Center, Meibergdreef 9, Amsterdam 1105 AZ, The Netherlands
* Corresponding author.
*E-mail address:* h.l.tan@amc.uva.nl

Card Electrophysiol Clin 6 (2014) 819–824
http://dx.doi.org/10.1016/j.ccep.2014.08.003

unfortunately does not help clinicians to sort out patients at risk of arrhythmia in most instances. This article provides the clinicians' view on sodium current disorders.

## SODIUM CURRENT DISORDERS: MISSING LINK FROM BENCH TO BEDSIDE

"Cardiac sodium current disorder" seems a simple nomenclature, but it includes diverse diseases, such as BrS, congenital LQTS, sick sinus syndrome (SSS), CCD, atrial fibrillation (AF), and DCM. Although these diseases commonly harbor a mutation in genes encoding an α- or β-subunit of the cardiac sodium channel, clinical manifestations vary among these diseases, and the mechanisms leading to different clinical phenotypes are poorly understood. The complexity of sodium current disorders is even evident within a single sodium current disease. For example, although BrS is considered to follow a mendelian autosomal-dominant inheritance pattern, studies in BrS families carrying a familial *SCN5A* mutation have repeatedly shown incomplete penetrance with variable expressivity. Thus, family members carrying the familial *SCN5A* mutation do not always manifest the same clinical features and may show different phenotypes, such as ventricular fibrillation (VF), cardiac conduction abnormality, or no symptom for life.[1,3] Such a phenomenon also has been reported in LQTS and DCM.[2,4] Another aspect of sodium current disorders is that, whereas conduction abnormality and the involvement of sodium channel–related genes are naturally expected to be involved in the pathogenesis of SSS, CCD, AF, or DCM, mutations in sodium channel–related genes are rarely found.[5–8] Because of an incomplete understanding of the mechanisms underlying sodium channel (dys) function, and of the ways in which it may be causal to the disease,[9,10] mutation carriership itself is currently of not much help in clinical practice, except for LQT3, in which genotype confirmation plays an important role in the choice of treatment.

Recent extensive clinical and experimental research has implicated that sodium current disorders may be not monogenic but may be more complex than previously expected.[10–14] For example, age and gender are well known modifiers of sodium current disorders,[9] but common gene variants have been additionally suggested to be involved in modifying the disease status.[11,13,15] Furthermore, the sodium channel has been revealed to be part of a macromolecular complex, and several interacting proteins are implicated in sodium channel function.[12,16] This suggests that genes encoding such proteins may be new candidates for mutation screening and subsequent functional testing.

At present, comprehension of the mechanisms underlying sodium current disorders is still largely dependent on bench work, and further research is mandatory before new diagnostic tools or therapy for patients with a sodium current disorder can be introduced.

## BRUGADA SYNDROME

From the clinicians' view, the most groundbreaking recent report on BrS is the successful elimination of recurrent VF episodes by epicardial ablation in the right ventricular outflow tract.[17] Abolishment of fragmented electrograms by ablation and the absence of VF recurrence during follow-up (except for one patient) strongly suggest the involvement of conduction abnormality in the pathogenesis of BrS. In that sense, it is natural to consider that genes encoding α- and β-subunits of the sodium channel or sodium channel interacting proteins (*SCN5A*, *SCN1B*, *SCN2B*, *SCN3B*, *GPD1L*, *RANGRF* [MOG1]) are involved in the pathogenesis of BrS. Carrying a mutation in one of such (putative) disease-causing genes is, however, not relevant for clinical decision making. As a matter of fact, mutations in SCN5A are found only in 20% of patients with BrS.[18] Mutations in *SCN5A* are most likely to be found in patients with BrS with long PR and QRS intervals on the electrocardiogram. Other genes have been found only in a few sporadic cases, except for *GPD1L*.[19] Clinical studies using a large cohort of patients with BrS have failed to show *SCN5A* mutation as a risk marker for future arrhythmic events.[20,21] Another point to keep in mind is that, in healthy subjects, a 2% to 5% background rate of rare variants was reported,[18] which implies that not all mutations found in BrS are causal for the disease. A recent clinical study by our group has raised additional doubts regarding the causality of *SCN5A* mutations in BrS.[10] In this study, we included 13 BrS families with more than five clinically affected individuals. In five families, one or two clinically affected individuals without the familial *SCN5A* mutation were observed,[10] suggesting that *SCN5A* mutations do not directly determine the BrS phenotype.[10] More recent genetic studies have implicated the involvement of common variants in the *SCN5A* promoter region or common variants in several genes (*SCN5A*, *SCN10A*, *HEY2*) in BrS.[11,15] At present, all patients with BrS, regardless of genotype or symptoms, are advised to avoid the use of sodium channel–inhibiting agents, as mentioned in the article by Postema and Woosley elsewhere in this issue. In addition, patients are to take measures (eg, antipyretics) to normalize body temperature in case of fever, factors that are known to decrease the conduction reserve and to cause arrhythmic events in BrS.[22]

## LONG QT SYNDROME

Congenital LQTS is a primary electrical disorder characterized by QT prolongation on the ECG and torsades de pointes type of ventricular tachycardia. There are four known LQTS subtypes that manifest QT prolongation through sodium channel dysfunction (gain-of-function) caused by a mutation in one of the sodium channel–controlling genes, namely *SCN5A*(LQT3), *CAV3*(LQT9), *SCN4B*(LQT10), and *SNTA1*(LQT12).[23–26] Patients with a *SCN5A* mutation are well characterized, whereas those with mutations in *CAV3*, *SCN4B*, and *SNTA1* less so, because they are very rare.[27]

Because LQT3 is known for its high risk of fatal consequences caused by VF, confirmation of *SCN5A* mutation carriership is important for the prevention of future fatal arrhythmic events. Treatment with β-blockers is essential for patients with recurrent arrhythmic events,[28] although β-blockers are less effective than in LQT1 or LQT2.[29] Patients who are not sufficiently protected and/or intolerant to β-blocker may benefit from mexiletine[30] or flecainide.[31] These drugs have been reported to be effective in treating patients with LQT3, but controversy exists because mexiletine has been reported to prolong QT interval in another study.[32] One of the most promising developments is the use of ranolazine, a late sodium current inhibitor.[33,34] Ranolazine has been reported to shorten QT interval[33] and alleviate symptoms[34] in a limited number of patients with LQT3. However, ranolazine also has a potential to prolong QT interval by blocking $I_{Kr}$ current. Although the recovery of $I_{Kr}$ channel block by ranolazine shows rapid kinetics,[35] careful observational studies in a larger number of patients are needed to establish the role of ranolazine for the treatment of LQT3. Currently, there are no large clinical studies showing the benefit of any of these drugs for the treatment of LQT3. Clearly, more evidence is needed before wide use in clinical practice may be considered.

## SICK SINUS SYNDROME/CARDIAC CONDUCTION DISEASE

Reports on SSS or CCD cases harboring an *SCN5A* mutation suggest the involvement of *SCN5A* in the development of the disease.[36–38] Of note, SSS and/or CCD in patients who carry an *SCN5A* mutation has been mostly reported as one of the clinical features in overlap syndrome,[39,40] and the role of *SCN5A* gene in the development of SSS/CCD is as yet unknown. Currently, there is no risk stratification for SSS or CCD according to the genotype.[22]

Clinically, both diseases develop at a later stage in life (around 70 years old),[41,42] and the consequences of developing SSS/CCD are not as devastating as the other sodium current disorders, such as BrS or LQT3. Pacemaker implantation is an established treatment in both diseases with a relatively low complication rate (excluding lead dislodgement), although patients are at risk of device infection or the development of heart failure.[41,43] Future direction may be to create biologic pacemakers using gene therapy.[44] However, significant challenges remain before such a therapy is introduced into clinical practice,[44] and a full mechanistic understanding of genes involved in the function of the conduction system is mandatory.

## ATRIAL FIBRILLATION

AF is the most common cardiac arrhythmia whose prevalence increases with advancing age. In most cases, such risk factors as hypertension, ischemic heart disease, valvular heart disease, and heart failure play a role in the development of AF. Yet, 10% to 20% of the patients harbor lone AF without apparent precipitating clinical factors.[45] Mendelian forms of lone AF have been described, and genes encoding cardiac ion channels or interacting proteins have been implicated as causal genes.[46] *SCN5A* is one such gene, but sequencing such candidate genes has found rare variants only in a minority of patients with lone AF (1.5%–3.8%)[8,47,48] or patients with AF and structural heart disease (<2.2%).[8] It should be kept in mind that the definition of minor allele frequency varied between the studies, which attempted to find relevant gene variants associated with AF. Furthermore, such variants cannot be called causal without a proof of cosegregation in a family.[47,48] Identifying rare or common variants associated with AF is an ongoing process, and causality of such variants remains largely unknown.[22] Thus, genetic testing in patients with AF is currently not recommended in clinical practice.[22]

## DILATED CARDIOMYOPATHY

DCM related to *SCN5A* mutations is characterized not only by the dilatation of left ventricle, but also by rhythm and conduction abnormalities.[2,49] In the report by McNair and colleagues,[6] which studied 338 patients with DCM, *SCN5A* mutation carriers were particularly characterized by a tendency for onset at younger age and the manifestation of arrhythmias including sinus node dysfunction, AF, ventricular tachycardia, and conduction disturbance. Clinical studies and experimental study suggest that *SCN5A* mutations are indeed involved in the disease development,[2,6,50,51] but much remains unknown with regards to the role of *SCN5A* mutations or the interaction of the genes implicated in the development of DCM. *SCN5A* is apparently not the major gene causing the disease considering that the number of *SCN5A* mutation carriers in DCM cohorts is low (1.7%–2.6%).[6,50] Because current knowledge on the genetic background of DCM and its causality is limited, the usefulness of genetic testing in clinical practice remains uncertain.[52,53] Genetic testing may be considered in familial DCM with rhythm disturbances and/or a family history of premature sudden cardiac death.[52]

## SUMMARY

The mechanism of sodium current disorders remains largely unknown and carriership of a mutation in one of the sodium channel–related genes has as yet no relevance for clinical decision making except for LQT3. Recent research results have shown the complexity of sodium current disorders but at the same time implicated the involvement of common/rare gene variants or newly found sodium channel interacting proteins. Such findings give possibilities to untangle the intricate mechanism of sodium current disorders. Further genetic and functional research on sodium current disorders may provide clinically relevant insights into sodium current disorders in the future.

## REFERENCES

1. Bezzina C, Veldkamp MW, van den Berg MP, et al. A single Na(+) channel mutation causing both long-QT and Brugada syndromes. Circ Res 1999;85:1206–13.
2. Olson TM, Keating MT. Mapping a cardiomyopathy locus to chromosome 3p22-p25. J Clin Invest 1996;97:528–32.
3. Giudicessi JR, Ackerman MJ. Determinants of incomplete penetrance and variable expressivity in heritable cardiac arrhythmia syndromes. Transl Res 2013;161:1–14.
4. Priori SG, Napolitano C, Schwartz PJ. Low penetrance in the long-QT syndrome: clinical impact. Circulation 1999;99:529–33.
5. Watanabe H, Darbar D, Kaiser DW, et al. Mutations in sodium channel beta1- and beta2-subunits associated with atrial fibrillation. Circ Arrhythm Electrophysiol 2009;2:268–75.
6. McNair WP, Sinagra G, Taylor MR, et al. SCN5A mutations associate with arrhythmic dilated cardiomyopathy and commonly localize to the voltage-sensing mechanism. J Am Coll Cardiol 2011;57:2160–8.
7. Ellinor PT, Nam EG, Shea MA, et al. Cardiac sodium channel mutation in atrial fibrillation. Heart Rhythm 2008;5:99–105.
8. Darbar D, Kannankeril PJ, Donahue BS, et al. Cardiac sodium channel (SCN5A) variants associated with atrial fibrillation. Circulation 2008;117:1927–35.
9. Remme CA. Cardiac sodium channelopathy associated with SCN5A mutations: electrophysiological, molecular and genetic aspects. J Physiol 2013;591(Pt 17):4099–116.
10. Probst V, Wilde AA, Barc J, et al. SCN5A mutations and the role of genetic background in the pathophysiology of Brugada syndrome. Circ Cardiovasc Genet 2009;2:552–7.
11. Bezzina CR, Barc J, Mizusawa Y, et al. Common variants at SCN5A-SCN10A and HEY2 are associated with Brugada syndrome, a rare disease with high risk of sudden cardiac death. Nat Genet 2013;45:1044–9.
12. Adsit GS, Vaidyanathan R, Galler CM, et al. Channelopathies from mutations in the cardiac sodium channel protein complex. J Mol Cell Cardiol 2013;61:34–43.
13. Crotti L, Monti MC, Insolia R, et al. NOS1AP is a genetic modifier of the long-QT syndrome. Circulation 2009;120:1657–63.
14. Chen LY, Ballew JD, Herron KJ, et al. A common polymorphism in SCN5A is associated with lone atrial fibrillation. Clin Pharmacol Ther 2007;81:35–41.
15. Bezzina CR, Shimizu W, Yang P, et al. Common sodium channel promoter haplotype in Asian subjects underlies variability in cardiac conduction. Circulation 2006;113:338–44.
16. Abriel H. Cardiac sodium channel Na(v)1.5 and interacting proteins: physiology and pathophysiology. J Mol Cell Cardiol 2010;48:2–11.
17. Nademanee K, Veerakul G, Chandanamattha P, et al. Prevention of ventricular fibrillation episodes in Brugada syndrome by catheter ablation over the anterior right ventricular outflow tract epicardium. Circulation 2011;123:1270–9.
18. Kapplinger JD, Tester DJ, Alders M, et al. An international compendium of mutations in the SCN5A-encoded cardiac sodium channel in patients referred for Brugada syndrome genetic testing. Heart Rhythm 2010;7:33–46.
19. Nielsen MW, Holst AG, Olesen SP, et al. The genetic component of Brugada syndrome. Front Physiol 2013;4:179.
20. Gehi AK, Duong TD, Metz LD, et al. Risk stratification of individuals with the Brugada electrocardiogram: a meta-analysis. J Cardiovasc Electrophysiol 2006;17:577–83.

21. Probst V, Veltmann C, Eckardt L, et al. Long-term prognosis of patients diagnosed with Brugada syndrome: results from the FINGER Brugada Syndrome Registry. Circulation 2010;121:635–43.
22. Ackerman MJ, Priori SG, Willems S, et al. HRS/EHRA expert consensus statement on the state of genetic testing for the channelopathies and cardiomyopathies this document was developed as a partnership between the Heart Rhythm Society (HRS) and the European Heart Rhythm Association (EHRA). Heart Rhythm 2011;8:1308–39.
23. Wang Q, Shen J, Li Z, et al. Cardiac sodium channel mutations in patients with long QT syndrome, an inherited cardiac arrhythmia. Hum Mol Genet 1995;4:1603–7.
24. Vatta M, Ackerman MJ, Ye B, et al. Mutant caveolin-3 induces persistent late sodium current and is associated with long-QT syndrome. Circulation 2006; 114:2104–12.
25. Medeiros-Domingo A, Kaku T, Tester DJ, et al. SCN4B-encoded sodium channel beta4 subunit in congenital long-QT syndrome. Circulation 2007; 116:134–42.
26. Ueda K, Valdivia C, Medeiros-Domingo A, et al. Syntrophin mutation associated with long QT syndrome through activation of the nNOS-SCN5A macromolecular complex. Proc Natl Acad Sci U S A 2008;105:9355–60.
27. Giudicessi JR, Ackerman MJ. Genotype- and phenotype-guided management of congenital long QT syndrome. Curr Probl Cardiol 2013;38:417–55.
28. Wilde A, Kaufman E, Shimizu W, et al. Sodium channel mutations, risk of cardiac events, and efficacy of beta-blocker therapy in type 3 long QT syndrome. Heart Rhythm 2012;9:S321.
29. Schwartz PJ, Priori SG, Spazzolini C, et al. Genotype-phenotype correlation in the long-QT syndrome: gene-specific triggers for life-threatening arrhythmias. Circulation 2001;103:89–95.
30. Schwartz PJ, Priori SG, Locati EH, et al. Long QT syndrome patients with mutations of the SCN5A and HERG genes have differential responses to Na+ channel blockade and to increases in heart rate. Implications for gene-specific therapy. Circulation 1995;92:3381–6.
31. Windle JR, Geletka RC, Moss AJ, et al. Normalization of ventricular repolarization with flecainide in long QT syndrome patients with SCN5A: deltakpq mutation. Ann Noninvasive Electrocardiol 2001;6: 153–8.
32. Ruan Y, Denegri M, Liu N, et al. Trafficking defects and gating abnormalities of a novel SCN5A mutation question gene-specific therapy in long QT syndrome type 3. Circ Res 2010;106:1374–83.
33. Moss AJ, Zareba W, Schwarz KQ, et al. Ranolazine shortens repolarization in patients with sustained inward sodium current due to type-3 long-QT syndrome. J Cardiovasc Electrophysiol 2008;19: 1289–93.
34. van den Berg MP, Van den Heuvel F, Van Tintelen JP, et al. Successful treatment of a patient with symptomatic long QT syndrome type 3 using ranolazine combined with a beta-blocker. Int J Cardiol 2014;171:90–2.
35. Antzelevitch C, Burashnikov A, Sicouri S, et al. Electrophysiologic basis for the antiarrhythmic actions of ranolazine. Heart Rhythm 2011;8:1281–90.
36. Benson DW, Wang DW, Dyment M, et al. Congenital sick sinus syndrome caused by recessive mutations in the cardiac sodium channel gene (SCN5A). J Clin Invest 2003;112:1019–28.
37. Schott JJ, Alshinawi C, Kyndt F, et al. Cardiac conduction defects associate with mutations in SCN5A. Nat Genet 1999;23:20–1.
38. Tan HL, Bink-Boelkens MT, Bezzina CR, et al. A sodium-channel mutation causes isolated cardiac conduction disease. Nature 2001;409: 1043–7.
39. Smits JP, Koopmann TT, Wilders R, et al. A mutation in the human cardiac sodium channel (E161K) contributes to sick sinus syndrome, conduction disease and Brugada syndrome in two families. J Mol Cell Cardiol 2005;38:969–81.
40. Makita N, Behr E, Shimizu W, et al. The E1784K mutation in SCN5A is associated with mixed clinical phenotype of type 3 long QT syndrome. J Clin Invest 2008;118:2219–29.
41. Riahi S, Nielsen JC, Hjortshoj S, et al. Heart failure in patients with sick sinus syndrome treated with single lead atrial or dual-chamber pacing: no association with pacing mode or right ventricular pacing site. Europace 2012;14:1475–82.
42. Lau CP, Tachapong N, Wang CC, et al. Prospective randomized study to assess the efficacy of site and rate of atrial pacing on long-term progression of atrial fibrillation in sick sinus syndrome: Septal Pacing for Atrial Fibrillation Suppression Evaluation (SAFE) Study. Circulation 2013;128:687–93.
43. Gillis AM, Russo AM, Ellenbogen KA, et al. HRS/ACCF expert consensus statement on pacemaker device and mode selection. Developed in partnership between the Heart Rhythm Society (HRS) and the American College of Cardiology Foundation (ACCF) and in collaboration with the Society of Thoracic Surgeons. Heart Rhythm 2012;9: 1344–65.
44. Morris GM, Boyett MR. Perspectives: biological pacing, a clinical reality? Ther Adv Cardiovasc Dis 2009;3:479–83.
45. Benjamin EJ, Wolf PA, D'Agostino RB, et al. Impact of atrial fibrillation on the risk of death: the Framingham Heart Study. Circulation 1998;98:946–52.
46. Parvez B, Darbar D. The "missing" link in atrial fibrillation heritability. J Electrocardiol 2011;44:641–4.

47. Weeke P, Parvez B, Blair M, et al. Candidate gene approach to identifying rare genetic variants associated with lone atrial fibrillation. Heart Rhythm 2014;11:46–52.
48. Olesen MS, Andreasen L, Jabbari J, et al. Very early onset lone atrial fibrillation patients have a high prevalence of rare variants in genes previously associated with atrial fibrillation. Heart Rhythm 2013; 11(2):246–51.
49. McNair WP, Ku L, Taylor MR, et al. SCN5A mutation associated with dilated cardiomyopathy, conduction disorder, and arrhythmia. Circulation 2004; 110:2163–7.
50. Olson TM, Michels VV, Ballew JD, et al. Sodium channel mutations and susceptibility to heart failure and atrial fibrillation. JAMA 2005;293:447–54.
51. Watanabe H, Yang T, Stroud DM, et al. Striking in vivo phenotype of a disease-associated human SCN5A mutation producing minimal changes in vitro. Circulation 2011;124:1001–11.
52. Yancy CW, Jessup M, Bozkurt B, et al. 2013 ACCF/AHA guideline for the management of heart failure: a report of the American College of Cardiology Foundation/American Heart Association Task Force on Practice Guidelines. J Am Coll Cardiol 2013;62: e147–239.
53. Gollob MH, Blier L, Brugada R, et al. Recommendations for the use of genetic testing in the clinical evaluation of inherited cardiac arrhythmias associated with sudden cardiac death: Canadian Cardiovascular Society/Canadian Heart Rhythm Society joint position paper. Can J Cardiol 2011;27:232–45.

# Sodium Current Disorders Geneticist's View

Silvia G. Priori, MD, PhD[a,b,*], Yanfei Ruan, MD[c], Sean O'Rourke, MD[d,†], Nian Liu, MD[c], Carlo Napolitano, MD, PhD[a,d]

**KEYWORDS**

• Genetics • Sodium • Ion channel

**KEY POINTS**

- Cardiac sodium channel function may be affected by mutations in several genes that cooperate to determine its function (multiple genes for the same phenotype).
- Cardiac sodium channel gene (*SCN5A*) is the most common cause of cardiac sodium channel dysfunction and is associated with multiple clinical phenotypes (multiple phenotypes for the same gene).
- Genetic testing for sodium channel–related disease has important diagnostic implications but, with the exception of long QT syndrome type 3 (LQT3), genotype-phenotype correlation and genotype-based clinical management are poorly defined.
- Distinguishing the true disease-causing mutations from rare variants is challenging and requires the use of multiple tools and specific training to maximize the interpretative skills and clinical applicability of the results of genetic testing.

## INTRODUCTION

In the past 20 years impressive advancements have occurred in the understanding of molecular genetics of cardiac rhythm disorders. With the discovery of the causative genes for major inherited diseases, diagnostic genotyping is introduced in the clinical practice. Genetic tests are performed not only for diagnostic purposes but also for risk stratification, assessment of drug treatment, and therapy strategy selection. In the field of inherited arrhythmogenic diseases, the identification of the genes responsible for cardiomyopathies and ion channel diseases has opened the molecular era in the understanding of the pathophysiology of inherited arrhythmogenic diseases and improved ability in prognosis and treatment. Although genetic tests are progressively entering the clinical practice, specific skills are needed to use the test results in a correct way to not lose potential benefits and to not stretch their indications. Performing genetic analyses without clear clinical indications and endpoints may bring about more problems than solutions.[1–3] This article summarizes the phenotypes associated with cardiac sodium channel mutations and related genes and outlines the possibilities and limitations of genetic testing.

## PHENOTYPES ASSOCIATED WITH SCN5A AND RELATED GENES

Since the first cardiac sodium channel mutation identified in long QT families, mutations of genes encoding alpha subunit of the human cardiac sodium channel $Na_v1.5$ have been associated with

Disclosures: None.

[a] Molecular Cardiology, IRCCS, Fondazione Salvatore Maugeri, Via Maugeri 10, Pavia 27100, Italy; [b] Department of Molecular Medicine, University of Pavia, Via Maugeri 10, Pavia 27100, Italy; [c] Department of Cardiology, Beijing An Zhen Hospital, Capital Medical University, 2 Anzhen Road, Beijing 100029, China; [d] Cardiovascular Genetics, Leon Charney Division of Cardiology, New York University, 522 First Avenue, New York, NY 10016, USA

[†] Deceased.

* Corresponding author. Molecular Cardiology, IRCCS Fondazione Salvatore Maugeri, Via Maugeri 10, Pavia 27100, Italy.
*E-mail address:* silvia.priori@fsm.it

Card Electrophysiol Clin 6 (2014) 825–833
http://dx.doi.org/10.1016/j.ccep.2014.08.002
1877-9182/14/$ – see front matter 

a spectrum of inherited arrhythmia syndromes, including LQT3, Brugada syndrome (BrS), cardiac conduction disease, dilated cardiomyopathy (DCM), sick sinus syndrome (SSS), and atrial fibrillation (AF).[4] From a genetic standpoint, several investigators have shown that cardiac sodium channel should be considered a macromolecular complex with several functionally related proteins that cooperate to control the opening and closing of the $Na^+$ conducting pore protein ($Na_v1.5$). This concept is well illustrated by the identification of $Na_v1.5$ regulatory gene mutations that affect cardiac sodium current in the absence of a mutation in the ion conducting channel ($Na_v1.5$) and cause clinical phenotypes almost undistinguishable from those described previously. The following paragraphs briefly summarize the phenotypes and their genetic determinants to highlight the genetic heterogeneity of sodium channel disorders. The second part of the article focuses on the clinical impact of such heterogeneity.

## *Long QT Syndrome Type 3*

LQT3 was the first phenotype associated with mutations in *SCN5A* encoding for $Na_v1.5$.[5] LQT3 accounts for 5% to 10% of long QT syndrome (LQTS) patients with identified mutations and its clinical presentation is described by Ruan and colleagues elsewhere in this issue.

The available data suggest high penetrance (80%) with heart rate corrected QT interval (QTc), often above 500 ms; a severe outcome; and reduced response to β-blockers.[6–8] It is important, however, to highlight that this typical LQT3 phenotype was outlined in cohorts with definite gain-of-function and pathogenetic mutations. The recent mounting drive to expanded indications for genetic testing toward subjects with borderline QT interval is having an impact on the average LQT3 patient profile. Subjects with borderline QTc and presumably low risk of events are being identified and current risk stratification schemes may not apply in these cases.

To generate an LQTS phenotype due to an abnormality of sodium current, a gain-of-function effect with a net increase of inward sodium current ($I_{Na}$) current has to be present. This can be obtained not only by genetic variants directly affecting the channel protein $Na_v1.5$, but also three other genes may cause LQTS through a gain-of-function effect on the cardiac sodium channel: LQTS type 9 (LQT9) caused by caveolin (*CAV3*) mutations, LQTS type 10 (LQT10) caused by sodium channel beta four subunit (*SCN4B*) mutations, and LQTS type 12 (LQT12) caused by syntrophin gene (*SNTA1*) mutations (**Table 1**). When mutated, these genes cause an increase in depolarizing $I_{Na}$ but this effect is reached through a variety of possible mechanisms. This evidence highlights the complexity of the pathophysiological mechanism that can lead to a genetic dysfunction of cardiac sodium current but it also has direct clinical implications. Cardiologists who want to approach genetic testing for suspected LQT3 (or related) patients need to have quantitative information on the sensitivity and clinical implications of the test.

The most relevant piece of information is the prevalence of these variants. An expert consensus document on genetic testing in inherited arrhythmogenic diseases[9] provided a systematic evaluation of the available evidence and produced lists of key genes, which are worth screening for clinical purposes. As for LQTS, the consensus is that the only relevant sodium-related gene is *SCN5A*, whereas all the others are considered too rare to justify systematic testing in the clinical setting.

## *Brugada Syndrome*

BrS is an arrhythmogenic disease characterized by ST segment elevation in right precordial leads and an increased risk of sudden cardiac death due to ventricular fibrillation. The clinical features are described by Ruan and colleagues elsewhere in this issue. As in the case of LQT3, BrS was initially linked to sodium channel mutations[10] but in this case the net functional consequence is that of a loss of function. Because $I_{Na}$ controls both action potential duration and conduction velocity, BrS patients show not only typical ST elevation but also conduction delay and a tendency to short action potential duration. This translates into a borderline short QT interval on the electrocardiogram. ST elevation seems due to a combination of delayed conduction in the right ventricular outflow tract and a transmural (epicardium vs endocardium) unbalance of inward and outward currents.[11]

With the progressive accumulation of knowledge, it has become clear that additional genes that alter the inward/outward current balance in the myocardium can cause BrS. The list of genes associated with BrS is continuously expanding. The cardiac sodium current remains, however, the most relevant culprit.[12] As in the case of LQT3, sodium current can be affected through a variety of mechanisms and genes involved in the sodium channel macromolecular complex (see **Table 1**). Reduced sodium current and a BrS phenotype can also be due to mutations in *SCN5A*-regulating genes: *GPD-1L*, *SCN1B*, *SCN2B*, *SCN3B*, and *MOG1*.

No study has systematically carried out parallel screening of all known BrS genes in a large cohort of clinically affected subjects, so precise estimate

**Table 1**
**Genes of the cardiac sodium channel macromolecular complex known to cause pathogenic alterations in $I_{Na}$**

| Gene | Protein | Effect of Mutation on $Na_v1.5$ | Clinical Phenotype(s) |
|---|---|---|---|
| Cardiac sodium channel subunits | | | |
| *SCN5A* | $Na_v1.5$, sodium channel alpha subunit | Gain of function<br>Loss of function | LQT3, DCM<br>BrS, PCCD, SSS, AF, DCM |
| *SCN1B* | Sodium channel $\beta_1$ subunit | Modulated $Na_v1.5$ expression and gating function | BrS, AFib |
| *SCN2B* | Sodium channel $\beta_2$ subunit | Reduced $Na_v1.5$ cell surface expression | BrS, AFib |
| *SCN3B* | Sodium channel $\beta_3$ subunit | Reduced $Na_v1.5$ cell surface expression | BrS |
| *SCN4B* | Sodium channel $\beta_4$ subunit | Reduced $\beta_4$ function as an open channel blocker enhances $Na_v1.5$ function | LQT10 |
| Other cardiac sodium channel macromolecular complex components | | | |
| *CAV3* | Cardiac caveolin gene | Altered gating kinetic of $Na_v1.5$ | LQT9 |
| *GDP-1L* | Glycerol-3-phosphate–like 1 | Reduced $Na_v1.5$ cell surface expression | BrS |
| *MOG-1* | Multicopy suppressor of GSP-1 | Reduced $Na_v1.5$ cell surface expression | BrS, AF |
| *SNTA1* | Syntrophin | Reduced $Na_v1.5$ nitrosylation | LQT12 |

of the yield of genetic testing is not available. It seems established that genetic screening of BrS has lower yield compared with other inherited arrhythmias. Current estimates suggest causative mutation can be identified in not more than 30% to 35% of patients. Moreover, besides *SCN5A*, none of the identified BrS genes reaches the 5% relative prevalence threshold considered sufficient to justify the screening.[9] The lower prevalence genes have been identified in only a few patients or in small families through candidate gene analysis.[13] Therefore, variants identified by next-generation sequencing technologies in these genes may be difficult to interpret and can be useless for clinical purposes, especially when associated with incomplete penetrance.[1] Thus, overall, genetic testing of BrS is indicated only for *SCN5A* (and possible calcium channel in the near future) in probands to confirm diagnosis but not exclude it. Once a mutation is identified, cascade familial screening is recommended.

The only consistent genotype-phenotype observation in BrS involved *SCN5A*. It has been suggested that the typical manifestation of BrS due to $I_{Na}$ impairment is that of conduction blocks, to a point that some investigators speculated that the most prominent phenotype associated with $I_{Na}$ mutations is progressive conduction defect and not BrS.[14] This finding has clinical implications because it may help indirect genetic testing and may support functional interpretation of mutants. For example, it is possible that a *SCN5A* mutation identified in an apparent BrS sporadic case does not cosegregate with ST elevation but it does with conduction defect(s) in relatives.

## *Progressive Cardiac Conduction Defect*

Progressive cardiac conduction defect (PCCD) is a serious disorder of the heart, which is characterized by prolonged impulse propagation, which progresses over time with an age-dependent penetrance. Patients may present various degrees of atrioventricular block, bundle branch block, tachyarrhythmia, and sudden death. The pathophysiological mechanisms underlying PCCD may be functional or structural, which cause PCCD without and with structural abnormalities. In recent 15 years, mutations of several genes have been associated with this disorder: *SCN5A*, *NKX2-5*, *PRKAG2*, *LMNA*, *TRPM4*, and *GJA5*.[15]

*SCN5A* is a major determinant of PCCD and the bench studies revealed that PCCD-associated *SCN5A* mutation causes loss-of-function in mutant channel, the same mechanism as the BrS-associated *SCN5A* mutations.[16] This finding explains the consistent overlap between BrS and PCCD.

*SCN5A* and *TRPM4* are the only common genes (defined as genes with causative mutation in >5% of affected individuals) for PCCD patients with a structurally intact heart.[17] According to a Heart Rhythm Society and European Heart Rhythm Association expert consensus statement on genetic testing, genetic testing may be considered as part of the diagnostic evaluation for patients with either isolated cardiac conduction defect (CCD) or CCD with concomitant congenital heart disease, especially when there is documentation of a positive family history of CCD.[9]

Because of the number of patients, currently there are no clear genotype-phenotype correlation and genotype-based risk stratifications for PCCD patients. There is a substantial incidence of sudden death in PCCD patients with first-degree AV block in association with bifascicular block and symptomatic, advanced AV block, so once cardiac involvement occurs, the clinician should maintain a low threshold to determine the need for pacemaker or implantable cardioverter-defibrillator implantation.[17] For these reasons, all family members and relatives should be tested for the same mutation once the mutation has been identified in the proband to recognize and follow-up those asymptomatic mutation carriers.

## Sick Sinus Syndrome

SSS is a group of abnormal heart rhythms caused by a malfunction of the sinus node. Manifestations include severe sinus bradycardia, sinus pauses or arrest, sinus node exit block, atrial tachyarrhythmia, alternating periods of atrial bradyarrhythmia, and tachyarrhythmia. The syndrome occurs in 1 of every 600 cardiac patients over the age of 65 years and accounts for approximately 50% of pacemaker implantations.[18]

Growing evidence has shown that genetic mutations in SCN5A channel may lead to familial SSS.[19,20] $Na_v1.5$ is present in the atrial muscle and the periphery of the node but absent from the center. In the center of the node, it is the L-type $Ca^{2+}$ current that is principally responsible for the action potential upstroke, which is slow compared with the upstroke elicited by $Na_v1.5$. $Na_v1.5$ is important, however, to provide sufficient depolarizing current to stimulate atrial myocytes, and this is the essential function of $Na_v1.5$ in the action potential conduction in the periphery of the sinoatrial node.[21] Electrophysiological studies demonstrated that SSS-associated *SCN5A* mutations cause loss of function in the mutant channel by altered channel kinetics properties or impaired cell surface localization, or both, the same mechanisms as BrS-associated mutation.[22] The initial evidence reported by Benson and colleagues,[19] however, showed that SSS-associated mutations seem to present a recessive pattern of inheritance. Whether this is a prerequisite for a loss-of-function mutation to cause a sinus node dysfunction and not BrS is currently unknown.

Due to the various causes of SSS and the limited *SCN5A*-associated SSS patients, currently genetic testing for SSS remains in the research field. The genotype-phenotype correlation, genotype-based prognosis, and management of SSS are issues await large cohort studies in the future.

## Dilated Cardiomyopathy

Currently 9 mutations in *SCN5A* gene have been associated with familial DCM. McNair and colleagues[23] reported that *SCN5A* mutations account for a modest proportion (1.7%) of familial DCM. Among these patients, 93% present arrhythmia phenotype, including sinus node dysfunction (33%), AF (60%), ventricular tachycardia (33%), and conduction defects (60%). The conduction disturbances seem unrelated to the degree of left ventricular dysfunction. The DCM phenotype presents age-related penetrance. Functional studies of these mutations demonstrated both gain of function and loss of function, which typically represent the mechanisms of LQT3 and BrS, respectively. Two-thirds of these mutations are located at the highly conserved homologous S3 and S4 transmembrane segments, suggesting a shared mechanism of disruption of the voltage-sensing mechanisms of cardiac sodium channel leading to DCM.

In an expert consensus statement on genetic testing,[9] *SCN5A* genetic testing is recommended for patients with DCM and significant cardiac conduction disease (first-, second-, or third-degree heart block) and/or family history of premature unexpected sudden death. Mutation-specific genetic testing should be performed in family members and relatives after the identification of the DCM-causing mutation in the index case. Given the limited number of identified mutations and reported patients, however, there is no clear genotype-based risk stratification of SCN5A-associated DCM.

## Atrial Fibrillation

AF is the most common sustained arrhythmia observed in clinical practice and it may be caused by genetic defects in a subset (10%–20%) of cases.[24] Multiple links between cardiac sodium channel and AF have been identified. LQT3 and BrS patients can present with AF,[25] and bench studies have showed increased atrial vulnerability associated with both gain- and loss-of-function mutations.[5,26] AF is a typical finding in BrS patients, with an incidence of approximately 20%.[27,28] On the other hand, screening of lone AF cohorts found a prevalence of *SCN5A* mutation of 4% to 8%.[25,29] Besides *SCN5A*, other sodium channel–related genes have been associated with AF: *SCN1B* and *SCN2B* encoding for beta-1 and beta-2 subunits of $Na_v1.5$[30] and MOG-1.[29] In all instances, functional characterization showed a reduction of the cardiac sodium current.

Overall, mechanisms of sodium-dependent AF seem complex because AF is found in conditions of both reduced and increased current; further studies are warranted. From a clinical standpoint, this observation has the consequence that possible onset of AF is to be carefully searched for in all patients presenting with cardiac sodium channel mutations, independently from the primary diagnosis.

The epidemiologic relevance of cardiac sodium channel defects (including all genes discussed previously), however, is currently considered too weak to justify systematic testing in patients presenting with lone AF.[9]

## THE COMPLEXITY OF SCN5A PHENOTYPES: IMPLICATIONS FOR GENETIC TESTING

### *Genetic Testing in Mendelian Traits Associated with Cardiac Sodium Channel*

Several clinical phenotypes have been associated with *SCN5A* (seen as a macromolecular complex) and specific indications for genetic testing have been outlined for each of them (**Box 1**). Even a perfect compliance with the current guidelines, however, written in the attempt to minimize the expected hurdles in interpretation of genetic testing, can result in interpretative uncertainties. This is true for all genetic testing but it is even more true in the case of cardiac sodium channel.

There are key issues that may imply interpretative problems: (1) the complexity of the biophysical consequences of *SCN5A* mutations, which determines the frequent appearance of overlap phenotypes; (2) incomplete penetrance that has an impact on risk stratification; (3) the lack of clear genotype-phenotype correlations, with the exception of few tens of well-characterized LQT3 mutations; (4) the role of common genetic variations (single nucleotide polymorphisms [SNPs]) and their modulatory role; (5) the consequences of genetic mutations in *SCN5A*-associated genes (beta subunits, Multicopy suppressor of GSP1 (MOG), caveolin-3 syntrophin, and so forth); and (6) the role of variants of unknown significance (VUS).

Among the most puzzling issues is how it is possible that a similar loss of function causes a spectrum of phenotypes. For example, it is not known whether the onset of a BrS versus DCM is dictated by the specific mutation (amino acid change) or by the coexistence of genetic modifiers or other unknown factors. Sorting out this aspect will be a major advancement of knowledge with profound clinical impact.

It follows that the interpretation and the predictive power of the reports issued by the genetic testing laboratories may be not straightforward. In general genetic testing of cardiac sodium channel, genetic defect is considered useful for diagnostic purposes. The implication in terms of risk stratification and therapeutic management, however, is more difficult to extrapolate.

When well-known and well-characterized mutations are identified, the clinical interpretation is usually nonproblematic. Novel or poorly characterized variants, however, are often found. In these cases, the DNA variant is defined as VUS. To distinguish between pathogenetic variants and nonsynonymous DNA variations without functional consequence is a primary endpoint. Publicly available databases (Exome Variant Server and 1000 Genomes) are routinely used to address whether the identified variant is also present in unselected genomes, which could suggest nonpathogenicity. These databases are often coupled with bioinformatic tools that attempt to predict the functional effect on the basis of amino acid change (SIFT, PolyPhen, and Provean). Finally, in vitro functional characterization may become required to place the result in a proper context, unless clear cosegregations are evident in a family under evaluation.

Even the most accurate assessment of a VUS, however, can be inconclusive. In silico algorithm may provide inconsistent results when testing the same variant. On the other hand, biophysics can provide broad information on whether a gain-of-function (long QT) or loss-of-function (BrS) type of clinical presentation can be expected or, in some cases, a combination of the two.[4] In other cases, in vitro expression can be used to predict response to therapy.[31,32] Nevertheless, when a reduction of $I_{Na}$ is identified in vitro, it is arduous to predict whether it will be associated with BrS, PCCD, or DCM or a combination of these. Therefore, in these cases, genetic testing should complement a thorough clinical evaluation and careful long-term clinical follow-up of the affected individuals. For example, a subject with a reduction of

**Box 1**
**Indications for genetic testing of inherited arrhythmias linked to sodium channel defects**

*Long QT syndrome*

Class I (is recommended)

- Comprehensive or LQT1-3 (KCNQ1, KCNH2, and SCN5A)–targeted LQTS genetic testing is recommended for any patient in whom a cardiologist has established a strong clinical index of suspicion for LQTS based on examination of a patient's clinical history, family history, and expressed electrocardiographic (resting 12-lead ECGs and/or provocative stress testing with exercise or catecholamine infusion) phenotype.
- Comprehensive or LQT1-3 (KCNQ1, KCNH2, and SCN5A)–targeted LQTS genetic testing is recommended for any asymptomatic patient with QT prolongation in the absence of other clinical conditions that might prolong the QT interval, such as electrolyte abnormalities, hypertrophy, bundle branch block, etc. (ie, otherwise idiopathic) on serial 12-lead ECGs defined as QTc 0.480 ms (prepuberty) or 0.500 ms (adults).
- Mutation-specific genetic testing is recommended for family members and other appropriate relatives subsequently after the identification of the LQTS-causative mutation in an index case.

Class IIb (may be considered)

- Comprehensive or LQT1-3 (KCNQ1, KCNH2, and SCN5A)–targeted LQTS genetic testing may be considered for any asymptomatic patient with otherwise idiopathic QTc values 0.460 ms (prepuberty) or 0.480 ms (adults) on serial 12-lead ECGs.

*Brugada syndrome*

Class I (is recommended)

- Mutation-specific genetic testing is recommended for family members and appropriate relatives after the identification of the BrS-causative mutation in an index case.

Class IIa (can be useful)

- Comprehensive or BrS1 (SCN5A)–targeted BrS genetic testing can be useful for any patient in whom a cardiologist has established a clinical index of suspicion for BrS based on examination of the patient's clinical history, family history, and expressed electrocardiographic (resting 12-lead ECGs and/or provocative drug challenge testing) phenotype.

Class III (is not indicated/recommended)

- Genetic testing is not indicated in the setting of an isolated type 2 or type 3 Brugada ECG pattern.

*Progressive cardiac conduction disease*

Class I (is recommended)

- Mutation-specific genetic testing is recommended for family members and appropriate relatives after the identification of the PCCD-causative mutation in an index case.

Class IIb (may be considered)

- Genetic testing may be considered as part of the diagnostic evaluation for patients with either isolated PCCD or CCD PCCD concomitant congenital heart disease, especially when there is documentation of a positive family history of PCCD.

*Atrial fibrillation*

Class III (is not indicated/recommended)

- Genetic testing is not indicated for AF at this time. SNP genotyping in general and SNP rs2200733 genotyping at the 4q25 locus in particular for AF is not indicated at this time based on the limited outcome data currently available.

*Dilated cardiomyopathy*

Class I (is recommended)

- Comprehensive or targeted (LMNA and SCN5A) DCM genetic testing is recommended for patients with DCM and significant cardiac conduction disease (ie, first-, second-, or third-degree heart block) and/or a family history of premature unexpected sudden death.
- Mutation-specific genetic testing is recommended for family members and appropriate relatives after the identification of a DCM-causative mutation in the index case.

Class IIa (can be useful)

- Genetic testing can be useful for patients with familial DCM to confirm the diagnosis, to recognize those who are at highest risk of arrhythmia and syndromic features, to facilitate cascade screening within the family, and to help with family planning.

*Adapted from* Ackerman MJ, Priori SG, Willems S, et al. HRS/EHRA expert consensus statement on the state of genetic testing for the channelopathies and cardiomyopathies: this document was developed as a partnership between the Heart Rhythm Society (HRS) and the European Heart Rhythm Association (EHRA). Heart Rhythm 2011;8:1308–39.

$Na_V1.5$ function and a BrS phenotype should be followed-up for possible development of atrioventricular blocks and should also regularly undergo cardiac imaging (echo or MRI) to exclude the presence of structural abnormalities[33] and their potential progressive worsening.

Overall, although in a majority of instances thorough assessment is able to establish/rule out the causative role of a putative mutation, in other cases, this objective cannot be reached. In this context, it is important to treat genetic testing as a probabilistic that requires additional information and specific expertise to be correctly interpreted.

### *The Role of Common Genetic Variations and Their Modulatory Role*

Dissecting the heritable nature of the electrocardiogram and the common genetic factors that may predispose to cardiac arrhythmias in the population has become a primary goal of genetic research in cardiology. Several candidate-gene or genome-wide association studies have identified several SNPs that modify QT interval[34–38] in the healthy population. The use of this information to detect genetic modifiers in inherited arrhythmia syndromes directly follows this line of research. Several SCN5A variants have been shown to act as modifiers.

The SCN5A-H558R was first identified as a modulator of the clinical expression of primary mutations.[22] Some investigators have reported that the effect of such common SNPs may be mutation specific. For example, the loss-of-function (Brugada-like) defect D1275N in SCN5A was rescued by R558 through enhancing cell surface targeting. In contrast, the defects of mutants E161K, P1298L, and R1632H were aggravated in the R558 background.[22] Additionally, H558R was shown to have different effects when present in cis (same allele) or in trans (different allele) of a primary mutation.[39] Another possible way to modulate cardiac sodium channel expression level is through the presence a set of SNPs (a haplotype) in the promoter region that reduces the amount of protein.[40]

Overall, these data suggest a role of SNP as modifiers in anecdotal cases but are far from bringing about implications for population-wide risk stratification. The effect of SNPs can be clinically evident, however, when multiple SNPs with an additive effect coexist to a point that multiple additive SNPs can cause a typical BrS phenotype.[41] Therefore, once the role of SNPs is clearly quantified, routine genotyping of SNPs (besides the standard genetic screening to identify the primary mutation) may become an important tool for diagnostic and prognostic purposes.

## SUMMARY

Cardiac sodium channel genetics is complex. Although pathophysiological knowledge has proceeded rapidly, the clinical implications of genetic testing are somewhat lagging behind. This is because the prevalence of mutations in each clinical phenotype associated with a sodium channel dysfunction is generally low. This limits the possibilities of genotype-based risk stratification. Once a mutation is found, specific expertise and trained personnel are required to provide correct interpretation of the finding. In the future, this complexity and interpretative difficulties are likely to become even more serious due to the progressive use of next-generation sequencing that allows low-cost genotyping and brings about a tendency of an incorrect use of genetic testing outside reasonable clinical indications. Nevertheless, an educated use of genetic testing of SCN5A coupled with high-level interpretative skill may support diagnosis and clinical management (including therapy selection) in several cases and allow reducing the number of DNA variations eventually labeled as VUS (ie, inconclusive results).

## REFERENCES


1. Napolitano C, Bloise R, Monteforte N, et al. Sudden cardiac death and genetic ion channelopathies: long QT, Brugada, short QT, catecholaminergic polymorphic ventricular tachycardia, and idiopathic ventricular fibrillation. Circulation 2012;125: 2027–34.
2. Priori SG. The fifteen years of discoveries that shaped molecular electrophysiology: time for appraisal. Circ Res 2010;107:451–6.
3. Priori SG, Napolitano C. Role of genetic analyses in cardiology: part I: mendelian diseases: cardiac channelopathies. Circulation 2006;113:1130–5.
4. Ruan Y, Liu N, Priori SG. Sodium channel mutations and arrhythmias. Nature reviews. Cardiology 2009; 6:337–48.
5. Wang Q, Shen J, Splawski I, et al. SCN5A mutations associated with an inherited cardiac arrhythmia, long QT syndrome. Cell 1995;80:805–11.
6. Napolitano C, Priori SG, Schwartz PJ, et al. Genetic testing in the long QT syndrome: development and validation of an efficient approach to genotyping in clinical practice. JAMA 2005;294:2975–80.
7. Priori SG, Napolitano C, Schwartz PJ, et al. Association of long QT syndrome loci and cardiac events among patients treated with beta-blockers. JAMA 2004;292:1341–4.
8. Priori SG, Schwartz PJ, Napolitano C, et al. Risk stratification in the long-QT syndrome. N Engl J Med 2003;348:1866–74.

9. Ackerman MJ, Priori SG, Willems S, et al. HRS/EHRA expert consensus statement on the state of genetic testing for the channelopathies and cardiomyopathies this document was developed as a partnership between the Heart Rhythm Society (HRS) and the European Heart Rhythm Association (EHRA). Heart Rhythm 2011;8:1308–39.
10. Chen Q, Kirsch GE, Zhang D, et al. Genetic basis and molecular mechanism for idiopathic ventricular fibrillation. Nature 1998;392:293–6.
11. Napolitano C, Antzelevitch C. Phenotypical manifestations of mutations in the genes encoding subunits of the cardiac voltage-dependent L-type calcium channel. Circ Res 2011;108:607–18.
12. Monteforte N, Napolitano C, Priori SG. Genetics and arrhythmias: diagnostic and prognostic applications. Rev Esp Cardiol (Engl Ed) 2012;65:278–86.
13. Nielsen MW, Holst AG, Olesen SP, et al. The genetic component of Brugada syndrome. Front Physiol 2013;4:179.
14. Probst V, Allouis M, Sacher F, et al. Progressive cardiac conduction defect is the prevailing phenotype in carriers of a Brugada syndrome SCN5A mutation. J Cardiovasc Electrophysiol 2006;17:270–5.
15. Smits JP, Veldkamp MW, Wilde AA. Mechanisms of inherited cardiac conduction disease. Europace 2005;7:122–37.
16. Bezzina CR, Rook MB, Groenewegen WA, et al. Compound heterozygosity for mutations (W156X and R225W) in SCN5A associated with severe cardiac conduction disturbances and degenerative changes in the conduction system. Circ Res 2003; 92:159–68.
17. Priori SG, Wilde AA, Horie M, et al. HRS/EHRA/APHRS expert consensus statement on the diagnosis and management of patients with inherited primary arrhythmia syndromes: document endorsed by HRS, EHRA, and APHRS in May 2013 and by ACCF, AHA, PACES, and AEPC in June 2013. Heart Rhythm 2013; 10:1932–63.
18. Adan V, Crown LA. Diagnosis and treatment of sick sinus syndrome. Am Fam Physician 2003;67: 1725–32.
19. Benson DW, Wang DW, Dyment M, et al. Congenital sick sinus syndrome caused by recessive mutations in the cardiac sodium channel gene (SCN5A). J Clin Invest 2003;112:1019–28.
20. Makita N, Sasaki K, Groenewegen WA, et al. Congenital atrial standstill associated with coinheritance of a novel SCN5A mutation and connexin 40 polymorphisms. Heart Rhythm 2005;2:1128–34.
21. Dobrzynski H, Boyett MR, Anderson RH. New insights into pacemaker activity: promoting understanding of sick sinus syndrome. Circulation 2007; 115:1921–32.
22. Gui J, Wang T, Jones RP, et al. Multiple loss-of-function mechanisms contribute to SCN5A-related familial sick sinus syndrome. PLoS One 2010;5: e10985.
23. McNair WP, Sinagra G, Taylor MR, et al. SCN5A mutations associate with arrhythmic dilated cardiomyopathy and commonly localize to the voltage-sensing mechanism. J Am Coll Cardiol 2011;57: 2160–8.
24. Darbar D, Roden DM. Genetic mechanisms of atrial fibrillation: impact on response to treatment. Nature reviews. Cardiology 2013;10:317–29.
25. Darbar D, Kannankeril PJ, Donahue BS, et al. Cardiac sodium channel (SCN5A) variants associated with atrial fibrillation. Circulation 2008;117:1927–35.
26. Blana A, Kaese S, Fortmuller L, et al. Knock-in gain-of-function sodium channel mutation prolongs atrial action potentials and alters atrial vulnerability. Heart Rhythm 2010;7:1862–9.
27. Natale A, Raviele A, Arentz T, et al. Venice Chart international consensus document on atrial fibrillation ablation. J Cardiovasc Electrophysiol 2007;18: 560–80.
28. Napolitano C. The contradictory genetics of atrial fibrillation: the growing gap between knowledge and clinical implications. J Cardiovasc Electrophysiol 2013;24:570–2.
29. Olesen MS, Yuan L, Liang B, et al. High prevalence of long QT syndrome-associated SCN5A variants in patients with early-onset lone atrial fibrillation. Circ Cardiovasc Genet 2012;5:450–9.
30. Watanabe H, Darbar D, Kaiser DW, et al. Mutations in sodium channel beta1- and beta2-subunits associated with atrial fibrillation. Circ Arrhythm Electrophysiol 2009;2:268–75.
31. Ruan Y, Denegri M, Liu N, et al. Trafficking defects and gating abnormalities of a novel SCN5A mutation question gene-specific therapy in long QT syndrome type 3. Circ Res 2010;106:1374–83.
32. Ruan Y, Liu N, Bloise R, et al. Gating properties of SCN5A mutations and the response to mexiletine in long-QT syndrome type 3 patients. Circulation 2007;116:1137–44.
33. Catalano O, Antonaci S, Moro G, et al. Magnetic resonance investigations in Brugada syndrome reveal unexpectedly high rate of structural abnormalities. Eur Heart J 2009;30:2241–8.
34. Arking DE, Pfeufer A, Post W, et al. A common genetic variant in the NOS1 regulator NOS1AP modulates cardiac repolarization. Nat Genet 2006; 38:644–51.
35. Marroni F, Pfeufer A, Aulchenko YS, et al. A genome-wide association scan of RR and QT interval duration in 3 European genetically isolated populations: the EUROSPAN project. Circ Cardiovasc Genet 2009;2:322–8.
36. Pfeufer A, Sanna S, Arking DE, et al. Common variants at ten loci modulate the QT interval duration in the QTSCD Study. Nat Genet 2009;41:407–14.

37. Smith JG, Lowe JK, Kovvali S, et al. Genome-wide association study of electrocardiographic conduction measures in an isolated founder population: Kosrae. Heart Rhythm 2009;6:634–41.
38. Wilton SB, Anderson TJ, Parboosingh J, et al. Polymorphisms in multiple genes are associated with resting heart rate in a stepwise allele-dependent manner. Heart Rhythm 2008;5:694–700.
39. Poelzing S, Forleo C, Samodell M, et al. SCN5A polymorphism restores trafficking of a Brugada syndrome mutation on a separate gene. Circulation 2006;114:368–76.
40. Bezzina CR, Shimizu W, Yang P, et al. Common sodium channel promoter haplotype in asian subjects underlies variability in cardiac conduction. Circulation 2006;113:338–44.
41. Bezzina CR, Barc J, Mizusawa Y, et al. Common variants at SCN5A-SCN10A and HEY2 are associated with Brugada syndrome, a rare disease with high risk of sudden cardiac death. Nat Genet 2013;45:1044–9.

# Index

*Note:* Page numbers of article titles are in **boldface** type.




Card Electrophysiol Clin 6 (2014) 835–840
http://dx.doi.org/10.1016/S1877-9182(14)00127-0
1877-9182/14/$ – see front matter 

Printed and bound by CPI Group (UK) Ltd, Croydon, CR0 4YY
03/10/2024
01040375-0019